Basic and Clinical Science Course
Section 6

Pediatric Ophthalmology and Strabismus

1999-2000

(Last major revision 1998-1999)

LIFELONG
EDUCATION FOR THE
OPHTHALMOLOGIST

American Academy of Ophthalmology

The Basic and Clinical Science Course is one component of the Lifelong Education for the Ophthalmologist (LEO) framework, which assists members in planning their continuing medical education. LEO includes an array of clinical education products that members may select to form individualized, self-directed learning plans for updating their clinical knowledge. Active members or fellows who use LEO components may accumulate sufficient CME credits to earn the LEO Award. Contact the Academy's Clinical Education Division for further information on LEO.

This CME activity was planned and produced in accordance with the ACCME Essentials.

The Academy provides this material for educational purposes only. It is not intended to represent the only or best method or procedure in every case, nor to replace a physician's own judgment or give specific advice for case management. Including all indications, contraindications, side effects, and alternative agents for each drug or treatment is beyond the scope of this material. All information and recommendations should be verified, prior to use, with current information included in the manufacturers' package inserts or other independent sources, and considered in light of the patient's condition and history. Reference to certain drugs, instruments, and other products in this publication is made for illustrative purposes only and is not intended to constitute an endorsement of such. Some material may include information on applications that are not considered community standard, that reflect indications not included in approved FDA labeling, or that are approved for use only in restricted research settings. The FDA has stated that it is the responsibility of the physician to determine the FDA status of each drug or device he or she wishes to use, and to use them with appropriate patient consent in compliance with applicable law. The Academy specifically disclaims any and all liability for injury or other damages of any kind, from negligence or otherwise, for any and all claims that may arise from the use of any recommendations or other information contained herein.

Each author states that he or she has no significant financial interest or other relationship with the manufacturer of any commercial product discussed in the chapters that he or she contributed to this publication or with the manufacturer of any competing commercial product.

Basic and Clinical Science Course

Thomas A. Weingeist, PhD, MD, Iowa City, Iowa
Senior Secretary for Clinical Education

Thomas J. Liesegang, MD, Jacksonville, Florida
Secretary for Instruction

M. Gilbert Grand, MD, St. Louis, Missouri
BCSC Course Chair

Section 6

Faculty Responsible for This Edition

M. Edward Wilson, MD, *Chair,* Charleston, South Carolina

Edward G. Buckley, MD, Durham, North Carolina

Jane D. Kivlin, MD, Milwaukee, Wisconsin

Mark S. Ruttum, MD, Milwaukee, Wisconsin

John W. Simon, MD, Albany, New York

Elbert H. Magoon, MD, Canton, Ohio
Practicing Ophthalmologists Advisory Committee for Education

Recent Past Faculty

Carol G. Blackwell, MD
Joseph H. Calhoun, MD
Monte A. Del Monte, MD
Allan M. Eisenbaum, MD
David S. Friendly, MD
J. Allen Gammon, MD
Mark J. Greenwald, MD
Marilyn B. Mets, MD

Marilyn T. Miller, MD
R. Hugh Minor, MD
Ronald L. Price, MD
James M. Richard, MD
Paul E. Romano, MD
William E. Scott, MD
Wilson K. Wallace, MD
Kenneth W. Wright, MD

In addition, the Academy gratefully acknowledges the
contributions of numerous past faculty and advisory
committee members who have played an important role in
the development of previous editions of the Basic and
Clinical Science Course.

American Academy of Ophthalmology Staff

Kathryn A. Hecht, EdD
Vice President, Clinical Education

Hal Straus
Director, Publications Department

Margaret Denny
Managing Editor

Fran Taylor
Medical Editor

Maxine Garrett
Administrative Coordinator

American Academy of Ophthalmology
655 Beach Street
Box 7424
San Francisco, CA 94120-7424

CONTENTS

GENERAL INTRODUCTION

The Basic and Clinical Science Course (BCSC) is designed to provide residents and practitioners with a comprehensive yet concise curriculum of the field of ophthalmology. The BCSC has developed from its original brief outline format, which relied heavily on outside readings, to a more convenient and educationally useful self-contained text. The Academy regularly updates and revises the course, with the goals of integrating the basic science and clinical practice of ophthalmology and of keeping current with new developments in the various subspecialties.

The BCSC incorporates the effort and expertise of more than 70 ophthalmologists, organized into 12 section faculties, working with Academy editorial staff. In addition, the course continues to benefit from many lasting contributions made by the faculties of previous editions. Members of the Academy's Practicing Ophthalmologists Advisory Committee for Education serve on each faculty and, as a group, review every volume before and after major revisions.

Organization of the Course

The 12 sections of the Basic and Clinical Science Course are numbered as follows to reflect a logical order of study, proceeding from fundamental subjects to anatomic subdivisions:

1. Update on General Medicine
2. Fundamentals and Principles of Ophthalmology
3. Optics, Refraction, and Contact Lenses
4. Ophthalmic Pathology and Intraocular Tumors
5. Neuro-Ophthalmology
6. Pediatric Ophthalmology and Strabismus
7. Orbit, Eyelids, and Lacrimal System
8. External Disease and Cornea
9. Intraocular Inflammation and Uveitis
10. Glaucoma
11. Lens and Cataract
12. Retina and Vitreous

In addition, a comprehensive Master Index allows the reader to easily locate subjects throughout the entire series.

References

Readers who wish to explore specific topics in greater detail may consult the journal references cited within each chapter and the Basic Texts listed at the back of the book. These references are intended to be selective rather than exhaustive, chosen by the BCSC faculty as being important, current, and readily available to residents and practitioners.

Related Academy educational materials are also listed in the appropriate sections. They include books, audiovisual materials, self-assessment programs, clinical modules, and interactive programs.

Study Questions and CME Credit

Each volume includes multiple-choice study questions designed to be used as a closed-book exercise. The answers are accompanied by explanations to enhance the learning experience. Completing the study questions allows readers both to test their understanding of the material and to demonstrate section completion for the purpose of CME credit, if desired.

The Academy is accredited by the Accreditation Council for Continuing Medical Education to sponsor continuing medical education for physicians. CME credit hours in Category 1 of the Physician's Recognition Award of the AMA may be earned for completing the study of any section of the BCSC. The Academy designates the number of credit hours for each section based upon the scope and complexity of the material covered (see the Credit Reporting Form in each individual section for the maximum number of hours that may be claimed).

Based upon return of the Credit Reporting Form at the back of each book, the Academy will maintain a record, for up to 3 years, of credits earned by Academy members. Upon request, the Academy will send a transcript of credits earned.

Conclusion

The Basic and Clinical Science Course has expanded greatly over the years, with the addition of much new text and numerous illustrations. Recent editions have sought to place a greater emphasis on clinical applicability, while maintaining a solid foundation in basic science. As with any educational program, it reflects the experience of its authors. As its faculties change and as medicine progresses, new viewpoints are always emerging on controversial subjects and techniques. Not all alternate approaches can be included in this series; as with any educational endeavor, the learner should seek additional sources, including such carefully balanced opinions as the Academy's Preferred Practice Patterns.

The BCSC faculty and staff are continuously striving to improve the educational usefulness of the course; you, the reader, can contribute to this ongoing process. If you have any suggestions or questions about the series, please do not hesitate to contact the faculty or the managing editor.

The authors, editors, and reviewers hope that your study of the BCSC will be of lasting value and that each section will serve as a practical resource for quality patient care.

OBJECTIVES FOR BCSC SECTION 6

Upon completion of BCSC Section 6, *Pediatric Ophthalmology and Strabismus*, the reader should be able to:

- Describe evaluation techniques for young children that provide the maximum gain of information with the least trauma and frustration
- Outline the anatomy and physiology of the extraocular muscles and their fascia
- Explain the classification, diagnosis, and treatment options for amblyopia
- Describe the commonly used diagnostic and measurement tests for strabismus
- Classify the various esodeviations and exodeviations and describe the management of each type
- Identify vertical strabismus and special forms of strabismus and formulate a treatment plan for each type
- List the possible complications of strabismus surgery and describe guidelines to minimize them
- Differentiate among various causes of congenital and acquired ocular infections in children and formulate a logical plan for the diagnosis and management of each type
- List the most common diseases and malformations of the cornea, lacrimal drainage system, anterior segment, and iris seen in children
- Describe the diagnostic findings and treatment options for childhood glaucoma
- Identify common types of childhood cataracts and other lens disorders
- Outline a diagnostic and management plan for childhood cataracts
- Identify appropriate diagnostic tests for pediatric uveitis
- Differentiate among various vitreoretinal diseases and disorders found in children
- List the characteristics of ocular tumors and phakomatoses seen in children
- Describe the characteristic findings of accidental and nonaccidental childhood trauma
- Outline the current joint policy statement regarding the role of vision in learning disabilities and dyslexia

Rapport With Children: Tips for A Productive Examination

The comprehensive ophthalmologist who only occasionally sees children may find the experience frustrating and unsatisfying. A positive attitude, the right equipment, and some knowledge of children can make the experience fruitful and enjoyable. Although no scientific data are available to help with this topic, a wealth of knowledge on child development can guide the ophthalmologist. Children should be approached in a manner consistent with their particular developmental stage. The younger the child, the more ingenious the examiner must be to engage and maintain the child's attention. It is especially important to work quickly with young children, who otherwise lose interest and become difficult to examine. For children under 3, a good general rule is "one toy—one look." Although accommodative targets at distance are ideal, it may be necessary to substitute a penlight at near in young or uncooperative patients. A small toy may be attached to a handheld light.

Checklist for Examining Children

The following is a general list of tips gleaned by ophthalmologists who deal frequently with children:

☐ Be yourself—children can spot a phony.

☐ Have fun, smile—try to make the encounter light and playful.

☐ Use the one toy–one look rule; have an array of age-appropriate toys.

☐ Greet the child and talk directly to him or her.

☐ Greet the adult with the child. The child's perception that you have parental approval is important to your rapport.

☐ If fusion (eye alignment) is in doubt, check it first before disrupting it with other tests.

☐ Go where the action is—you may only have a few moments of cooperation, so it's best to check what you most need to see at the beginning of the examination.

☐ Use positive phraseology and avoid negative suggestions. Say something will be "comfortable" rather than "it will not hurt." Say "I want to show you something" rather than "I want to examine your eyes," giving the patient a shared expectation of something interesting rather than scary or invasive.

☐ Be prepared to abandon or repeat the examination if building rapport is more important. But be persistent when dealing with a life- or vision-threatening problem and even use sedation or anesthesia if necessary.

- Be honest—nothing destroys your credibility quicker than telling a child something won't hurt when you know it will. If drops are necessary, an anesthetic drop first will minimize discomfort.
- Consider a pediatric corner in your waiting room or at least a few things for children to play with there.
- Consider removing your white coat for children. They associate white coats with other doctors who give shots, not nice ophthalmologists who are fun to visit.
- Try to make verbal contact by inducing the patient to speak. Asking a question that the child can answer such as "What grade are you in?" or "How old are you?" is a good place to start. Sometimes you can show a child a picture and ask what's in it as a way to break the ice.
- Establish physical contact with some friendly gesture. Some ophthalmologists greet a child by saying "Give me five" and holding out their hand. Asking the child to hold something such as your penlight or occluder or to touch a picture may help.
- Cultivate special vocabulary such as "magic glasses" for the polaroid lenses.
- Consider obtaining a VCR-driven TV and moving animals controlled by foot pedals. They can make fixation much easier and be a great delight to a child and parent.
- Use small finger puppets, which are inexpensive and interesting to children, and other targets (Fig 1).

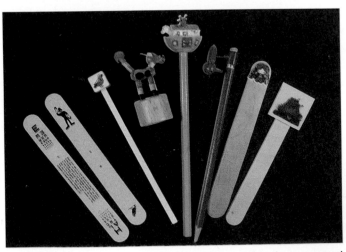

FIG 1—Small toys, pictures, and reduced letter and E charts are used as near fixation targets. (Reproduced with permission from Haldi BA, Mets MB. Nonsurgical treatment of strabismus. In: *Focal Points: Clinical Modules for Ophthalmologists.* San Francisco: American Academy of Ophthalmology; 1997;15:4. Photograph courtesy of Betty Anne Haldi, CO.)

□ Try the blue and green lights of the ophthalmoscope and slit lamp to help gain a child's attention; they are less threatening than the bright white light.

□ Use the indirect ophthalmoscope with the lowest illumination level needed to see details in the fundus.

□ Make a game of the ophthalmoscope by asking the patient to look at a distant object "even if I get in the way with my bright light."

□ Increase your energy level a little but without hurrying or being phony. You can't hope to match children's energy level, but you may be able to keep their attention with a brisk pace and several toys and activities.

□ By contrast, if a procedure that might provoke anxiety is planned, slow down the pace. A sense of calm and quiet may be helpful in achieving the proper mood.

Use of Anesthesia for Foreign Body Removal

Procedures that are anxiety provoking or painful can be better accomplished if the child knows that it is possible to numb the area. For example, the following process to remove foreign bodies can comfort the child:

1. Explain to the child that the eyes can be made numb.

2. Show the child that you have a drop that is cold, but most children say it is also comfortable. You can call it a "magic drop." Drop it on the back of the child's hand first, before putting it in the eye. Tell the patient he or she might have felt that first drop but probably won't notice a second drop so much because the eye is already numb.

3. Demonstrate with a second drop that the eye has become numb. Show the child that a soft cotton-tip applicator with drops on it can touch the eye without hurting or even being felt.

4. Instruments for foreign body removal can then be introduced in a similar fashion.

Examining the Child for Strabismus

Using the one toy–one look rule, the examiner checks on the first look to see whether the corneal reflexes are in exactly the same position, and whether they are in the center of the eye or toward one side. If the corneal reflexes are equal, the patient either has straight eyes or an extremely small deviation. If the reflexes are not equal, the examiner should then determine which eye is fixating.

The eye will be turned in the direction opposite the position of the displaced corneal reflex; if the problem is esotropia, the reflection from the deviated eye is temporal to where it would be if the eye were straight (the terminology and concepts mentioned in this introduction are defined and discussed in depth in chapters I through XIV). The image of the fixation light then falls on the nasal retina, thereby localizing it from the patient's reference point as coming from the temporal visual field. Thus, a patient with an esotropic eye sees the image appearing to come from the temporal side.

If the patient is being tested with prisms to measure the amount of deviation, the base of the prism is held temporally, i.e., base out. So if the eye is turned in, the corneal reflex is out, the image is out, and the base of the correcting prism is held out. Another way to remember which way to position the prism is that the prism apex is pointed in the direction of the deviation.

If the first look indicates that the patient has, for example, a right esotropia, then on the second look the examiner should determine whether or not the patient can alternate fixation and maintain it. The fixating left eye is covered, so that the deviated right eye will be forced to abduct in order to fixate the target. The cover is then removed from the left eye. If the patient is now capable of maintaining fixation with the right eye, he or she has an alternating esotropia, most likely with roughly equal visual acuity in both eyes. A patient who cannot maintain fixation with the right eye (is not able to alternate fixation) will revert to fixation with the left eye and right esotropia. This patient probably has some degree of amblyopia of the right eye. If the patient's corneal reflexes appeared equal on the first look, the cover-uncover test is performed to detect any phoria.

Tests and measurements should be done both at distance viewing (6 m or 20 ft) and at near viewing (0.3 m or 13 in). Refractive correction should be in place when appropriate.

Day S. History, examination and further investigation. In: Taylor D, ed. *Pediatric Ophthalmology.* 2nd ed. Cambridge, MA: Blackwell; 1996.

McKeown CA. The pediatric eye examination. In: Albert DM, Jakobiec FA, eds. *Principles and Practice of Ophthalmology.* 2nd ed. Philadelphia: Saunders; 1994.

Moody E. Ophthalmic examinations of infants and children. In: Nelson LB, Calhoun JH, Harley RD, eds. *Pediatric Ophthalmology.* 3rd ed. Philadelphia: Saunders; 1991.

Preferred Practice Patterns Committee, Pediatric Ophthalmology Panel. *Pediatric Eye Evaluations.* San Francisco: American Academy of Ophthalmology; 1997.

PART 1

STRABISMUS

CHAPTER I

Anatomy of the Extraocular Muscles and Their Fascia

Origin, Course, Insertion, Innervation, and Action of the Extraocular Muscles

There are seven extraocular muscles: the four rectus muscles, the two oblique muscles, and the levator palpebrae superioris muscle. Cranial nerve VI (abducens) innervates the lateral rectus muscle; cranial nerve IV (trochlear) innervates the superior oblique muscle; and cranial nerve III (oculomotor) innervates the levator palpebrae, superior rectus, medial rectus, inferior rectus, and inferior oblique muscles. CN III has an upper and lower division: the upper division supplies the levator palpebrae and superior rectus muscles; the lower division supplies the medial rectus, inferior rectus, and inferior oblique muscles. The parasympathetic innervation of the sphincter pupillae and ciliary muscle travels with the branch of the lower division of cranial nerve III that supplies the inferior oblique muscle. BCSC Section 5, *Neuro-Ophthalmology,* discusses the ocular motor nerves in more detail, and Section 2, *Fundamentals and Principles of Ophthalmology,* provides extensive illustration of the anatomical structures mentioned in this chapter.

When the eye is directed straight ahead, and the head is also straight, it is said to be in *primary position.* The *primary action* of a muscle is its major effect on the position of the eye when the muscle contracts while the eye is in primary position. The *secondary* and *tertiary actions* of a muscle are the additional effects on the position of the eye in primary position. The globe usually can be moved about 50° in each direction from primary position. Under normal viewing circumstances, however, the eyes move only about 15°–20° from primary position before head movement occurs.

Horizontal Rectus Muscles

The horizontal rectus muscles are the medial and lateral rectus muscles. Both arise from the annulus of Zinn. The *medial rectus muscle* courses along the medial orbital wall and inserts 5.5 mm from the limbus; the *lateral rectus muscle* inserts 6.9 mm from the limbus after coursing along the lateral orbital wall. The medial and lateral rectus muscles have only horizontal action: the medial rectus is an adductor and the lateral rectus is an abductor (Fig I-1).

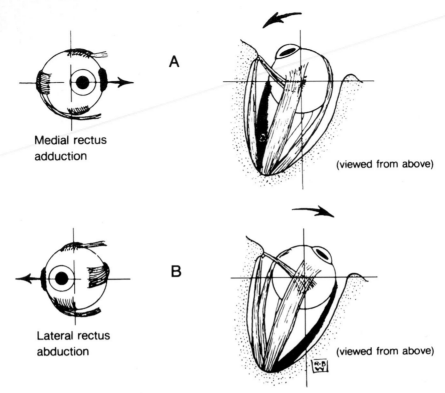

Medial rectus
adduction

A

(viewed from above)

B

Lateral rectus
abduction

(viewed from above)

FIG I-1—The right horizontal rectus muscles. *A,* Right medial rectus muscle. *B,* Right lateral rectus muscle. (Reprinted from von Noorden GK. *von Noorden–Maumenee's Atlas of Strabismus.* 3rd ed. St Louis: Mosby; 1977.)

Vertical Rectus Muscles

The vertical rectus muscles are the superior and inferior rectus muscles. The *superior rectus muscle* originates from the annulus of Zinn and courses anteriorly, upward over the eyeball, and laterally, forming an angle of 23° with the visual axis of the eye in primary position. It inserts 7.7 mm from the limbus. The superior rectus muscle's primary action is elevation; secondary actions are adduction and intorsion (incycloduction) (Fig I-2).

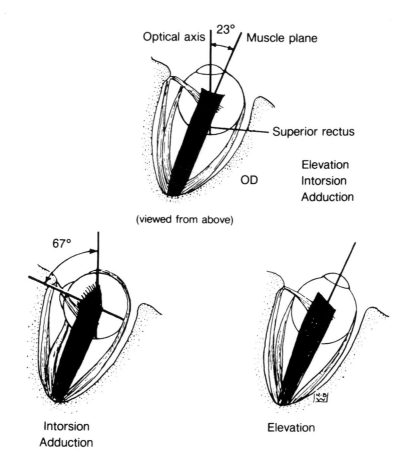

Optical axis | 23° / Muscle plane

Superior rectus

Elevation
Intorsion
Adduction

OD

(viewed from above)

67°

Intorsion
Adduction

Elevation

FIG I-2—The right superior rectus muscle. (Reprinted from von Noorden GK. *von Noorden–Maumenee's Atlas of Strabismus.* 3rd ed. St Louis: Mosby; 1977.)

The *inferior rectus muscle* also arises from the annulus of Zinn, and it then courses anteriorly, downward, and laterally along the floor of the orbit, forming an angle of 23° with the visual axis of the eye in primary position. It inserts 6.5 mm from the limbus. The inferior rectus muscle's primary action is depression; secondary actions are adduction and extorsion (excycloduction) (Fig I-3).

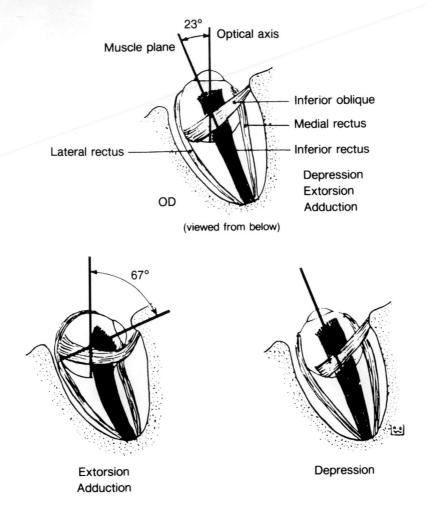

FIG I-3—The right inferior rectus muscle, viewed from below. (Reprinted from von Noorden GK. *von Noorden–Maumenee's Atlas of Strabismus.* 3rd ed. St Louis: Mosby; 1977.)

Oblique Muscles

The *superior oblique muscle* originates from the orbital apex above the annulus of Zinn and passes anteriorly and upward along the superomedial wall of the orbit. It becomes tendinous before passing through the *trochlea,* a pulley made of cartilage located on the nasal side of the superior orbital rim and connected to the superior oblique tendon by fine fibrils of connective tissue. The tendon is then reflected inferiorly, posteriorly, and laterally, forming an angle of 51° with the visual axis of the eye in primary position. It inserts in the posterosuperior quadrant of the eyeball, almost or entirely lateral to the midvertical plane or center of rotation, passing under

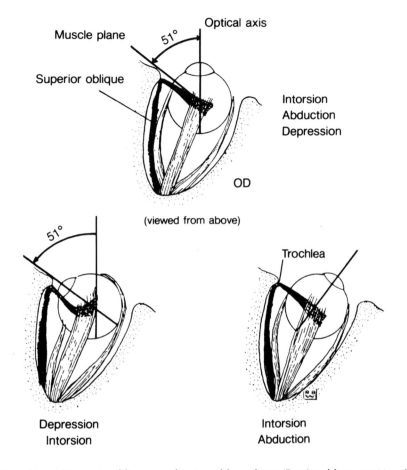

Muscle plane

Superior oblique

51°

Optical axis

Intorsion
Abduction
Depression

OD

(viewed from above)

51°

Depression
Intorsion

Trochlea

Intorsion
Abduction

FIG I-4—The right superior oblique muscle, viewed from above. (Reprinted from von Noorden GK. *von Noorden–Maumenee's Atlas of Strabismus.* 3rd ed. St Louis: Mosby; 1977.)

the superior rectus muscle. The primary action of the superior oblique muscle is intorsion (incycloduction); secondary actions are depression and abduction (Fig I-4).

The *inferior oblique muscle* originates from the periosteum of the maxillary bone, just posterior to the orbital rim and lateral to the orifice of the lacrimal fossa. It passes laterally, superiorly, and posteriorly, going inferior to the inferior rectus muscle and inserting under the lateral rectus muscle in the posterolateral portion of the globe, in the area of the macula. It forms an angle of 51° with the visual axis of the eye in primary position. The primary action of the inferior oblique muscle is extorsion (excycloduction); secondary actions are elevation and abduction (Fig I-5).

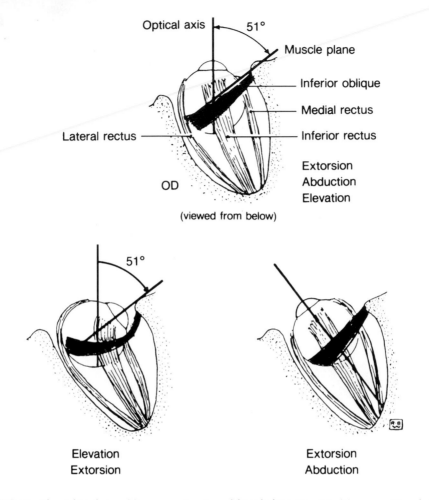

Optical axis   51°

Muscle plane

Inferior oblique

Medial rectus

Lateral rectus

Inferior rectus

Extorsion
Abduction
Elevation

OD

(viewed from below)

51°

Elevation
Extorsion

Extorsion
Abduction

FIG I-5—The right inferior oblique muscle, viewed from below. (Reprinted from von Noorden GK. *von Noorden–Maumenee's Atlas of Strabismus.* 3rd ed. St Louis: Mosby; 1977.)

Levator Palpebrae Superioris Muscle

The levator palpebrae superioris muscle arises at the apex of the orbit from the lesser wing of the sphenoid bone just superior to the annulus of Zinn. The origin of this muscle blends with the superior rectus muscle inferiorly and with the superior oblique muscle medially. It passes anteriorly, lying just above the superior rectus muscle; the fascial sheaths of these two muscles are connected. The levator palpebrae superioris muscle becomes an aponeurosis in the region of the superior fornix. It has both a cutaneous and tarsal insertion. BCSC Section 7, *Orbit, Eyelids, and Lacrimal System,* discusses this muscle in detail.

TABLE I-1

EXTRAOCULAR MUSCLES

MUSCLE	APPROX. LENGTH OF ACTIVE MUSCLE (mm)	ORIGIN	ANATOMIC INSERTION	DIREC-TION OF PULL*	TENDON LENGTH (mm)	ARC OF CONTACT (mm)	ACTION FROM PRIMARY POSITION	INNERVA-TION
Medial rectus (MR)	40	Annulus of Zinn	5.5 mm from medial limbus	90°	4.5	7	Adduction	Lower CN III
Lateral rectus (LR)	40	Annulus of Zinn	6.9 mm from lateral limbus	90°	7	12	Abduction	CN VI
Superior rectus (SR)	40	Annulus of Zinn	7.7 mm from superior limbus	23°	6	6.5	Elevation Intorsion Adduction	Upper CN III
Inferior rectus (IR)	40	Annulus of Zinn	6.5 mm from inferior limbus	23°	7	6.5	Depression Extorsion Adduction	Lower CN III
Superior oblique (SO)	32	Orbit apex above annulus of Zinn (functional origin at the trochlea)	Posterior to equator in superotemporal quadrant	51°	26	7–8	Intorsion Depression Abduction	CN IV
Inferior oblique (IO)	37	Behind lacrimal fossa	Macular area	51°	1	15	Extorsion Elevation Abduction	Lower CN III
Levator palpebrae superioris (LPS)	40	Orbit apex above annulus of Zinn	Septa of pretarsal orbicularis and anterior surface of tarsus	—	14–20	—	Eyelid elevation	Upper CN III

*relative to visual axis in primary position

Table I-1 summarizes the characteristics of the extraocular muscles and shows their relationship to one another (Fig I-6).

Insertion Relationships of the Rectus Muscles

Starting at the medial rectus and proceeding to inferior rectus, lateral rectus, and superior rectus muscles, the rectus muscle tendons insert progressively farther from the limbus. A continuous curve drawn through these insertions yields a spiral, known as the *spiral of Tillaux*. The temporal side of the vertical rectus muscle insertion is farther from the limbus (i.e., more posterior) than is the nasal side (Fig I-7).

Apt L. An anatomical reevaluation of rectus muscle insertions. *Trans Am Ophthalmol Soc.* 1980;78:365–375.

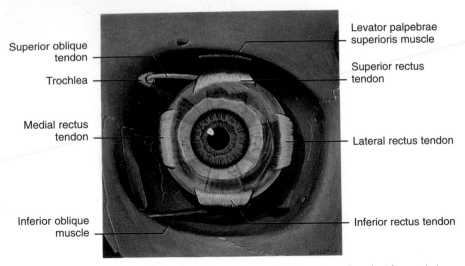

Levator palpebrae
superioris muscle

Superior oblique
tendon

Superior rectus
tendon

Trochlea

Medial rectus
tendon

Lateral rectus tendon

Inferior oblique
muscle

Inferior rectus tendon

FIG I-6—Extraocular muscles, frontal composite view, left eye. (Reproduced with permission from Dutton JJ. *Atlas of Clinical and Surgical Orbital Anatomy.* Philadelphia: Saunders; 1994:23.)

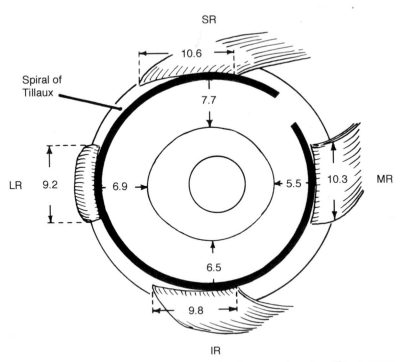

SR

10.6

Spiral of
Tillaux

7.7

LR   9.2

6.9

5.5   10.3   MR

6.5

9.8

IR

FIG I-7—Spiral of Tillaux, right eye. Note: the distances given in millimeters are averages only and may vary greatly in individuals. (Reprinted from von Noorden GK. *von Noorden–Maumenee's Atlas of Strabismus.* 3rd ed. St Louis: Mosby; 1977.)

Blood Supply of the Extraocular Muscles

Arterial System

The muscular branches of the ophthalmic artery provide the most important blood supply for the extraocular muscles. The *lateral muscular branch* supplies the lateral rectus, superior rectus, superior oblique, and levator palpebrae superioris muscles; the *medial muscular branch,* the larger of the two, supplies the inferior rectus, medial rectus, and inferior oblique muscles.

The lateral rectus muscle is partially supplied by the *lacrimal artery;* the *infraorbital artery* partially supplies the inferior oblique and inferior rectus muscles.

The muscular branches give rise to the *anterior ciliary arteries* accompanying the rectus muscles; each rectus muscle has from one to three anterior ciliary arteries. These pass to the episclera of the globe and then supply blood to the anterior segment. The superior and inferior rectus muscles carry the bulk of the blood supply.

Venous System

The venous system parallels the arterial system, emptying into the *superior* and *inferior orbital veins.* Generally, four *vortex veins* are located posterior to the equator; these are usually found near the nasal and temporal margins of the superior rectus and inferior rectus muscles.

Fine Structure of the Extraocular Muscles

The ratio of nerve fibers to eye muscle fibers in the extraocular muscles is high (1:3–1:5) compared to that found in other skeletal muscles (1:50–1:125), allowing for more accurate control. Extraocular muscle is a specialized form of skeletal muscle that incorporates several different fiber types from a slow, tonic type resistant to fatigue and active in holding gaze straight ahead to the type adapted for rapid (saccadic) eye movements. Intermediate fiber types also exist.

Fiber Types

Felderstruktur muscle fibers are unique to the extraocular muscles. These are slow, tonic, "stamina-oriented" muscle fibers that tend to be superficial in the muscle, near the orbital wall, and smaller in size. They usually have aerobic metabolism, many mitochondria, high capillary density, oxidative enzymes, innervation by multiple *en grappe* endings, and small nerve fibers. They contract slowly, smoothly, and with a graded response, depending on repetitive stimuli, and participate in smooth pursuit.

Fibrillenstruktur muscle fibers, the usual type of fiber seen in skeletal muscle, correspond to striated muscles of the body. These fast, phasic fibers tend to be deeper in the center of the muscle and larger in size; they usually have *en plaque* nerve endings, glycolytic enzymes, large nerve fibers that are myelinated, and fewer mitochondria. These muscle fibers contract rapidly as a fast twitch in response to a single stimulus and function in saccadic movements of the eye.

Orbital and Fascial Relationships

Tenon's Capsule (the Fascia Bulbi)

Tenon's capsule is an envelope of elastic connective tissue that is attached to the optic nerve posteriorly and becomes fused with the intermuscular membrane 3 mm from the limbus, to which it is attached anteriorly. Posterior to the equator, Tenon's capsule is a fibrous condensation that separates the orbital fat inside the muscle cone from the sclera, thereby keeping fat out of the sclera. Anterior to the equator, Tenon's capsule extends forward over the extraocular muscles and separates them from the orbital fat and structures lying outside the muscle cone. Six extraocular muscles penetrate Tenon's capsule; the levator palpebrae superioris is the only one that does not.

Muscle Cone

The muscle cone lies posterior to the equator. It consists of the extraocular muscles, the extraocular muscle sheaths, and the intermuscular membrane. The muscle cone extends posteriorly to the annulus of Zinn in the orbital apex.

Muscle Capsule

Each rectus muscle has a surrounding fascial capsule that extends with the muscle from its origin to its insertion. These capsules are thin posteriorly, but near the equator they thicken as they pass through Tenon's capsule, continuing anteriorly with the muscles to their insertions. Anterior to the equator between the undersurface of the muscle and the sclera there is almost no fascia, only connective tissue footplates that connect the muscle to the globe.

Intermuscular Septum (Membrane)

The four rectus muscles are connected by a thin layer of tissue that underlies the conjunctiva. This is the intermuscular septum, which spans between rectus muscles and fuses with the conjunctiva 3 mm posterior to the limbus.

"Check Ligaments"

The term *check ligaments* was originally proposed because it was thought that these structures limited the excursion of the extraocular muscles. However, these fascial extensions neither check the motion of the globe nor are they ligaments. Beginning anterior to the equator, they extend from the muscle sheath, pass through the overlying Tenon's capsule, and insert on the corresponding orbital wall. They are slightly more well developed for the horizontal rectus muscles, and they function as support structures for the globe and its surrounding tissue. These fascial attachments limit motility only when they are scarred.

Lockwood's Ligament

The muscle capsule of the inferior oblique muscle (but not the muscle itself) is bound to the inferior rectus muscle capsule. This fusion is called *Lockwood's ligament,* and it connects the lower eyelid retractors.

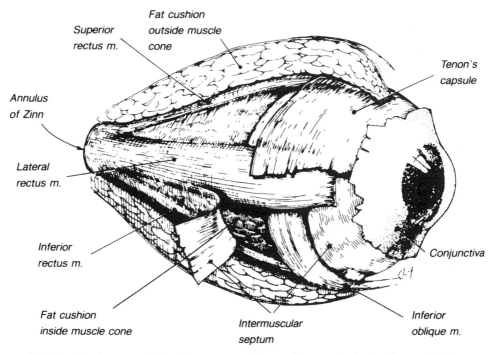

FIG I-8—Muscle cone relationships. (Reprinted from Parks MM. *Ocular Motility and Strabismus*. Hagerstown, MD: Harper & Row; 1975.)

Adipose Tissue

The eye is supported and cushioned in the orbit by a large amount of fatty tissue. External to the muscle cone, fatty tissue comes forward with the rectus muscles, stopping about 10 mm from the limbus. Fatty tissue is also present inside the muscle cone, kept away from the sclera by Tenon's capsule (Fig I-8). If Tenon's capsule is cut or torn, fat can prolapse inside Tenon's capsule and may form a firm adhesion to sclera, muscle, intermuscular membrane, and/or conjunctiva (see p 152).

Anatomical Implications

The nerves to the rectus muscles and the superior oblique muscle enter the muscles about one third of the distance from the origin to the insertion (or trochlea, in the case of the superior oblique muscle) (Fig I-9). Damaging these nerves during anterior surgery is difficult, but not impossible. An instrument thrust more than 26 mm posterior to the rectus muscle's insertion may cause injury to the nerve.

The nerve supplying the inferior oblique muscle enters the lateral portion of the muscle where it crosses the inferior rectus muscle; the nerve can be damaged by surgery in this area. Since the parasympathetic innervation to the sphincter pupillae and ciliary muscle accompanies the nerve to the inferior oblique muscle, surgery in this area may also result in pupillary abnormalities.

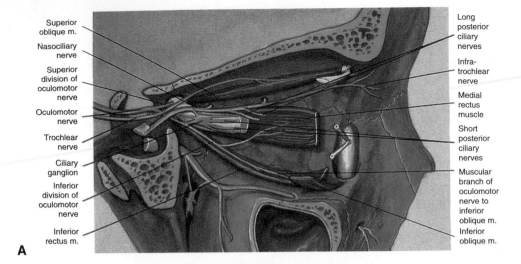

A

Superior oblique m.
Nasociliary nerve
Superior division of oculomotor nerve
Oculomotor nerve
Trochlear nerve
Ciliary ganglion
Inferior division of oculomotor nerve
Inferior rectus m.

Long posterior ciliary nerves
Infra-trochlear nerve
Medial rectus muscle
Short posterior ciliary nerves
Muscular branch of oculomotor nerve to inferior oblique m.
Inferior oblique m.

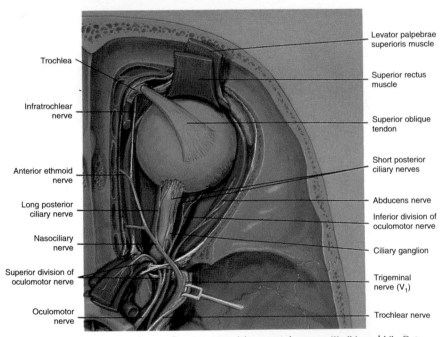

B

Trochlea
Infratrochlear nerve
Anterior ethmoid nerve
Long posterior ciliary nerve
Nasociliary nerve
Superior division of oculomotor nerve
Oculomotor nerve

Levator palpebrae superioris muscle
Superior rectus muscle
Superior oblique tendon
Short posterior ciliary nerves
Abducens nerve
Inferior division of oculomotor nerve
Ciliary ganglion
Trigeminal nerve (V₁)
Trochlear nerve

FIG I-9—The extraocular muscles are innervated by cranial nerves III, IV, and VI. Cutaway views facing nasally *(A)* and down *(B)* show the course of these ocular motor nerves. *CN III* (oculomotor) divides into a superior and inferior division in the cavernous sinus or at the superior orbital fissure. The superior division innervates the superior rectus and levator muscles. The inferior division sends branches to the medial rectus, inferior rectus, and inferior oblique muscles and the ciliary ganglion. *CN IV* (trochlear) enters the orbit through the superior orbital fissure, crosses over the superior rectus and levator muscle complex, and runs along the external surface of the superior oblique muscle, entering in the posterior one third. *CN VI* (abducens) enters the orbit through the superior orbital fissure and annulus of Zinn to supply the lateral rectus muscle. (Reproduced with permission from Buckley EG, Freedman S, Shields MB. *Atlas of Ophthalmic Surgery.* Vol III: *Strabismus and Glaucoma.* St Louis: Mosby; 1995:11.)

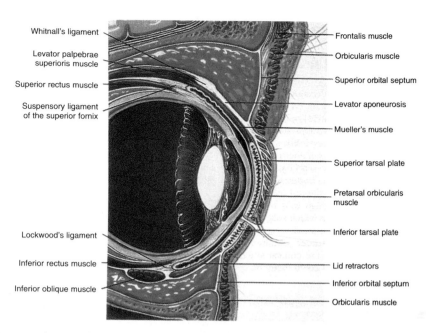

Whitnall's ligament

Levator palpebrae
superioris muscle

Superior rectus muscle

Suspensory ligament
of the superior fornix

Lockwood's ligament

Inferior rectus muscle

Inferior oblique muscle

Frontalis muscle

Orbicularis muscle

Superior orbital septum

Levator aponeurosis

Mueller's muscle

Superior tarsal plate

Pretarsal orbicularis
muscle

Inferior tarsal plate

Lid retractors

Inferior orbital septum

Orbicularis muscle

FIG I-10—Attachments of the upper and lower eyelids to the vertical rectus muscles. Superiorly, the suspensory ligament acts to connect the superior rectus and levator, which facilitates movement of the eyelid on attempted upgaze. Large recessions of the superior rectus muscle can result in upper eyelid retraction, while resections can create a ptosis. Surgery on the inferior rectus can also cause changes in position of the lower eyelid because of the presence of Lockwood's ligament. A recession of the inferior rectus muscle can result in lower eyelid retraction, while a resection of the inferior rectus muscle can result in advancement of a lower eyelid and a narrowing of the palpebral fissure. (Reproduced with permission from Buckley EG, Freedman S, Shields MB. *Atlas of Ophthalmic Surgery.* Vol III: *Strabismus and Glaucoma.* St Louis: Mosby; 1995:15.)

The inferior rectus muscle is distinctly bound to the lower eyelid by the fascial extension from its sheath. Recession, or weakening, of the inferior rectus muscle tends to widen the palpebral fissure with an associated lower lid droop; and resection, or strengthening, of the inferior rectus muscle tends to narrow the fissure by elevating the lower eyelid. Therefore, any alteration of the inferior rectus muscle may be associated with palpebral fissure change (Fig I-10).

The superior rectus muscle is loosely bound to the levator palpebrae superioris muscle. The eyelid may be pulled forward following resection of the superior rectus muscle, thus narrowing the palpebral fissure, and pulled upward with a recession, widening the fissure. In hypotropia a pseudoptosis may be present since the upper eyelid tends to follow the superior rectus.

The blood supply to the extraocular muscles provides almost all of the temporal half of the anterior segment circulation and the majority of the nasal half of the anterior segment circulation, which also receives some blood from the long posterior ciliary artery. Therefore, simultaneous surgery on three rectus muscles may induce anterior segment ischemia, particularly in older patients (see p 153).

Whenever muscle surgery is performed, special care must be taken to avoid penetration of Tenon's capsule. As discussed above, if the integrity of Tenon's capsule 10 mm posterior to the limbus is violated, fatty tissue may prolapse through the capsule and form a restrictive adhesion, limiting ocular motility.

When surgery is performed in the domain of the vortex veins, accidental severing of a vein is possible. The procedures that present the greatest risk for damaging a vortex vein are inferior rectus and superior rectus muscle recession or resection, inferior oblique muscle weakening procedures, and exposure of the superior oblique muscle tendon.

The sclera is thinnest just posterior to the four rectus muscle insertions. This area is the site for most muscle surgery, especially for recession procedures. Therefore, the risk of scleral perforation is always present during eye muscle surgery. This risk can be minimized by

- Using spatulated needles with swedged sutures
- Working with a clean, dry, and blood-free surgical field
- Using loupe magnification or the operating microscope
- Employing a head-mounted fiberoptic light source in addition to the overhead operating lights

Chapter XIII, Surgery of the Extraocular Muscles, discusses these procedures and complications in greater detail.

Bron AJ, Tripathi RC, Tripathi BJ, eds. *Wolff's Anatomy of the Eye and Orbit.* 8th ed. London: Chapman and Hall; 1997.

Buckley EG, Freedman S, Shields MB. *Atlas of Ophthalmic Surgery.* Vol III: *Strabismus and Glaucoma.* St Louis: Mosby; 1995.

Koornneef L. *Spatial Aspects of Orbital Musculofibrous Tissue in Man.* Amsterdam: Swets & Zeitlinger; 1977.

Parks MM. Ocular motility and strabismus. In: *Duane's Clinical Ophthalmology.* Philadelphia: Lippincott; 1993; vol. 1:1–20.

CHAPTER II

Motor Physiology

Basic Principles and Terms

Axes of Fick, Center of Rotation, Listing's Plane, and Median Plane

The movement of the eye around a theoretic center of rotation is explained with specific terminology. Two helpful concepts are the axes of Fick and Listing's plane (Fig II-1). The *axes of Fick* are designated as x, y, and z. The *x axis* is a transverse axis passing through the center of the eye at the equator; voluntary vertical rotations of the eye occur about this axis. The *y axis* is a sagittal axis passing through the pupil; involuntary torsional rotations occur about this axis. The *z axis* is a vertical axis; voluntary horizontal rotations occur about this axis. *Listing's equatorial plane* passes through the center of rotation and includes the x and z axes. The y axis is perpendicular to Listing's plane.

Another helpful term for defining ocular movement is the median plane. The *median plane* is a sagittal plane that passes anteroposteriorly through the body, bisecting the head into symmetric parts (Fig II-2).

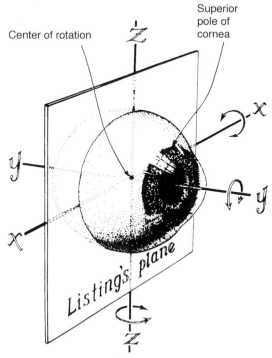

Center of rotation

Superior
pole of
cornea

Listing's plane

FIG II-1—Axes of Fick, center of rotation, Listing's plane. (Reprinted from Parks MM. *Atlas of Strabismus*. Philadelphia: Harper & Row; 1983.)

Positions of Gaze

Positions of gaze are also discussed in detail in chapter VI. The following is basic terminology:

□ *Primary position* is straight ahead

□ *Secondary positions* are straight up, straight down, right gaze, and left gaze

□ *Tertiary positions* are the four oblique positions of gaze: up and right, up and left, down and right, and down and left

□ *Cardinal positions* are up and right, up and left, right, left, down and right, down and left

Arc of Contact

As the eye rotates, the extraocular muscle involved and the sclera act like a rope and pulley. The point of effective, or physiologic, insertion is the tangential point where the muscle first contacts the globe. The action of the eye muscle may be considered a vector of force that acts at this tangential point to rotate the eye. The length of muscle actually in contact with the globe constitutes the arc of contact.

Primary, Secondary, and Tertiary Action

With the eye in primary position, the horizontal rectus muscles are purely horizontal movers around the z (vertical) axis, and they have a primary action only. The vertical rectus muscles have a direction of pull that is mostly vertical as their primary

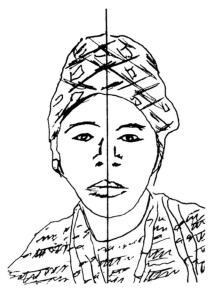

FIG II-2—Median plane.

action, but the angle of pull from origin to insertion is 23° inclined to the visual axis, giving rise also to *torsion,* which is defined as any rotation of the vertical corneal meridians. Intorsion (also called incycloduction) is the secondary action for the superior rectus; extorsion (also called excycloduction) is the secondary action for the inferior rectus; and adduction is the tertiary action for both muscles. Because the oblique muscles are inclined 51° to the visual axis, torsion is their primary action. Vertical rotation is their secondary and horizontal rotation is their tertiary action (Table II-1).

Field of Action

The term *field of action* is used in two ways to describe entirely separate and distinct concepts:

□ To indicate the direction of rotation of the eye when a muscle contracts

□ To refer to the gaze position in which the effect of the muscle is most readily observed

For the lateral rectus muscle these two movements are both abduction; for the medial rectus they are both adduction. However, the two are not the same for all muscles. For example, the inferior oblique muscle creates some vertical, torsional, and horizontal movement whenever it contracts. Furthermore, the amount of vertical, horizontal, and torsional change depends on the position of the eye. Only attempted elevation of the eye increases inferior oblique muscle activity; it does not increase with attempted abduction. Thus, a field of action is not a single unvarying movement for the inferior oblique muscle.

Field of activation would perhaps be a better term for this concept of what a muscle does. For example, the inferior oblique muscle is usually tested by its contribution to vertical eye movement in the adducted position because this is its field of greatest vertical action.

TABLE II-1

ACTION OF THE EXTRAOCULAR MUSCLES FROM PRIMARY POSITION

MUSCLE*	PRIMARY	SECONDARY	TERTIARY
Medial rectus	Adduction	—	—
Lateral rectus	Abduction	—	—
Inferior rectus	Depression	Extorsion	Adduction
Superior rectus	Elevation	Intorsion	Adduction
Inferior oblique	Extorsion	Elevation	Abduction
Superior oblique	Intorsion	Depression	Abduction

*The superior muscles are intortors; the inferior muscles are extortors. The vertical rectus muscles are adductors; the oblique muscles are abductors.

Thus, evaluation of fields of action must involve three separate aspects:

☐ The plane of the muscle action
☐ The gaze direction, which increases or decreases the innervation to the muscle
☐ The vector distribution of the muscle's force (vertical, horizontal, torsional) in various gaze positions

The importance of fields of action is that a deviation *(strabismus)* that increases with gaze in some directions may be a result of the weakness of the muscle normally pulling the eye in that direction. For example, esotropia increasing with gaze to the right may be the result of right lateral rectus muscle weakness.

Changing Muscle Action With Different Gaze Positions

The horizontal rectus muscles are the chief movers for horizontal gaze in all gaze positions. The vertical rectus muscles are the chief movers for vertical gaze in all gaze positions because of their greater size and power. When the eye abducts about 23°, it is perpendicular to the line of pull of the vertical rectus muscles, and these muscles then primarily affect vertical rotation. In this position the oblique muscles are now almost perpendicular to the y axis and function chiefly by cycloduction of the globe (see Figures I-2 and I-3).

In adduction of 51° the oblique muscles are nearly pure vertical rotators of the globe. The transverse x axis of the eye has been rotated to be almost perpendicular to their plane of muscle action; the vertical rectus muscles have become partial adductors and produce some increased torsional effect (Fig II-3). (See also Figures I-4 and I-5).

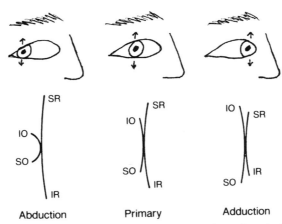

| Abduction | Primary | Adduction |

FIG II-3—The contribution of oblique muscles and vertical rectus muscles to vertical ductions is represented for the right eye. In abduction the rectus muscles contribute nearly the entire movement; in adduction both rectus and oblique muscles contribute. In abduction the superior rectus muscle is practically a pure elevator while the inferior oblique muscle is almost a pure tortor.

Physiology of Muscle Contraction

Position of rest   The position of each eye in the orbit without any innervation to the extraocular muscles is described as the position of rest. The position of each eye is slightly divergent in normal persons.

Motor units   An individual motor nerve fiber and its several muscle fibers is a motor unit. *Electromyography* records motor unit electrical activity. An electromyogram is useful in investigating normal and abnormal innervation and can be helpful in documenting paralysis, recovery from paralysis, and abnormalities of innervation in myasthenia gravis and muscle atrophy. However, this test is not helpful in ordinary comitant strabismus, as it is difficult to perform.

Recruitment during fixation or following movement   As the eye moves farther into abduction, for example, more and more lateral rectus motor units are activated and brought into play by the brain to help pull the eye. This process is called *recruitment*. In addition, as the eye fixates farther into abduction, the frequency of activity of each motor unit increases until it reaches a peak (for some motor units, several hundred contractions per second).

Saccades   Saccadic movements require a sudden, strong pulse of force from the extraocular muscles in order to move the eye rapidly against the viscosity produced by the fatty tissue and fascia in which the globe lies. For example, abducting the eye in a saccade requires a sudden great increase in lateral rectus muscle activity to get the eye moving and, at the same time, a total inhibition of the medial rectus muscle until the eye is again stabilized in the new gaze position. Velocity is nearly proportional to the size of saccade and can be 10°–400°/sec. The velocity of the saccadic movement and the high forces that must be produced are affected by muscle paresis, and study of saccadic velocity is of practical value in determining paresis of muscles and abnormal innervation. BCSC Section 5, *Neuro-Ophthalmology,* discusses saccades in detail.

Jampel RS. The fundamental principle of the action of the oblique ocular muscles. *Am J Ophthalmol.* 1970;69:623–638.

Metz HS, Scott AB, O'Meara D, et al. Ocular saccades in lateral rectus palsy. *Arch Ophthalmol.* 1970;84:453–460.

Scott AB. Ocular motility. In: Tasman W, Jaeger EA, eds. *Biomedical Foundations of Ophthalmology.* Philadelphia: Lippincott; 1997; vol 2.

Scott AB, Collins CC. Division of labor in human extraocular muscle. *Arch Ophthalmol.* 1973;90:319–322.

Eye Movements

Monocular Eye Movements (Ductions)

Ductions are monocular rotations of the eye. *Adduction* is movement of the eye nasally, while *abduction* is movement of the eye temporally. *Elevation* (supraduction or sursumduction) is an upward rotation of the eye; *depression* (infraduction or deorsumduction) is a downward rotation of the eye. *Intorsion* (incycloduction) is defined as a nasal rotation of the superior portion of the vertical corneal meridian. *Extorsion* (excycloduction) is a temporal rotation of the superior portion of the vertical corneal meridian.

The following are also important terms relating to the muscles used in monocular eye movements:

□ *Agonist:* the primary muscle moving the eye in a given direction

□ *Synergist:* the muscle in the same eye as the agonist that acts with the agonist to produce a given movement; e.g., the inferior oblique muscle is a synergist with the agonist superior rectus muscle for elevation of the eye

□ *Antagonist:* the muscle in the same eye as the agonist that acts in the direction opposite to that of the agonist; the medial rectus and lateral rectus muscles are antagonists

Sherrington's law of reciprocal innervation states that increased innervation and contraction of a given extraocular muscle are accompanied by a reciprocal decrease in innervation and contraction of its antagonist. For example, as the right eye abducts, the right lateral rectus muscle receives increased innervation while the right medial rectus receives decreased innervation.

Binocular Eye Movements (Versions and Vergences)

When binocular eye movements are conjugate and the eyes move in the same direction, such movements are called *versions.* When the eye movements are disjugate and the eyes move in opposite directions, such movements are known as *vergences* (e.g., convergence and divergence).

Versions: conjugate binocular eye movements   *Right gaze* (dextroversion) is movement of both eyes to the patient's right. *Left gaze* (levoversion) is movement of both eyes to the patient's left. *Elevation,* or *upgaze* (sursumversion), is an upward rotation of both eyes; *depression,* or *downgaze* (deorsumversion), is a downward rotation of both eyes. In *dextrocycloversion* both eyes rotate so that the superior portion of the vertical corneal meridian moves to the patient's right. Similarly, *levocycloversion* is movement of both eyes so that the superior portion of the vertical corneal meridian rotates to the patient's left.

The term *yoke muscles* is used to describe two muscles (one in each eye) that are the prime movers of their respective eyes in a given position of gaze. For example, when the eyes move or attempt to move into right gaze, the right lateral rectus muscle and the left medial rectus muscle are simultaneously innervated and contracted. These muscles are said to be "yoked" together.

Each extraocular muscle in one eye has a yoke muscle in the other eye. Because the effect of a muscle is usually best seen in a given direction of gaze, the concept of yoke muscles is used to evaluate the contribution of each extraocular muscle to eye movement. The six positions of gaze in which one muscle of each eye is the prime mover are known as the *cardinal positions of gaze.* Table II-2 and Figure II-4 give these six cardinal positions of gaze and the yoke muscles whose primary actions are in that field of gaze.

Hering's law of motor correspondence states that equal and simultaneous innervation flows to synergistic muscles concerned with the desired direction of gaze. This law has its most useful application in evaluating binocular eye movements and, in particular, the yoke muscles involved.

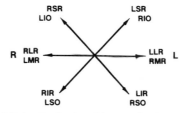

FIG II-4—Cardinal positions and yoke muscles.

TABLE II-2

YOKE MUSCLES IN CARDINAL POSITIONS OF GAZE

Eyes up and right
(dextrosursumversion) . . . . RSR and LIO

Eyes up and left
(levosursumversion) . . . . LSR and RIO

Eyes right
(dextroversion) . . . . RLR and LMR

Eyes left
(levoversion) . . . . LLR and RMR

Eyes down and right
(dextrodeorsumversion) . . . . RIR and LSO

Eyes down and left
(levodeorsumversion) . . . . LIR and RSO

RSR=right superior rectus; LIO=left inferior oblique; LSR=left superior rectus; RIO=right inferior oblique;
RLR=right lateral rectus; LMR=left medial rectus; LLR=left lateral rectus; RMR=right medial rectus;
RIR=right inferior rectus; LSO=left superior oblique; LIR=left inferior rectus; RSO=right superior oblique

Hering's law has important clinical implications, especially when dealing with a paralytic strabismus (see chapter V). Since the amount of innervation to both eyes is always determined by the fixating eye, the angle of deviation will vary depending on which eye is fixating. When the normal eye is fixating, the amount of misalignment is called the *primary deviation*. When the paretic eye is fixating, the amount of misalignment is called the *secondary deviation*. The secondary deviation is often larger than the primary deviation.

Hering's law is also necessary to explain the following example. If a patient has a right superior oblique muscle paresis and fixates with the right eye an object that is located up and to the patient's left, the innervation of the right inferior oblique muscle required to move the eye into this gaze position is reduced, because the RIO does not have to overcome the normal antagonistic effect of the right superior oblique muscle. Therefore, according to Hering's law, less innervation is also received by the right inferior oblique muscle's yoke muscle, the left superior rectus muscle. This decreased innervation could lead to the incorrect impression that the left superior rectus muscle is paretic (Fig II-5).

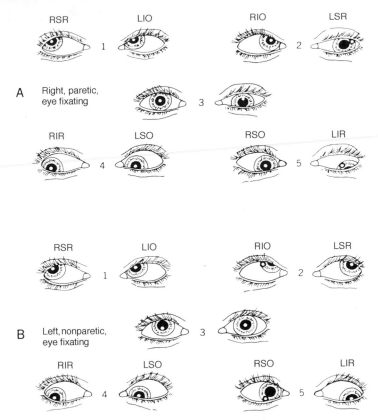

FIG II-5—Paresis of right superior oblique muscle. *A*, With right paretic eye fixating, little or no vertical difference appears between the two eyes in the right (uninvolved) field of gaze *(1* and *4)*. In primary position *(3)* a left hypotropia may be present since the right elevators require less innervation and thus the left elevators will receive less than normal innervation. When gaze is up and left *(2)*, the RIO needs less than normal innervation to elevate OD, since its antagonist, the RSO, is paretic. Consequently, its yoke, the LSR, will be apparently underacting, and pseudoptosis with pseudoparesis of the LSR will be present. When gaze is toward the field of action of the paretic muscle *(5)*, maximal innervation is required to move OD down during adduction, and thus the LIR will be overacting. *B*, With left sound eye fixating, no vertical difference appears in the right field of gaze *(1* and *4)*. In primary position *(3)*, OD is elevated because of unbalanced elevators. When gaze is up and left *(2)*, the RIO shows marked overaction, since its antagonist is paretic and there is contracture of the unopposed muscle. Normal action of the LSR is seen. When gaze is down and left *(5)*, normal innervation required by the fixating normal eye does not suffice to fully move the paretic eye. (Reprinted from von Noorden GK. *Atlas of Strabismus.* 4th ed. St Louis: Mosby; 1983:24–25.)

The above example is said to involve an inhibitional paresis of the contralateral antagonist when the paretic eye is fixating. However, the term *contralateral antagonist,* when used in conjunction with the concept of inhibitional paresis, is a contradiction. A more accurate description would be an inhibitional paresis of the antagonist (left superior rectus muscle) of the *yoke muscle* (left inferior rectus muscle) of the paretic muscle (right superior oblique muscle).

Vergences: disjugate binocular eye movements   *Convergence* is movement of both eyes nasally relative to a given position; *divergence* is movement of both eyes temporally relative to a given position. *Incyclovergence* is a rotation of both eyes so that the superior portion of each vertical corneal meridian rotates toward the median plane; *excyclovergence* is a rotation of both eyes so that the superior portion of each vertical corneal meridian rotates away from the median plane. *Vertical vergence* movement, though less frequently encountered, can also occur; here one eye moves upward, and the other downward. Other important terms and concepts related to vergences include the following:

- *Tonic convergence* represents the constant innervational tone to the extraocular muscles when an individual is awake and alert. As a result of the anatomical shape of the bony orbits and the position of the rectus muscle origins, the alignment of the eyes under complete muscle paralysis is divergent. Therefore, convergence tone is necessary in the awake state to maintain straight eyes even in the absence of strabismus.

- *Accommodative convergence* of the visual axes occurs as part of the synkinetic near reflex. A fairly consistent increment of accommodative convergence (AC) occurs for each diopter of accommodation (A), giving the *accommodative convergence/accommodation ratio (AC/A).*

   Abnormalities of this ratio are common, and they are an important cause of strabismus. With an abnormally high AC/A ratio, the excess convergence tends to produce esotropia during accommodation on near targets. An abnormally low AC/A ratio will tend to make the eyes exotropic when the individual looks at near targets. For techniques of measuring the accommodative convergence/accommodation ratio, see p 66.

- *Voluntary convergence* is a voluntary stimulation of the near reflex.

- *Proximal (instrument) convergence* is an induced convergence movement caused by a psychologic awareness of near; it is seen particularly when a person looks through an instrument such as a binocular microscope.

- *Fusional convergence* is an optomotor reflex to converge and position the eyes so that similar retinal images project on corresponding retinal areas. Fusional convergence is accomplished without changing the refractive state of the eyes and is prompted by bitemporal retinal image disparity.

- *Fusional divergence* is the only form of divergence that has clinical significance. It is an optomotor reflex to diverge and align the eyes so that similar retinal images project on corresponding retinal areas. Fusional divergence is accomplished without changing the refractive state of the eyes and is prompted by binasal retinal image disparity.

Supranuclear Control Systems for Eye Movement

There are five supranuclear eye movement systems:

☐ The *saccadic system* generates all fast (up to 400°–500°/sec) eye movements, or eye movements of refixation. It functions to place an object of interest on the fovea or to move the eyes from one object to another. Saccades are initiated by burst cells within the paramedian pontine reticular formation (PPRF). Their activation requires suppression of pause cell activity. Pause cells are inhibited by corticobulbar projections from the frontal lobe.

☐ The *smooth pursuit system* generates all following, or pursuit, eye movements. Pursuit latency is shorter than for saccades, but the maximum peak velocity of these slow pursuit movements is limited to 30°–60° per sec. The pathway starts with the striate cortex, which receives input from the lateral geniculate bodies. Extrastriate visual areas then receive input and project ipsilaterally to the dorsolateral pontine nuclei. Ultimately, the vestibular nuclei receive the input (probably through the cerebellar flocculus and dorsal vermis) and transmit it to ocular motor nuclei of cranial nerves III, IV, and VI.

☐ The *vergence system* controls disjugate eye movement, as in convergence or divergence. Supranuclear control of vergence eye movements is not yet fully understood.

☐ The *position maintenance system* maintains a specific gaze position, allowing an object of interest to remain on the fovea. The site of this system is not known.

☐ The *nonoptic reflex systems* integrate eye movements and body movements. The most clinically important system is the labyrinthine reflex system involving the semicircular canals of the inner ears. Other, less important, systems involve the utricle and saccule of the inner ears. The cervical, or neck, receptors also provide input for this nonoptic reflex control.

These systems are discussed in depth in BCSC Section 5, *Neuro-Ophthalmology.*

CHAPTER III

Sensory Physiology and Pathology

Objective visual space consists of actual visual objects in physical space outside of, and independent of, our visual system. *Subjective visual space* is our conscious awareness of these visual objects and their relationships to us as perceived and interpreted by the brain.

Physiology of Normal Binocular Vision

If an area of the retina is stimulated by any means—externally by light or internally by mechanical pressure or electrical processes—the resulting sensation will always be one of *light,* and the light will be subjectively localized as coming from a specific visual direction in space. This directional value of the retinal elements is an intrinsic physiologic property of the retina and the brain. Thus, the stimulation of any retinal area results in a visual sensation from a subjective visual direction relative to the visual direction of the fovea. The visual direction of the fovea is termed the *visual axis,* and normally, with central fixation, it is subjectively localized straight ahead. BCSC Section 12, *Retina and Vitreous,* illustrates and discusses in depth the anatomy and physiology of the retina.

Correspondence

If retinal areas in the two eyes share a common subjective visual direction, that is, if their simultaneous stimulation results in the subjective sensation that the stimulating target or targets come from the same direction in space, these retinal areas or points are said to be *corresponding.* If the simultaneous stimulation of retinal areas in the two eyes results in the sensation of two separate visual directions, or diplopia, these retinal areas or points are said to be *noncorresponding,* or *disparate.* If corresponding retinal areas in the two eyes bear identical relationships to the fovea in each eye—e.g., both corresponding areas are located equidistantly to the right or left of and above or below the fovea—then *normal retinal correspondence* (NRC) exists. Dissimilar relationships between two corresponding retinal areas and their respective foveas indicate *anomalous retinal correspondence* (ARC), which is discussed in detail on pp 40–42.

If the two eyes have normal retinal correspondence and each fovea fixates an identical point, this point will be seen singly. Points to both sides of this fixation point will likewise fall on corresponding retinal areas and will also be seen singly, as long as these points lie on a horizontal plane known as the *Vieth-Müller circle.* This circle passes through the optical centers of each eye and the point of fixation. When attempts are made to duplicate the Vieth-Müller circle experimentally, the

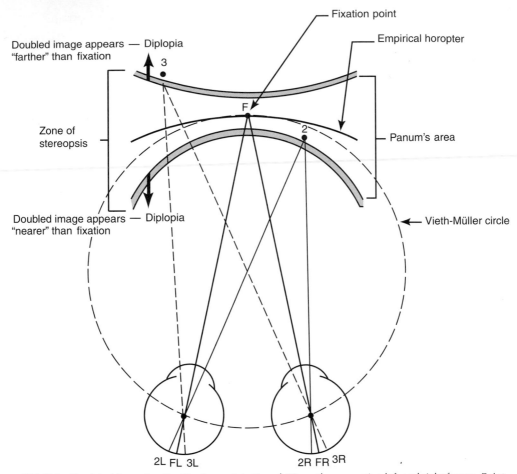

Fixation point

Empirical horopter

Doubled image appears — Diplopia
"farther" than fixation

3

F

Zone of
stereopsis

2

Panum's area

Doubled image appears — Diplopia
"nearer" than fixation

Vieth-Müller circle

2L FL 3L   2R FR 3R

FIG III-1—Empirical horopter. F = Fixation point; FL and FR are the respective left and right foveas. Point 2, falling within Panum's area, is seen singly and stereoscopically. Point 3 falls outside of Panum's area and is therefore seen double.

locus of all points seen singly falls not on the circle but on a curved surface called the *empirical horopter* (Fig III-1). The horopter exists not only in two dimensions but is actually a three-dimensional space obtained by rotating the horizontal horopter around an axis connecting the centers of rotation of the two eyes. The geometric figure thus formed is a *torus*.

Each fixation point determines a specific horopter. By definition, all points lying on the horopter curve will stimulate corresponding retinal elements and thus be seen singly. All points not lying on the horopter will mathematically fall on disparate retinal elements and would therefore be expected to create double vision. However, double vision does not occur physiologically within a limited area surrounding the horopter curve, because the visual system fuses the two disparate retinal images, resulting in single binocular vision with *stereopsis*. The slightly different images caused by the three-dimensional object stimulate stereoscopic perception.

The areas near the fovea allow very little overlap (small receptive fields) before diplopia is elicited, whereas more overlap (larger receptive fields) is tolerated farther toward the periphery of vision. Figure III-1 shows objects in this space that fall mathematically on disparate retinal areas but are physiologically seen singly. This space is called *Panum's area of single binocular vision*. Objects outside of Panum's area fall on widely disparate retinal areas and are seen as coming from two different visual directions, causing diplopia.

A three-dimensional object will be partly in front of and partly behind the empirical horopter and will thus stimulate disparate retinal points and be seen stereoscopically. As long as the three-dimensional object falls entirely within Panum's area, it will be seen singly. Objects that fall outside of Panum's area are seen double, because the images are too disparate to be fused cortically into a single image. Stereopsis is a response to horizontally disparate retinal stimulation. The zone of stereopsis is actually wider than Panum's fusional area, creating a zone in front of and behind Panum's space where double images can still be perceived as being farther away or closer than the object of regard (see Figure III-1).

Fusion

Fusion is the cortical unification of visual objects into a single percept that is made possible by the simultaneous stimulation of corresponding retinal areas. For retinal images to be fused, they must be similar in size and shape. Fusion has been artificially divided into sensory fusion, motor fusion, and stereopsis.

Sensory fusion   This form of fusion is based on the innate orderly topographic relationship between the retinas and the visual cortex whereby corresponding retinal points project to the same cortical locus, and corresponding adjacent retinal points have adjacent cortical representations.

Motor fusion   This type of fusion is a vergence movement that causes similar retinal images to fall and be maintained on corresponding retinal areas even though natural (e.g., phorias) or artificial causes tend to induce disparities. For example, if progressive base-out prism is introduced before both eyes while a target is viewed, the retinal images would move temporally over both retinas if the eyes remained in fixed position. However, fusional convergence movements occur to maintain similar retinal images on corresponding retinal areas, and the eyes will be observed to converge. This response is called *fusional convergence*. Motor fusion may be thought of as a diplopia-avoidance mechanism. Fusional vergence amplitudes can be measured with rotary prisms, by major haploscopes, and by other devices. Representative normal values are given in Table III-1. Fusional vergences are also discussed in chapter VI.

Stereopsis   Stereopsis should not be thought of as a form of simple fusion. As discussed, it occurs when retinal disparity is too great to permit the simple superimposition or fusion of the two visual directions but is not great enough to elicit diplopia. Stereopsis is, therefore, a bridge between simple sensory and motor fusion and

TABLE III-1

AVERAGE NORMAL FUSIONAL AMPLITUDES IN PRISM DIOPTERS (Δ)

TESTING DISTANCE	CONVERGENCE FUSIONAL AMPLITUDES	DIVERGENCE FUSIONAL AMPLITUDES	VERTICAL FUSIONAL AMPLITUDES
6 m	14Δ	6Δ	2.5Δ
25 cm	38Δ	16Δ	2.6Δ

diplopia. It is a relative or subjective ordering of visual objects in depth, or three dimensions.

Stereopsis and *depth perception* should not be considered synonymous terms. Monocular clues contribute to depth perception. These monocular clues include object overlap, relative object size, highlights and shadows, motion parallax, and perspective. Stereopsis is a binocular sensation of relative depth caused by horizontal retinal image disparity. Nasal disparity between two similar retinal images is interpreted by the brain as farther away from the fixation point, temporal disparity as nearer. At distances farther than 20 feet, we rely almost entirely on monocular clues for depth perception.

Retinal Rivalry

The rapid alternation in the perceived image of two dissimilar objects presented to the foveal areas of each eye simultaneously is called *retinal rivalry*. For example, if two dissimilar objects, each consisting of thin lines but differing in directional orientation, are viewed by each fovea separately and simultaneously, the binocular impression is one of a constantly changing mosaic. Retinal rivalry occurs because of the physiologic inability of the two foveas to simultaneously perceive dissimilar objects.

Selected Neurophysiological Aspects

M- and P-Cell Neurophysiology

Neurophysiological animal studies have identified two specific pathways used to process visual information, which arise from different populations of retinal ganglion cells. Ganglion cell stimulation from a retinal image results in simultaneous parallel processing through these two different pathways. Nuclei in the lateral geniculate body can be divided into *parvocellular* (*P-cells*, or small cells) and *magnocellular* (*M-cells*, or large cells). P-cell neurons are more sensitive to color, high spatial frequencies, fine two-point discrimination, and fine stereopsis, and they project to areas of the central visual field and fovea. M-cell neurons are sensitive to direction, motion, speed, flicker, gross binocular disparities, and gross stereopsis. They project to parafoveal and more peripheral retina. M-cell neurons are used for determining *where*, whereas P-cell neurons examine static objects and determine *what*.

Even though the two pathways are distinct, they overlap, and both systems interact to process visual information. In the striate cortex parvo- and magno-recipient lamellae are segregated; however, there are interconnecting pathways, so information commingles. From the striate cortex information from M-cells goes predominantly to parieto-occipital areas, while information from P-cells goes to temporo-occipital areas.

Pattern deprivation amblyopia, which is a failure to develop fine two-point discrimination, is probably associated predominantly with abnormal P-cell development. M-cell development is also affected, especially if the retinal image disparity is quite large. M-neuron maldevelopment occurs predominantly in cases of strabismus and may contribute to associated motor abnormalities such as the latent nystagmus and asymmetrical horizontal smooth pursuit often seen in patients with congenital or infantile strabismus.

The maldevelopment of M versus P pathways secondary to strabismus or to anisometropia and a blurred retinal image is currently being studied. The exact neurologic ramifications of a blurred retinal image and strabismus on the developing visual system are also under investigation. See also BCSC Section 5, *Neuro-Ophthalmology.*

Tychsen L. Binocular vision. In: Hart WM, ed. *Adler's Physiology of the Eye: Clinical Applications.* 9th ed. St Louis: Mosby; 1992:773–853.

van Essen DC, Maunsell JH. Hierarchical organization and functional streams in the visual cortex. *Trends Neuroscience.* 1983;6:370–395.

Monocular Deprivation

Eyelid suturing of one eye of a kitten during the first 2 or 3 months of life produces atrophy (reduced cell size) of cell bodies in the lateral geniculate laminae that receive input from the deprived eye and a nearly complete loss of cortical input from that eye. Experimentally induced anisometropia and nonalternating esotropia produce similar effects, although usually not as severe. Alternate occlusion or the severing of both medial rectus muscles (thereby producing alternating exotropia) causes the striate cortical cells to be influenced almost exclusively by one or the other eye; binocular input is lost.

Hubel DH, Wiesel TN. Binocular interaction in striate cortex of kittens reared with artificial squint. *J Neurophysiol.* 1965;28:1041–1057.

von Noorden GK. Mechanisms of amblyopia. *Adv Ophthalmol.* 1977;34:93–115.

For kittens and monkeys the sensitive period during which deprivation and strabismic amblyopia can be produced is approximately the first 3 months of life. Experimental amblyopia cannot be induced after this age. The comparable sensitive period for humans is not as well documented but probably extends to at least the age of 5–10 years. Amblyopia is discussed in detail in the next chapter.

von Noorden GK. Application of basic research data to clinical amblyopia. *Ophthalmology.* 1978;85:496–504.

Laboratory observations on experimental animals must not be uncritically transferred to humans. However, the clinical implication of these laboratory findings is that unilateral opacities in infants should be corrected as soon as possible after birth,

since such lesions would be expected to produce the most profound type of amblyopia, *deprivation amblyopia,* as they have been shown to do. Strabismic and anisometropic amblyopia should likewise be treated as soon as practicable by patching
as well as by correction of the deviation and/or refractive error. Prolonged alternate
patching should probably be avoided, since it would be expected to decrease the
number of binocularly driven cortical cells.

Abnormalities of Binocular Vision

It is important to realize that pathologic suppression, amblyopia, and anomalous
retinal correspondence develop only in young children. After the age of 6 or 7 years,
the development of these abnormalities is rare.

Diplopia and Confusion

Diplopia   Double vision, or diplopia, usually results from an acquired misalignment of the visual axes that causes an image to fall simultaneously on the fovea of
one eye and on a nonfoveal point in the other eye. The object that falls on these noncorresponding points must be outside Panum's area to be seen double. The same
object is seen as having two different locations in subjective space, and the foveal
image is always clearer than the nonfoveal image. The symptomatology of diplopia
depends on the age at onset, duration, and subjective awareness. The younger the
child, the greater the ability to suppress, or inhibit, the nonfoveal image.

Central fusional disruption (horror fusionis) is an intractable diplopia that features both an absence of suppression and a loss of fusional amplitudes to maintain
fusion. The angle of strabismus may be small or variable. Horror fusionis can occur
in a number of clinical settings: after disruption of fusion for a prolonged period;
after head trauma; and, rarely, in long-standing strabismus. The management of these
patients can be frustrating.

Confusion   *Visual confusion,* like diplopia, is associated with ocular misalignment;
however, confusion is very rare. Most adult patients with acquired ocular misalignment see two of the same image. Rarely, however, patients will describe the simultaneous perception of two different images superimposed on each other. Because the
eyes are misaligned, dissimilar images fall on corresponding retinal areas, causing
visual confusion. Objects that are physically separated in objective space are seen
as having the same location in subjective space. Since the two foveas are physiologically incapable of simultaneous perception of dissimilar objects, confusion may
represent a phenomenon of nonfoveal retinal areas only. This theory would explain
why clinically significant visual confusion is so rare.

Suppression

Suppression is the alteration of visual sensation that occurs when the images from
one eye are inhibited or prevented from reaching consciousness. *Pathologic suppression* results from strabismic misalignment of the visual axes. It can be seen as an
adaptation of a visually immature brain to avoid diplopia. *Physiologic suppression* is
the mechanism that prevents physiologic diplopia from reaching consciousness.

The following is a useful classification of suppression for the clinician:

□ *Central versus peripheral. Central suppression* is the term used to describe the mechanism that keeps the foveal image of the deviating eye from reaching consciousness, thereby preventing confusion. However, since the two foveas cannot simultaneously perceive dissimilar objects, this central scotoma of the nonfixating fovea is considered by many clinicians to be a physiologic form of suppression rather than a pathologic one. In addition, this scotoma of the deviated eye can be documented immediately after onset of ocular misalignment even in new-onset strabismus in a visually mature adult. Despite complaining about diplopia, adults with new-onset strabismus fixate with one eye at a time and demonstrate a small scotoma of the nonfixating fovea, preventing central visual confusion. This response to adult-onset strabismus supports the opinion that central suppression should be classified as physiologic rather than pathologic, since pathologic suppression can develop only in an immature visual system.

   Peripheral suppression is the mechanism that eliminates diplopia by preventing awareness of the image that falls on the peripheral retina in the deviating eye and resembles the image falling on the fovea of the fixating eye. This form of suppression is clearly pathologic and develops as a cortical adaptation only within an immature visual system. Adults cannot develop peripheral suppression and therefore cannot eliminate the peripheral second image of the object viewed by the fixating eye (the *object of regard*) without closing or occluding the deviating eye.

□ *Monocular versus alternating.* If suppression is unidirectional, or always causes the image from the dominant eye to predominate over the image from the deviating eye, the suppression is *monocular*. This type of mechanism may lead to the establishment of strabismic amblyopia. If the process is bidirectional, or switches over a period of time between the images of the two eyes, the suppression is described as *alternating.*

□ *Facultative versus obligatory.* Suppression may be considered *facultative* if present only when the eyes are in the deviated state and absent in all other states. Patients with intermittent exotropia, for instance, often have suppression when the eyes are divergent but enjoy high-grade stereopsis when the eyes are straight. In contrast, *obligatory suppression* is present at all times, whether the eyes are deviated or aligned. The suppression scotomata in the deviating eye may be either relative in the sense of permitting some visual sensation or absolute, permitting no perception of light.

Tests of suppression   If a patient with strabismus and normal retinal correspondence does not have diplopia, suppression is present provided the sensory pathways are intact. In less clear-cut situations several simple tests are available for clinical diagnosis of suppression.

   In the *Worth four-dot test* a red lens is worn in front of one eye, and a green lens in front of the other. The eye behind the red lens can see red light but not green light, because the red lens blocks these wavelengths. Similarly, the eye behind the green lens can see green light but not red light. If a target consisting of two green lights, one red light, and one white light is viewed, the patient with normal ocular alignment will report a total of four lights. The white light is usually reported to undergo color rivalry; however, only one light is seen in the position of the white light. If the eye behind the green lens is suppressed, a total of two lights is reported. If the eye behind the red lens is suppressed, a total of three lights is reported. If the patient reports five lights, diplopia is present. A report of more than five lights is likely to be factitious. A polarized Worth four-dot test is now available, which is administered and interpreted much like the traditional test except that polarized glasses are worn rather than red and green ones.

In the *red lens test* a red lens is placed before one eye as the patient fixates a light. If only one light is seen (either red or white), suppression is present. It is possible to use prisms placed in any direction to move the image out of the suppression scotoma of the deviating eye until two lights are seen. Bagolini lenses may also be used to test for suppression (see Figure III-3 and discussion on p 42).

Management of suppression Therapy for suppression often involves the treatment of the strabismus itself:

□ Proper refractive correction

□ Occlusion to permit equal and alternate use of each eye and to overcome any amblyopia that may be present

□ Alignment of the visual axes to permit simultaneous stimulation of corresponding retinal elements by the same object

Orthoptic exercises may be attempted to overcome the tendency of the image from one eye to suppress the image from the other eye when both eyes are open. These exercises are designed to first make the patient aware of diplopia, then of simultaneous perception, then of fusion on both an instrument and in free space. The role of orthoptics in the therapy of suppression is controversial. In treatment of patients with esotropia, antisuppression therapy can cause intractable diplopia as suppression disappears. Antisuppression therapy is safer in patients with intermittent exotropia, but the results have received mixed reviews. Patients with no fusion potential should *never* undergo antisuppression therapy.

Anomalous Retinal Correspondence

In young children with long-standing ocular deviations a sensory shift in retinal correspondence may develop so that retinal areas that receive the same images—as determined by the angle of the strabismus—develop a common visual direction. Such a shift implies a reordering of inputs into the visual cortex. This adaptation is thought to enable the development of a crude type of binocularity in the presence of strabismus.

Several tests for anomalous retinal correspondence (ARC) have been developed, but they can basically be divided into two groups: those that stimulate the fovea of one eye and an extrafoveal area of the other eye, and those that stimulate the foveal area in each eye. Note that ARC is a binocular phenomenon, tested and documented in both eyes simultaneously. Eccentric fixation is a monocular phenomenon found on testing one eye alone, and it is not in any way related to ARC. However, since many tests for ARC depend on stimulating each fovea separately, the presence of eccentric fixation can significantly affect the test results.

Diplopia test The diplopia test (red lens test) involves stimulating the fovea of the fixating eye and an extrafoveal area of the other eye. The test can be done at both distance and near. The patient's deviation is measured objectively. Then a red lens is placed before the deviating eye while the patient fixates a white light. Diplopia is present if the patient notes both a red light (through the filter) and a white light.

Often, recognition of diplopia will be facilitated by the addition of a 5Δ or 10Δ (prism diopter) vertical prism in front of the red glass in order to place the image of the fixation light out of the suppression scotoma. The following responses are possible:

□ The patient may see a red light and a white light. If the patient has esotropia, the images appear uncrossed; e.g., the red light is to the right of the white light with the red lens over the right eye. This response is known as *homonymous, or uncrossed, diplopia*. If the patient has exotropia, the images appear crossed; e.g., the red light is to the left of the white light with the red lens over the right eye. This response is known as *heteronymous, or crossed, diplopia*. If the measured separation between the two images equals the previously determined deviation, then the patient has *normal retinal correspondence*.

□ If the patient sees the two lights superimposed so that they appear pinkish despite a measurable esotropia or exotropia, then an abnormal localization of retinal points is present. This condition is known as *harmonious anomalous retinal correspondence*.

□ If the patient sees two lights (with uncrossed diplopia in esotropia, and crossed diplopia in exotropia), but the separation between the two images is found to be less than the previously determined deviation, then the patient has *unharmonious anomalous retinal correspondence*. Some investigators consider unharmonious ARC to be an artifact of the testing situation.

The Worth four-dot can be used instead of the red lens test.

Afterimage test   The afterimage test involves stimulation of the macula of each eye. Since the light flash stimulation necessary for this test is done for each eye separately, the presence of eccentric fixation in one eye will significantly affect the results. This test involves the stimulation, or "labeling," of each eye with a different linear afterimage, one horizontal and one vertical. Since suppression scotomata extend along the horizontal retinal meridian and may obscure most of a horizontal afterimage, the vertical afterimage is placed on the deviating eye and the horizontal afterimage on the fixating eye simply by having each eye fixate the linear light filament separately.

The central zone of the linear light is occluded to allow for the fovea to fixate and remain "unlabeled." The patient is then asked to draw the relative positions of the perceived afterimages. Possible perceptions are the following (Fig III-2):

□ If the patient has normal retinal correspondence, the two afterimages will be seen as a cross with a single gap (which corresponds to the fovea of each eye) in the center.

□ If the patient has an esotropia and anomalous retinal correspondence, the afterimages from both eyes will be seen as crossed.

□ If the patient has a left exotropia and anomalous retinal correspondence, the afterimages from both eyes will be seen as uncrossed.

Amblyoscope   With the amblyoscope the examiner determines the *objective angle,* at which the targets imaged on the two foveas will produce no movement with alternate target presentation. If the images are seen superimposed, with the angle between the arms of the amblyoscope equal to the objective angle, correspondence is normal; if not, correspondence is anomalous. The patient is then asked to superimpose the two targets. If superimposition occurs with the amblyoscope arms set at

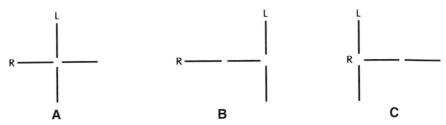

FIG III-2—*A,* Patient with normal retinal correspondence sees afterimages as a cross. *B,* Patient with esotropia and ARC sees afterimages side by side and crossed. *C,* Patient with left exotropia and ARC sees afterimages side by side and uncrossed.

0 angle (arms parallel), the patient shows harmonious anomalous retinal correspondence. If the arms are set somewhere between 0 and the objective angle of squint, unharmonious anomalous retinal correspondence is present theoretically. The reader is reminded that unharmonious ARC may be an artifact of the testing situation.

Bagolini test The *Bagolini striated glasses* are lenses with no dioptric power that have many narrow striations running parallel in one meridian. For testing purposes these lenses may be placed at 135° in front of the right eye and at 45° in front of the left eye. The advantage of the Bagolini glasses is that they afford the most lifelike situation for testing retinal correspondence. Figure III-3 summarizes some of the possible subjective results from this test.

Monofixation Syndrome

A patient with monofixation syndrome usually has a small-angle esotropia, but there may be exotropia or even no manifest deviation. A small-angle strabismus (usually less than 8Δ) usually can be detected under binocular conditions. These patients are sometimes said to have *microtropias*. A central scotoma and peripheral fusion are present with binocular viewing. Amblyopia is a common finding; usually it is slight, but it may be profound. Fixation can be central or eccentric, stereo acuity is reduced, and horizontal fusional amplitudes are present. Anomalous retinal correspondence is found on some sensory tests.

Patients with monofixation syndrome may have latent phoria in excess of a manifest microtropia. When this occurs, the alternate prism cover test measurement will exceed the simultaneous prism cover test measurement. This tropia with overlying phoria combination is only found in patients with monofixation syndrome.

Monofixation syndrome may be a primary condition, although it is often a consequence of esotropia treatment with glasses and/or surgery. It can also result from anisometropia or macular lesions. It can be the cause of unilaterally reduced vision when no obvious strabismus is present. If amblyopia is clinically significant, occlusion therapy is indicated.

Diagnosis To accurately diagnose monofixation syndrome the clinician must demonstrate both the absence of central binocular vision *(bifixation)* and the presence of peripheral binocular vision *(peripheral fusion).* Documentation of a macular scotoma in the nonfixating eye during binocular viewing is needed to verify the

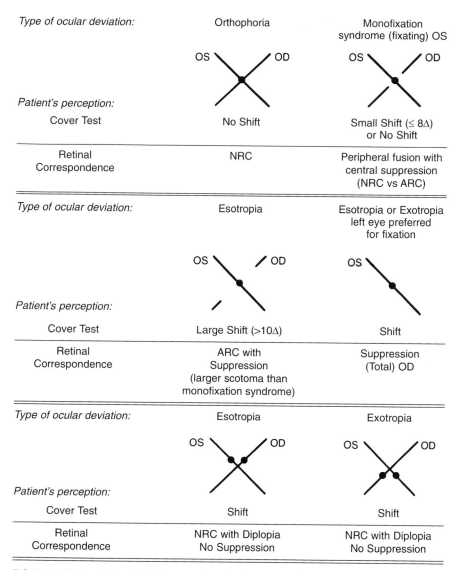

Type of ocular deviation:	Orthophoria	Monofixation syndrome (fixating) OS
Patient's perception:		
Cover Test	No Shift	Small Shift (≤ 8Δ) or No Shift
Retinal Correspondence	NRC	Peripheral fusion with central suppression (NRC vs ARC)
Type of ocular deviation:	Esotropia	Esotropia or Exotropia left eye preferred for fixation
Patient's perception:		
Cover Test	Large Shift (>10Δ)	Shift
Retinal Correspondence	ARC with Suppression (larger scotoma than monofixation syndrome)	Suppression (Total) OD
Type of ocular deviation:	Esotropia	Exotropia
Patient's perception:		
Cover Test	Shift	Shift
Retinal Correspondence	NRC with Diplopia No Suppression	NRC with Diplopia No Suppression

FIG III-3—The Bagolini striated glass test for retinal correspondence and suppression. For these figures, the Bagolini lens is oriented at 135° in front of the right eye and at 45° in front of the left eye. The perception of the oblique lines seen by each eye under binocular conditions is shown. Examples of the types of strabismus in which these responses are commonly found are given.

absence of bifixation. Several binocular perimetric techniques have been described to plot the monofixation scotoma. However, they are rarely used clinically. Patients can be taught to recognize their own scotoma when viewing a handheld light through Bagolini striated glasses. The central scotoma is perceived as a gap in one of the lines surrounding the fixation light (see Figure III–3). Patients can then be encouraged to switch fixation to the nonpreferred eye and observe the scotoma move to the other light streak.

Vectographic projections of Snellen letters can be used clinically to document the facultative scotoma of the monofixation syndrome. Snellen letters are viewed through polarized analyzers (AO Vectograph Project-O Chart slide) or goggles equipped with liquid crystal shutters (BVAT II BVS, Mentor O and O) in such a way that some letters are seen with only the right eye, some with only the left eye, and some with both eyes. Patients with monofixation syndrome delete letters that are imaged only in the nonfixating eye.

The red lens or polarized Worth four-dot test can be used to demonstrate both the presence of peripheral fusion and the absence of bifixation. The standard Worth four-dot flashlight projects onto a central retinal area of 1° or less when viewed at 10 feet, well within the 3°–5° scotoma characteristic of monofixation syndrome. Therefore, patients with monofixation syndrome will report two or three lights when viewing at 10 feet, depending on their ocular fixation preference. Bifixators will report four lights. As the Worth four-dot flashlight is brought closer to the patient, the dots begin to project onto peripheral retina outside of the central monofixation scotoma until a fusion response (four lights) is obtained. This usually occurs between 2 and 3 feet.

Testing stereo acuity is a very important part of the monofixation syndrome evaluation. Any amount of gross stereopsis confirms the presence of peripheral fusion. Most patients with monofixation syndrome will demonstrate 200–3000 seconds of arc stereopsis. However, since some monofixation syndrome patients will have no demonstrable stereopsis, other tests for peripheral fusion must be used in conjunction with stereo acuity measurement. Fine stereopsis (40 seconds of arc or better) is present only in patients with bifixation.

Another diagnostic maneuver available to document the presence of a facultative scotoma is the *4Δ base-out prism test*. The prism is quickly placed before one eye and then the other during binocular viewing, and motor responses are observed. Patients with bifixation usually show a version (bilateral) movement away from the eye covered by the prism followed by a unilateral fusional convergence movement of the eye not behind the prism. A similar response occurs regardless of which eye the prism is placed over. Often no movement is seen in patients with monofixation syndrome when the prism is placed before the nonfixating eye. A refixation version movement is seen when the prism is placed before the fixating eye, but the expected fusional convergence does not occur.

The 4Δ base-out prism test is the least reliable method used to document the presence of a macular scotoma. An occasional bifixation patient will recognize diplopia when the prism is placed before an eye but make no convergence movement to correct for it. Monofixation syndrome patients may switch fixation each time the prism is inserted and show no movement, regardless of which eye is tested.

Lang J. Evaluation in small angle strabismus or microtropia. In: Aruga A, ed. *Strabismus Symposium*. Basel: Karger; 1968:219–222.

Parks MM. Sensory adaptations in strabismus. In: Nelson LB, Calhoun JH, Harley RD, eds. *Pediatric Ophthalmology*. 3rd ed. Philadelphia: Saunders; 1991:122–127.

Parks MM. The monofixation syndrome. *Trans Am Ophthalmol Soc*. 1969;67:609–657. (This classic thesis outlines early studies of small-angle deviations and central versus peripheral binocular vision. The development of the various terms used to describe these conditions is also covered in detail.)

CHAPTER IV

Amblyopia

Amblyopia is a unilateral or bilateral reduction of best-corrected visual acuity that cannot be attributed directly to the effect of any structural abnormality of the eye or the posterior visual pathway. It is caused by abnormal visual experience early in life, usually resulting from one of the following:

□ Ocular misalignment

□ Uncorrected refractive error

□ Other disorders that degrade the quality of images transmitted to the brain from the eye

Amblyopia is primarily a defect of central vision; the peripheral visual field nearly always remains normal.

Amblyopia is responsible for more unilaterally reduced vision of childhood onset than all other causes combined, with a prevalence of 2%–4% in the North American population. This fact is particularly distressing because, in principle, nearly all amblyopic visual loss is preventable or reversible with timely, appropriate intervention. Children with amblyopia or at risk for developing it at a young age, when the prognosis for successful treatment is best, can now be identified with screening methods such as photorefraction that can be used in primary care medical offices or community-based programs. Consensus has not yet emerged, however, regarding the best way to deal with this important public health problem.

Day SH, Norcia AM. Photographic detection of amblyogenic factors. *Ophthalmology.* 1986;93:25–28.

Ehrlich MI, Reinecke RD, Simons K. Preschool vision screening for amblyopia and strabismus. Programs, methods, guidelines. *Surv Ophthalmol.* 1983;28:145–163.

Although understanding of the neurophysiologic mechanisms that underlie amblyopia is far from complete, the study of experimental modification of visual experience in animals and laboratory testing of amblyopic humans have provided some insights. Animal models have revealed that a variety of profound disturbances of visual system neuron function may develop as a result of abnormal early visual experience. Cells of the primary visual cortex can completely lose their innate ability to respond to stimulation of one or both eyes, and cells that remain responsive may show significant functional deficiencies. Abnormalities also occur in neurons in the lateral geniculate body. Evidence concerning involvement at the retinal level remains inconclusive; if present, changes in the retina make at most a minor contribution to the overall visual defect.

Several findings from both animals and humans, such as increased spatial summation and lateral inhibition when light detection thresholds are measured using different-sized spots, suggest that the receptive fields of neurons in the amblyopic visual system are abnormally large. This disturbance may account for the *crowding phenomenon* (also known as *contour interaction*), whereby Snellen letters or equivalent symbols of a given size become more difficult to recognize if they are closely surrounded by similar forms, such as a full line or chart of letters. Crowding phenomenon sometimes causes the measured "linear" acuity of an amblyopic eye to drop several lines below that measured with isolated letters.

Greenwald MJ, Parks MM. Amblyopia. In: Tasman W, Jaeger EA, eds. *Duane's Clinical Ophthalmology.* Philadelphia: Lippincott; 1990; vol 1, chap 10, 1–22.

von Noorden GK. Amblyopia: a multidisciplinary approach. Proctor lecture. *Invest Ophthalmol Vis Sci.* 1985;26:1704–1716.

Classification

Amblyopia has traditionally been subdivided in terms of the major disorders that may be responsible for its occurrence.

Strabismic Amblyopia

The most common form of amblyopia develops in the consistently deviating eye of a child with ocular misalignment. Constant, nonalternating tropias (typically esodeviations) are most likely to cause significant amblyopia. Strabismic amblyopia is thought to result from competitive or inhibitory interaction between neurons carrying the nonfusible inputs from the two eyes, which leads to domination of cortical vision centers by the fixating eye and chronically reduced responsiveness to the nonfixating eye's input. It has been suggested, but not proved, that this same mechanism is responsible for eliminating diplopia in strabismic children through suppression. Amblyopia itself does not as a rule prevent diplopia, however. Older patients with long-standing deviations frequently develop double vision after strabismus surgery, despite the presence of substantial amblyopic acuity reduction.

Several features of typical strabismic amblyopia are uncommon in other forms of amblyopia. *Grating acuity,* the ability to detect patterns composed of uniformly spaced stripes, which normally corresponds closely to Snellen acuity, is often reduced considerably less than Snellen acuity in strabismic amblyopia. Apparently, forms are seen by the affected eye in a twisted or distorted manner that interferes more with letter recognition than with the simpler task of determining whether a grating pattern is present. This discrepancy must be considered when the results of tests based on grating detection, such as Teller card preferential looking (a method of estimating acuity in infants and toddlers), are interpreted.

When illumination is reduced, the acuity of an eye with strabismic amblyopia tends to decline less sharply than that of a normal or organically diseased eye. This phenomenon is sometimes referred to as the *neutral-density filter effect* after the device classically used to demonstrate it. In dim light the normal eye may see no better than its amblyopic fellow.

Eccentric fixation   Eccentric fixation refers to the consistent use of a nonfoveal region of the retina for monocular viewing by an amblyopic eye. Minor degrees of eccentric fixation, detectable only with special tests such as visuscopy, Haidinger's brushes, or Maxwell's spot, are seen in many patients with strabismic amblyopia and relatively mild acuity loss. Clinically evident eccentric fixation, detectable by observing the noncentral position of the corneal reflection from the amblyopic eye while it fixates a light with the dominant eye covered, generally implies visual acuity of 20/200 or worse. See chapter VI for clinical testing. Use of nonfoveal retina for fixation cannot in general be regarded as the primary cause of reduced acuity in affected eyes. The mechanism of this interesting phenomenon, long a source of speculation, remains unknown.

Anisometropic Amblyopia

Second in frequency to strabismic amblyopia, anisometropic amblyopia develops when unequal refractive error in the two eyes causes the image on one retina to be chronically defocused. It is believed to result partly from the direct effect of image blur on the development of visual acuity in the involved eye and partly from interocular competition or inhibition similar (but not necessarily identical) to that responsible for strabismic amblyopia. Relatively mild degrees of hyperopic or astigmatic anisometropia (1–2 D) can induce mild amblyopia. Mild myopic anisometropia (less than –3 D) usually does not cause amblyopia, but unilateral high myopia (–6 D) often results in severe amblyopic visual loss. Unless strabismus is associated, which is not uncommon, the eyes of a child with anisometropic amblyopia look normal to the family and primary care physician; detection and treatment are often delayed until school age, when the prognosis for recovery of vision is guarded.

Isoametropic Amblyopia

A bilateral reduction in acuity that is usually relatively mild, isoametropic amblyopia results from large, approximately equal, uncorrected refractive errors in both eyes of a young child. Its mechanism involves the effect of blurred retinal images alone. Hyperopia exceeding about +5 D and myopia in excess of –10 D carry a risk of inducing bilateral amblyopia. Uncorrected bilateral astigmatism in early childhood may result in loss of resolving ability limited to the chronically blurred meridians (meridional amblyopia). The degree of cylindrical ametropia necessary to produce meridional amblyopia is not known; many normal infants show astigmatic refractive errors up to about 3 D that resolve spontaneously without apparent sequelae.

Deprivation Amblyopia

The old terms amblyopia ex anopsia or disuse amblyopia are sometimes still used for this type of amblyopia, which is usually caused by congenital or early acquired media opacities. This form of amblyopia is the least common but most damaging and difficult to treat. Amblyopic visual loss resulting from a unilateral lack of form vision tends to be worse than that produced by bilateral deprivation of similar degree, because interocular effects add to the direct developmental impact of severe image degradation. Even in bilateral cases, however, acuity of 20/200 or worse can occur.

In general, dense congenital cataracts that occupy the central 3 mm or more of the lens must be considered capable of causing severe amblyopia. Similar lens opacities acquired during childhood (up to age 8–10 years) can be almost as harmful. Small polar cataracts, around which retinoscopy can be readily performed, and lamellar cataracts, through which a reasonably good view of the fundus can be obtained, may cause mild to moderate amblyopia or may have no effect on visual development. Occlusion amblyopia is a form of deprivation amblyopia caused by excessive therapeutic patching.

Diagnosis

Amblyopia is diagnosed when evidence of reduced visual acuity that cannot be explained entirely on the basis of physical abnormalities is found in association with a history or finding of a condition known to be capable of causing amblyopia. Reliable differentiation of amblyopia from other forms of visual loss on the basis of the characteristics of vision alone is not generally possible at present. The crowding phenomenon, for example, is typical of amblyopia but not uniformly demonstrable. Afferent pupillary defects are characteristic of optic nerve disease but occasionally appear to be present with amblyopia. Amblyopia sometimes coexists with visual loss directly caused by an uncorrectable structural abnormality of the eye such as optic nerve hypoplasia or coloboma, which may in fact be its underlying cause. When such a situation is encountered in a young child, it is appropriate to undertake a trial of occlusion therapy; improvement in vision confirms that amblyopia was indeed present.

Multiple assessments using a variety of tests or performed on different occasions are sometimes required to make a final judgment concerning the presence and severity of amblyopia. General techniques for visual acuity assessment in children are discussed in chapter VI, but the clinician trying to determine the degree of amblyopic visual loss in a young patient should keep certain special considerations in mind. The *binocular fixation pattern,* which indicates strength of preference for one eye or the other under binocular viewing conditions, is a test generally relied upon for estimating the relative level of vision in the two eyes for children with strabismus under about 3 years old. This test is quite sensitive for detecting amblyopia, but it is sometimes falsely positive, showing a strong preference when vision is equal or nearly equal in the two eyes, particularly with small-angle strabismic deviations.

Acuity can usually be measured directly in children 3–6 years old using modified Snellen technique. But often only isolated letters can be used, which may lead to measurement underestimating amblyopic visual loss. Crowding bars may help alleviate this problem (Fig IV-1). In addition, the young child's brief attention span frequently results in measurements that fall short of the true limits of acuity; these results can mimic bilateral amblyopia or obscure or falsely suggest a significant interocular difference.

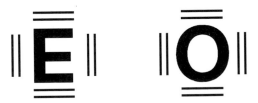

FIG IV-1—Crowding bars, or contour interaction bars, allow the examiner to test the crowding phenomenon with isolated optotypes. Lines surrounding the optotype mimic the full row of optotypes to the amblyopic child. (Reproduced with permission from Coats DK, Jenkins RH. Vision assessment of the pediatric patient. *Refinements.* San Francisco: American Academy of Ophthalmology; 1997;1:1.)

Treatment

Treatment of amblyopia involves the following steps:

□ Eliminating if possible any obstacle to vision such as a cataract

□ Correcting refractive error

□ In most unilateral or asymmetric cases forcing use of the poorer eye by limiting use of the better eye

Cataract Removal

Cataracts capable of producing amblyopia must be operated on without unnecessary delay. Removal of significant congenital lens opacities during the first 2–3 months of life is necessary for optimal recovery of vision. In symmetric bilateral cases the interval between operations on the first and second eyes should be no more than 1–2 weeks. Acutely developing severe traumatic cataracts in children under 8–10 years old should be removed within a few weeks of injury if possible. Significant cataracts with uncertain time of onset also deserve prompt and aggressive treatment during childhood if recent development is at least a possibility (for example, in the case of an opacity that appears to have originated from a posterior lenticonus deformity). BCSC Section 11, *Lens and Cataract,* discusses the special considerations of cataract surgery in children; see also chapter XXII of this volume.

Refractive Correction

Optical prescription for amblyopic eyes should in general correct the full refractive error as determined with cycloplegia. Because the amblyopic eye's ability to control accommodation tends to be impaired, it cannot be relied upon to compensate for uncorrected hyperopia as would the normal child's eye. Refractive correction for aphakia following cataract surgery in childhood must be provided promptly to avoid compounding the visual deprivation effect of the lens opacity with that of a severe optical deficit. Both anisometropic and isoametropic amblyopia may improve considerably with refractive correction alone over a period of several months.

Occlusion and Optical Degradation

Full-time total occlusion of the sound eye is the most powerful means of treating amblyopia by enforced use of the defective eye. This treatment is usually done with commercially available adhesive patches; the patch can either be left in place at night or removed at bedtime. Spectacle-mounted occluders or special opaque contact lenses can be used as an alternative to full-time patching if skin irritation or poor adhesion proves to be a significant problem, provided that close supervision ensures that they remain in place consistently. (Most skin-related problems can be eliminated by switching to a different brand of patch or by preparing the skin with tincture of benzoin or ostomy adhesive before application.) Full-time patching should generally be employed only in cases where the presence of constant strabismus eliminates any possibility of useful binocular vision. The child whose eyes are consistently or intermittently straight needs to be given some opportunity to see binocularly.

Part-time occlusion can usually achieve the same results as full-time occlusion. One to several days of patching can alternate with one to several of no patch, or patching can be done daily for periods ranging from 1 or 2 hours to all but 1 or 2 waking hours. The relative duration of patch-on and patch-off intervals should reflect the degree of amblyopia; for moderate to severe deficits at least half-time occlusion is preferred. If constant strabismus is present, some clinicians routinely patch the amblyopic eye during periods when the dominant eye is in use, but consensus is lacking on the value of this practice. The child undergoing part-time occlusion should be kept as visually active as possible when the patch is in place, but no specific visual exercises have been shown convincingly to be of particular benefit.

Other methods of amblyopia treatment involve *optical degradation* of the better eye's image to the point that it becomes inferior to the amblyopic eye's, an approach often referred to as *penalization*. Use of the amblyopic eye is thus promoted within the context of binocular seeing. A cycloplegic agent (usually atropine drops or ointment, 0.5% or 1.0%) is regularly administered (generally once daily) to the better eye so that it is unable to accommodate and suffers from blur with near viewing. When uncorrected hyperopia is present, the effect is amplified. Some practitioners concurrently administer a miotic (such as echothiophate iodide 1/8%) to the amblyopic eye to potentiate its near vision.

Atropinization offers the particular advantage of being difficult to thwart even if the child objects. Alternative methods of treatment based on the same principle involve spherical lenses or diffusing filters. These methods avoid potential pharmacologic side effects and may be capable of inducing greater blur. If the child is wearing glasses, application of translucent tape or a thick uneven layer of clear nail polish to the spectacle lens can be tried. Proper utilization (no peeking!) of spectacle-borne devices must be closely monitored.

Another benefit of atropinization and other methods of penalization is that the eyes can work together, a great practical advantage in children with latent nystagmus and, theoretically, an advantage in all patients.

When a therapeutic approach other than occlusion is initiated, it must be established that the better eye's vision has in fact been sufficiently degraded. In the strabismic patient this is easily done by noting an immediate switch of fixation preference. When the eyes are straight, preference for use of the amblyopic eye over its blurred fellow eye should be demonstrated with the aid of a vertical prism that optically induces ocular misalignment. (Reduction of the preferred eye's measured acuity below the amblyopic eye's level does not by itself provide adequate assurance that treatment will be effective.)

Complications of Therapy

Any form of amblyopia therapy introduces the possibility that overtreatment can lead to amblyopia in the originally better eye. Full-time occlusion carries the greatest risk of this complication and requires very close monitoring, especially in the younger child. The first follow-up visit after initiation of treatment should occur within 1 week for an infant and after an interval corresponding to 1 week per year of age for the older child (e.g., 4 weeks for a 4-year-old). Subsequent visits can be scheduled at longer intervals based on early response. Part-time occlusion and optical degradation methods allow for less frequent observation, but regular follow-up is still critical. The parents of a strabismic child should be instructed to watch for a switch in fixation preference and to report its occurrence promptly. If iatrogenic amblyopia develops, it can nearly always be treated successfully with judicious patching of the newly better eye or alternating occlusion. Sometimes simply stopping treatment altogether for a few weeks leads to equalization of vision.

The desired end point of therapy for unilateral amblyopia is free spontaneous alternation of fixation, although one eye may still be used somewhat more frequently than the other, and/or linear Snellen acuity that differs by no more than one line between the two eyes. The time required for completion of treatment depends on the following:

□ Degree of amblyopia

□ Choice of therapeutic approach

□ Compliance with the prescribed regimen

□ Age of the patient

More severe amblyopia, less complete obstruction of the dominant eye's vision, and older age are all associated with a need for more prolonged treatment. Full-time occlusion during infancy may reverse substantial strabismic amblyopia in 1 week or less. In contrast, an older child who wears a patch only after school and on weekends may require a year or more of treatment to overcome a moderate deficit.

Compliance issues   Lack of compliance with the inevitably unpleasant therapeutic regimen is a common problem that can prolong the period of treatment or lead to outright failure. If difficulties derive from a particular treatment method, a suitable alternative should be sought. Families who appear to lack sufficient motivation need to be counseled concerning the importance of the project and the need for firmness in carrying it out. They can be reassured that once an appropriate routine is established and maintained for a short time, the daily effort required is likely to diminish.

The problems associated with an unusually resistant child vary according to age. In infancy restraining the child through physical methods such as arm splints or mittens or merely making the patch stick tighter with tincture of benzoin may be useful. For children more than 3 years old creating goals and offering rewards tends to work well, as does linking patching to play activities (e.g., decorating the patch each day). Authoritative words directed specifically toward the child by the doctor may also help. The toddler period (1–3 years) is particularly challenging; sometimes, the best solution is to back off and renew efforts when the child becomes 3.

Unresponsiveness   In some cases even conscientious application of an appropriate therapeutic program fails to improve vision at all or beyond a certain level. Complete or partial unresponsiveness to treatment is occasionally found in younger children, but it is most often seen in patients more than 5 years old. Conversely, significant improvement in vision may be achievable with protracted effort even in adolescents. The decision whether to initiate or continue treatment in a prognostically unfavorable situation should take into account the wishes of the patient and family. Primary therapy should generally be terminated if there is a lack of demonstrable progress over a period of 3–6 months with good compliance.

Before it is concluded that intractable amblyopia is present, refraction should be carefully rechecked, and the macula and optic nerve critically inspected for subtle evidence of hypoplasia or other malformation that might have been previously overlooked. Amblyopia associated with unilateral high myopia and extensive myelination of retinal nerve fibers is a specific syndrome in which treatment failure is particularly common.

Recurrence When amblyopia treatment is discontinued after fully or partially successful completion, approximately one half of patients will show some degree of recurrence, which can nearly always be reversed with renewed therapeutic effort. Repeated backsliding can be prevented by an acuity maintenance regimen, typically patching for 1–3 hours per day or the equivalent. It may be judged advantageous in some cases to institute maintenance patching immediately upon completion of primary treatment. An alternative strategy is to gradually diminish the daily patching period to the minimum that preserves optimal acuity. Once the need for maintenance occlusion is established, it often must be continued until 8–10 years of age. As long as vision remains stable, intervals of up to 6 months between follow-up visits are acceptable.

Lambert SR, Boothe RG. Amblyopia: basic and clinical science perspectives. In: *Focal Points: Clinical Modules for Ophthalmologists.* San Francisco: American Academy of Ophthalmology; 1994;12:8.

Preferred Practice Patterns Committee, Pediatric Ophthalmology Panel. *Amblyopia.* San Francisco: American Academy of Ophthalmology; 1997.

CHAPTER V

Introduction to Strabismus

Terminology

The term *strabismus* is derived from the Greek word *strabismos,* "to squint, to look obliquely or askance." Strabismus means ocular misalignment, whether caused by abnormalities in binocular vision or by anomalies of neuromuscular control of ocular motility. Many terms are employed in discussing strabismus, and unless they are used correctly and uniformly, confusion and misunderstanding can occur.

Orthophoria is the ideal condition of ocular balance. In reality, orthophoria is seldom encountered, as a small heterophoria can be documented in most individuals, at least in certain gaze positions, using Maddox rod testing (see chapter VI). Some ophthalmologists therefore consider "orthophoria" to mean *essentially* straight eyes, even if a small heterophoria is present.

Heterophoria is an ocular deviation kept latent by the fusional mechanism (latent strabismus). *Heterotropia* is a deviation that is manifest and not kept under control by the fusional mechanism (manifest strabismus).

A detailed nomenclature has evolved to describe types of ocular deviations. This vocabulary uses many prefixes and suffixes based on the relative positions of the visual axes of both eyes to account for the multiple strabismic patterns encountered. Abbreviations commonly used in describing strabismus are listed in Table V-1.

TABLE V-1

COMMON STRABISMUS ABBREVIATIONS

HORIZONTAL DEVIATION	DISTANCE (6 m)	NEAR (33 cm)
Exophoria	X	X'
Esophoria	E	E'
Exotropia	XT	XT'
Esotropia	ET	ET'
Intermittent exotropia	X(T)	X(T)'
Intermittent esotropia	E(T)	E(T)'

VERTICAL DEVIATION	DISTANCE (6 m)	NEAR (33 cm)
Right hypertropia	RHT	RHT'
Left hypertropia	LHT	LHT'
Right hypotropia	RHoT (R Hypo T)	RHoT'
Left hypotropia	LHoT (L Hypo T)	LHoT'

Prefixes

- *Eso-:* The eye is rotated so that the cornea is deviated nasally and the fovea is rotated temporally. This is also known as a *convergent horizontal strabismus.*
- *Exo-:* The eye is rotated so that the cornea is deviated temporally and the fovea is rotated nasally. This is also known as a *divergent horizontal strabismus.*
- *Hypo-:* The eye is rotated so that the cornea is deviated inferiorly and the fovea is rotated superiorly. This is also known as a *vertical strabismus.*
- *Hyper-:* The eye is rotated so that the cornea is deviated superiorly and the fovea is rotated inferiorly. This is also known as a *vertical strabismus.*
- *Incyclo-:* The eye is rotated so that the superior portion of the vertical meridian is torted nasally and the inferior portion of the vertical meridian is torted temporally. This is also known as a *torsional strabismus.*
- *Excyclo-:* The eye is rotated so that the superior portion of the vertical meridian is torted temporally and the inferior portion of the vertical meridian is torted nasally. This is also known as a *torsional strabismus.*

Suffixes

- *-phoria:* A latent deviation that is controlled by the fusional mechanism so that under normal binocular vision the eyes remain aligned
- *-tropia:* A manifest deviation that exceeds the control of the fusional mechanism so that the eyes are not aligned

Usage

For all of the above deviations (eso-, exo-, hyper-, hypo-, incyclo-, and excyclo-), it is assumed that the deviating eye is the one that is not fixating, as the fixating eye should be directed at the fixation target. In some instances it is important to identify the deviating eye, especially when seeking to call attention to the "offending" eye as causing the deviation. This usage is particularly helpful when dealing with vertical deviations, restrictive or paretic strabismus, or amblyopia in a preverbal child.

Classification

No classification is perfect or all-inclusive, and several methods of classifying eye alignment and motility disorders are used. Certain types of strabismus are more easily classified one way, whereas other types lend themselves to a different classification. Several useful classifications follow. By applying the appropriate classification from each of the categories listed below, it is possible to describe more clearly a patient's particular form of strabismus.

Fusional Status

- *Phoria:* A latent deviation in which fusional control is always present
- *Intermittent tropia:* Fusional control is present part of the time
- *Tropia:* A manifest deviation in which fusional control is not present

Variation of the Deviation with Gaze Position or Fixating Eye

□ *Comitant (concomitant):* The deviation does not vary with direction of gaze or fixating eye.

□ *Incomitant (noncomitant):* The deviation varies with direction of gaze or fixating eye. Most incomitant strabismus is *paralytic,* or *restrictive.* Especially if acquired, incomitant strabismus may indicate neurologic or orbital disease.

Fixation

□ *Alternating:* Spontaneous alternation of fixation from one eye to the other
□ *Monocular:* Definite preference for fixation with one eye

Age of Onset

□ *Congenital:* A deviation documented in early infancy, presumably related to a defect present at birth; the term *infantile* might be more appropriate

□ *Acquired:* A deviation with later onset, after a period of apparently normal visual development

Type of Deviation

□ *Horizontal:* Esodeviation or exodeviation
□ *Vertical:* Hyperdeviation or hypodeviation
□ *Torsional:* Incyclodeviation or excyclodeviation
□ *Combined:* Horizontal, vertical, and/or torsional

CHAPTER VI

Diagnostic Techniques for Strabismus and Amblyopia

History and Characteristics of the Presenting Complaint

The motility examination begins with the patient's history. Because children become increasingly impatient during an examination, an experienced ophthalmologist will take advantage of the opportunity to observe the child while taking the history. The ophthalmologist should attempt to establish rapport with the patient and, if examining a child, with the parent(s) as well. See the Introduction for a detailed discussion on examining the child.

Especially when the patient is a child, it is important to obtain information regarding the mother's pregnancy, paying close attention to maternal health, gestational age at time of birth, birth weight, and neonatal history. The physician should also ask about the child's developmental milestones.

It is desirable to document the age of onset of a deviation or symptom, and old photographs are invaluable for this purpose. Baby pictures, grade-school snapshots, graduation photographs, and driver license pictures can impart critical information. In addition, the physician should seek to answer the following questions about the deviation or symptom:

☐ Is it associated with trauma or emotional or physical stress?

☐ Is the deviation constant or intermittent?

☐ Is the deviation present for distance, near, or both?

☐ Is it unilateral or alternating?

☐ Is it present only when the patient is inattentive or fatigued?

☐ Does one eye have a tendency to close when the patient is outside in bright sunlight?

Earlier treatment should be reviewed, including any previous management such as occlusion therapy, spectacle correction, use of miotics, orthoptic therapy, or prior eye muscle surgery. While obtaining the history, the physician should observe the patient continually, noting such behaviors as head posturing, head movement, attentiveness, and motor control.

Past and present medications should be recorded, along with drug sensitivities and/or allergic responses. It is also important to document previous surgeries, anesthetic methods used and their results, and a detailed family history of strabismus or other eye disorders.

Assessment of Visual Acuity

Distance Visual Acuity

Numerous tests are available for distance visual acuity determination: Snellen letters, including matching games such as HOTV; Allen pictures; "illiterate Es"; and Lea symbols are the most commonly encountered tests for visual acuity. Table VI-1 lists the standards of acuity for various tests at different ages.

Visual acuity is determined, by convention, first for the right eye and then for the left. A patch or occluder is used in front of the left eye as the acuity of the right eye is checked, then vice versa. An adhesive patch is both the most effective occluder and, unfortunately, the most objectionable from the child's point of view. The line with the smallest figures in which the majority of letters can be read accurately is recorded; if the patient misses a few of the figures on a line, a notation is made. If the patient does not have corrective lenses, a pinhole may be used to estimate the best visual acuity potential. However, the use of pinholes in children is cumbersome and often inconclusive.

Patients with poor vision may need to walk to the chart until they can see the big E or equivalent (20/400 line). In such cases visual acuity is recorded as the distance in feet/size of the letter; e.g., if the patient is able to read the big E at 5 feet, the acuity would be recorded as 5/400. Because the selection of large figures is limited, it is advisable to confirm measurements slightly closer to the chart using figures that can be changed.

The visual acuity assessment in children is often difficult, and the clinician must resort to various means of evaluation. In preverbal or nonverbal children, acuity can be evaluated by the *CSM method. C* refers to the location of the corneal light reflex as the patient fixates the examiner's light under monocular conditions (opposite eye covered). Normally, the reflected light from the cornea is near the *center* of the cornea, and it should be positioned symmetrically in both eyes. If the fixation target is viewed eccentrically, fixation is termed *uncentral* (UC). *S* refers to the *steadiness* of fixation on the examiner's light as it is held motionless and also as it is slowly moved about. The *S* evaluation is also done under monocular conditions. *M* refers to the ability of the strabismic patient to *maintain* alignment first with one eye, then

TABLE VI-1

NORMAL VISUAL ACUITY USING VARIOUS TESTS IN CHILDREN

AGE (YEARS)	VISION TEST	NORMAL
0–2	Visual evoked potential (VEP)	20/30 (age 1)
0–2	Preferential looking	20/30 (age 2)
0–2	Fixation behavior	CSM (see text)
2–5	Allen pictures	20/40–20/20
2–5	HOTV	20/40–20/20
2–5	E-game	20/40–20/20
5+	Snellen	20/30–20/20

with the other, as the opposite eye is uncovered. Maintenance of fixation is evaluated under binocular conditions. Inability to maintain fixation with either eye with the opposite eye uncovered is presumptive evidence of a difference in acuity between the two eyes. Thus, preverbal or nonverbal patients with strong fixation preference in one eye should be suspected of having amblyopia in the other eye. An exotropic eye that has eccentric fixation and nystagmoid movements when attempting fixation might be designated uncentral, unsteady, and unmaintained (UC, US, UM).

In children with straight eyes it is impossible to tell if the patient will maintain fixation with either eye unless he or she is tested with the *vertical prism,* or *induced tropia, test.* This test is performed by placing a moderate-sized prism (10–15Δ) base down over one eye to induce a vertical deviation. An alternate method includes the use of a larger prism held base out. The patient is then tested for the ability to maintain fixation with either eye under binocular, albeit dissociated, viewing conditions. It is important to determine whether each eye can maintain fixation through smooth pursuit or a blink; strong fixation preference for one eye indicates amblyopia in the nonpreferred eye.

Occasionally, avoidance movements can be demonstrated when the good eye is occluded. The patient may attempt to maneuver around the occluder when the good eye is covered but not when the poorly seeing eye is covered. A child with poor vision in the right eye, for example, might be noted to "fix and follow" (F and F) more poorly using that eye and to object to an occlusion of the left eye.

The visual acuity of older children can be tested using illiterate Es (the "E-game"), pictures, symbols, letters, or numbers. Often a child will be cooperative enough to allow use of the Allen pictures, which include common items such as a car, a horse, and a handprint. Very young children may be able to match the distant picture with a similar figure on a near card, the same method used with the HOTV system. The child being tested with the E game is asked to point his or her hand (or fingers) in the direction of the E. This test can be difficult to use because of age, developmental status, or lack of cooperation.

The type of test used should be identified along with the results to facilitate comparisons with measurements taken at other times. Most pediatric ophthalmologists consider Snellen acuity most reliable, followed by HOTV, Lea symbols, E-game, Allen pictures, and fixation behavior. The most reliable test which the child can perform should be used in each case. Preferential looking techniques using Teller acuity cards can be a useful adjunctive test for comparing visual acuity between fellow eyes in infants and preverbal children.

Patients with latent nystagmus may show better visual acuity with both eyes open than with one eye occluded. To assess this situation it may be helpful to place a +5.00 D sphere lens in front of the eye not being tested.

Near Visual Acuity

Tests of near visual acuity include reading cards with graduated, small standardized print. With a near card, visual acuity at 14 inches (35 cm) is recorded. Again, both uncorrected and corrected visual acuity are determined. Because of inaccuracy related to viewing distance, near visual acuities should never be compared with distance acuities in children.

Assessment of Eye Movements

Generally, versions are tested first. The examiner should pay particular attention to the movements of both eyes into the nine diagnostic positions of gaze. Limitations of movement into these positions and asymmetry of excursion of the two eyes should be noted. Spinning the child, or provoking the doll's head phenomenon, may be helpful in eliciting the vestibular-stimulated eye movements. If versions are not full, duction movements should be tested for each eye separately. BCSC Section 5, *Neuro-Ophthalmology,* also discusses testing of the ocular motility system.

The examiner must use ingenuity to keep the patient's attention, and such tricks as brightly colored toys, pictures, and storytelling about the objects are essential. A well-prepared examiner will always have several toys or pictures at hand (see the Introduction, Rapport With Children, on pp 3–6).

Tests of Ocular Alignment

Ocular alignment tests can be grouped into four basic types: cover tests, corneal light reflex tests, dissimilar image tests, and dissimilar target tests.

Cover tests Eye movement capability, image formation and perception, foveal fixation in each eye, attention, and cooperation are all necessities for cover testing. If the patient is unable to maintain constant fixation on an accommodative target, the results of cover testing may not be valid, and this battery of tests therefore should not be used.

There are three types of cover tests: the cover-uncover test, the alternate cover test, and the simultaneous prism-cover test. All can be performed with fixation at distance or near. Some deviations (e.g., intermittent exotropia) may be more evident at distance, while others (e.g., accommodative esotropia) may be more evident at near.

The monocular *cover-uncover test* is the most important test to differentiate a phoria from a tropia (Fig VI-1). As one eye is covered, the examiner watches carefully for any movement in the opposite, *noncovered* eye; such movement indicates the presence of a tropia. Movement of the *covered* eye just after the cover is removed indicates a phoria that becomes manifest only when binocularity is interrupted. If the patient has a phoria, the eyes will be straight before *and* after the cover-uncover test; the deviation that appears during the test is a result of interruption of binocular vision and the inability of the fusional mechanism to operate. A patient with a tropia, however, starts out with a deviated eye and also ends up after the test with either the same or the opposite eye deviated (if the opposite eye is the deviated one, the condition is termed *alternating heterotropia*). Some patients may have straight eyes and start out with a phoria prior to the cover-uncover test; but after prolonged testing, and therefore prolonged interruption of binocular vision, complete dissociation into a manifest tropia can occur.

The *alternate cover test (prism and cover test)* measures the total deviation, both latent and manifest (Fig VI-2). It does not specify how much of which type of deviation is present; i.e., it does not separate the phoria from the tropia. The cover is placed alternately in front of each eye several times to dissociate the eyes and maximize the deviation; it is important to quickly transfer the occluder from one eye to the other to prevent fusion from occurring. This test must be done at both distance and near fixation, with and without glasses. Once dissociation is achieved, the amount of deviation is measured using prisms to eliminate the eye movement as the cover is alternately switched from one eye to the other. It may be necessary to use

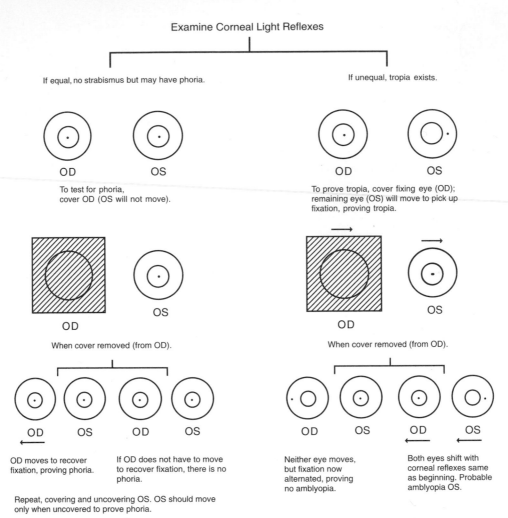

Examine Corneal Light Reflexes

If equal, no strabismus but may have phoria.

If unequal, tropia exists.

OD   OS

OD   OS

To test for phoria,
cover OD (OS will not move).

To prove tropia, cover fixing eye (OD);
remaining eye (OS) will move to pick up
fixation, proving tropia.

OS

OD

OS

OD

When cover removed (from OD).

When cover removed (from OD).

OD   OS   OD   OS

OD   OS   OD   OS

OD moves to recover
fixation, proving phoria.

If OD does not have to move
to recover fixation, there is no
phoria.

Neither eye moves,
but fixation now
alternated, proving
no amblyopia.

Both eyes shift with
corneal reflexes same
as beginning. Probable
amblyopia OS.

Repeat, covering and uncovering OS. OS should move
only when uncovered to prove phoria.

FIG VI-1—The monocular cover-uncover test.

both horizontally and vertically placed prisms. The amount of prism power required is the measure of deviation. Stacking the prisms one on top of the other, rather than placing the required amount divided before both eyes, can induce large measurement errors. However, it is appropriate to "stack" horizontal and vertical prisms before the same eye if necessary.

Whereas the alternate cover test measures the total deviation (phoria and tropia), the *simultaneous prism-cover test* is helpful in determining the actual heterotropia present when both eyes are uncovered (tropia alone). The test is performed by covering the fixating eye at the same time the prism is placed in front of the deviating eye. The test is repeated using increasing prism powers until the deviated eye no longer shifts. Again, the power of the prism is the measure of deviation. This test

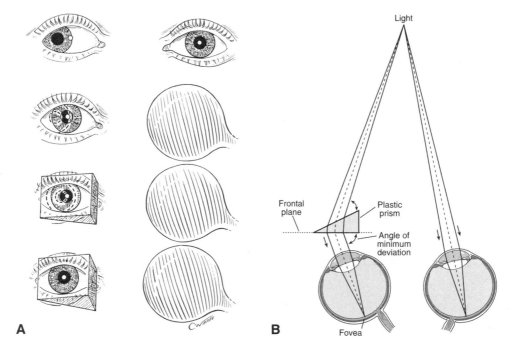

A   **B**

FIG VI-2—*A,* In the top row the child is seen to have a right exotropia. In the second row the cover test shows movement of the right eye to fixate when the left eye is covered. In the third row a small prism introduced before the right eye begins to neutralize the deviation. In the bottom row the correct prism has been introduced, and no more movement is seen when the cover is alternated between eyes. *B,* The diagram shows how the prism eliminates movement on cover testing by aligning rays of light from the fixation target with the fovea in the exotropic right eye. The size of the prism gives a measurement of the exotropia. (Reproduced with permission from Simon JW, Calhoun JH. *A Child's Eyes: A Guide to Pediatric Primary Care.* Gainesville, Fla: Triad Publishing Co; 1997:72.)

has special application in monofixation syndrome, which may include a small-angle heterotropia. Patients with this condition may reduce the amount of deviation measured in the alternate cover test by exerting at least partial control of a coexisting phoria through peripheral fusion when both eyes are open. In this instance the simultaneous prism-cover test measures the amount of tropia in a deviation that has a superimposed phoria.

Corneal light reflex tests These tests are useful in assessing ocular alignment in patients who cannot cooperate sufficiently to allow cover testing or who have poor fixation. The main tests of this type are the Hirschberg, modified Krimsky, Bruckner, and major amblyoscope methods.

Hirschberg's method is based on the premise that 1 mm of decentration of the corneal light reflection corresponds to about 7°, or 15Δ, of ocular deviation of the visual axis. Therefore, a light reflex at the pupillary margin is about 2 mm from the pupillary center, which corresponds to 15°, or 30Δ, of deviation. A reflex in the mid-iris region is about 4 mm from the pupillary center, which is roughly 30°, or 60Δ, of deviation; similarly, a reflex at the limbus is about 45°, or 90Δ, of deviation (Fig VI-3).

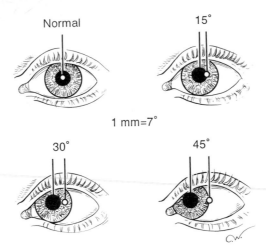

Normal   15°

1 mm=7°

30°   45°

FIG VI-3—Hirschberg test. The extent to which the corneal light reflex is displaced from the center of the pupil provides an approximation of the angular size of the deviation (in this example, a left esotropia). (Reproduced with permission from Simon JW, Calhoun JH. *A Child's Eyes: A Guide to Pediatric Primary Care.* Gainesville, Fla: Triad Publishing Co; 1997:72.)

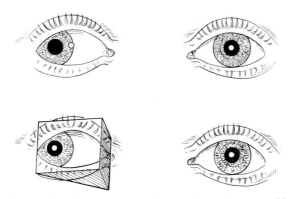

FIG VI-4—Krimsky test. The right exotropia in the top picture is measured by the size of the prism required to center the pupillary reflexes, as shown at bottom. (Reproduced with permission from Simon JW, Calhoun JH. *A Child's Eyes: A Guide to Pediatric Primary Care.* Gainesville, Fla: Triad Publishing Co; 1997:72.)

Krimsky's method uses reflections produced on both corneas by a penlight. The original method involved placing prisms in front of the deviating eye. More common modifications involve prisms held before the fixing eye, or split between the two eyes. By adjusting the prisms so as to center the corneal reflection in the deviated eye, it is possible to approximate and quantitate the deviation (Fig VI-4).

The *Bruckner test* is performed by using the direct ophthalmoscope to obtain a red reflex simultaneously in both eyes. If strabismus is present, the deviated eye will have a lighter and brighter reflex than the fixating eye. Note that this test detects, but does not measure, the deviation. This test will also identify opacities in the visual axis and moderate to severe anisometropia.

The *major amblyoscope method* uses separate target illumination, which can be moved to center the corneal light reflection. The amount of deviation is then read directly from the scale of the amblyoscope.

Dissimilar image tests   These tests are based on the patient's response to diplopia created by two dissimilar images. The three major types are the Maddox rod test, the double Maddox rod test, and the red filter test.

The *Maddox rod test* uses a specially constructed device consisting of a series of parallel cylinders. It converts a point source of light into a line image. The optical properties of the cylinders cause the streak of light to be situated 90° to the orientation of the parallel cylinders. Since fusion is precluded by the Maddox rod, no differentiation between heterophorias and heterotropias can be made. The Maddox rod can be used to test for horizontal, vertical, and (when used in conjunction with another Maddox rod) cyclodeviations. To test for horizontal deviations, the Maddox rod is placed in front of the right eye with the cylinders in the horizontal direction. The patient fixates a point source of light and then sees a vertical line with the right eye and a white light with the left eye. If the light bisects the line, orthophoria is present; if the light is on the left side of the line, an esodeviation is present; and if the light is on the right side of the line, an exodeviation is present. A similar procedure with the cylinders aligned vertically is used to test for vertical deviations. To measure the amount of deviation present, the examiner holds prisms of different powers until the line crosses the point source. The Maddox rod test is not a satisfactory test for horizontal deviations, however, since accommodative convergence cannot be controlled.

The *double Maddox rod test* is used for determination of cyclodeviations. A Maddox rod is placed in front of each eye. Frequently, the rods are placed in a trial frame with the rods aligned vertically so that the patient sees horizontal line images. The patient is asked to rotate the axes of the rods until the lines are parallel. In order to facilitate the patient's recognition of the two lines, it is often helpful to dissociate the lines by placing a small prism base up or base down in the trial frame in front of one eye. The total number of degrees of deviation and the direction (incyclo or excyclo) can be determined by the angle of rotation that causes the line images to appear horizontal and parallel. Traditionally, a red Maddox rod was placed before the right eye and a white Maddox rod before the left, but recent evidence suggests the different colors can cause fixation artifacts that do not occur if the same color is used bilaterally.

Simons K, Arnoldi K, Brown MH. Color dissociation artifacts in double Maddox rod cyclodeviation testing. *Ophthalmology.* 1994;101:1897–1901.

In the *red filter test* a red filter is placed in front of the right eye. This test is used for the same purpose as the Maddox rod test, but it is not applicable to cyclodeviations. As in the Maddox rod test, prisms are used to eliminate the horizontal or vertical diplopia, and the amount of deviation is recorded.

Dissimilar target tests   These tests are based on the patient's response to the dissimilar images created by each eye viewing a different target; the deviation is measured first with one eye fixating and then with the other. Several tests of this type have been devised, but the three most frequently encountered are the Lancaster red-green projection test, the Hess screen test, and the major amblyoscope test.

The *Lancaster red-green test* uses red-green goggles that can be reversed, a red slit projector, a green slit projector, and a screen ruled into squares of 7 cm. At the test distance of 2 m each square subtends 2°. The patient's head is held steady; by convention the test is begun with the red filter in front of the right eye. The examiner projects a red slit onto the screen and the patient is asked to place the green slit so that it appears to coincide with the red slit. The relative positions of the two streaks are then recorded. The test is repeated for the diagnostic positions of gaze (see p 65), and the goggles are then reversed so that the deviation with the fellow eye fixating might be recorded. This test dissociates the eyes; it is useful only in those patients who have normal retinal correspondence.

The *Hess screen test* is also useful in evaluating patients with paretic or paralytic strabismus who have normal retinal correspondence. The test uses red-green goggles, a special screen that has a red dot (or light) in 8 inner positions and 16 outer positions, and a green slit projector. At a test distance of 50 cm, the patient is asked to place the green slit light so that it appears to coincide with the individual red dots (or lights). The relative positions are connected by a straight line; usually just the eight inner dots (or lights) and the central point of fixation are plotted. The goggles are then reversed so the deviation with the other eye fixating can be recorded.

Major amblyoscope testing uses dissimilar targets that the patient is asked to superimpose. If the patient has normal retinal correspondence, the horizontal, vertical, and torsional deviations can be read directly from the calibrated scale of the amblyoscope.

Complications With Ocular Alignment Assessment

Two potential pitfalls in the evaluation of ocular alignment are the conditions of pseudostrabismus and angle kappa. *Pseudostrabismus* is the appearance of strabismus despite normal alignment. The most common form is pseudoesotropia, which results from coverage of the nasal sclera by the wide, flat nasal bridge and epicanthal folds so common in infancy. Because no real deviation exists, both corneal light reflex testing and cover testing will be normal. The appearance of crossing should gradually improve during infancy and early childhood. If it does not, repeat examination is warranted.

Angle kappa is the angle between the visual axis and the anatomic pupillary axis of the eye. If the fovea is temporal to the pupillary axis (as is usually the case), the corneal light reflection will be slightly nasal to the center of the cornea. This is termed *positive angle kappa*, and it will simulate exodeviation. If the position of the fovea is nasal to the pupillary axis, the corneal light reflection will be slightly temporal to the center of the cornea. This is termed *negative angle kappa*, and it will simulate esodeviation (Fig VI-5). One cause for a positive angle kappa is retinopathy of prematurity (ROP) with temporal dragging of the macula. Although affected patients appear to be exotropic, the eye continues to appear abducted even when fixing under monocular conditions.

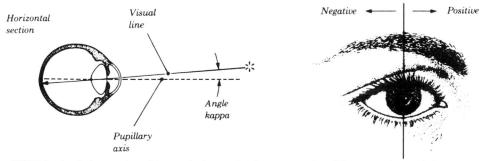

FIG VI-5—Angle kappa. A positive angle kappa simulates exotropia, while a negative angle kappa simulates esotropia. (Reprinted from Parks MM. *Ocular Motility and Strabismus*. Hagerstown, MD: Harper & Row; 1975.)

Positions of Gaze

The *primary position of gaze* is the position of the eyes when fixating an object at infinity straight ahead. For practical purposes infinity is considered to be 20 ft (6 m), and for this position the head should be straight. If the patient's problem has a vertical component, the definition of primary position is expanded to include the eyes fixating straight ahead at a distant object with the head tilted to the right and to the left.

Cardinal positions are those six positions of gaze in which the prime mover is one muscle of each eye, together called *yoke muscles* (see Table II-3 and Figure II-4, p 29). *Midline positions* are straight up and straight down from primary position. These two gaze positions help determine the elevating and depressing capabilities of the eye, but they do not isolate any one muscle since two elevator and two depressor muscles affect midline gaze positions.

The phrase *diagnostic positions of gaze* has been applied to the composite of these nine gaze positions: the six cardinal positions, straight up and down, and primary position. Several schemes have been devised to record the results of ocular alignment and motility in the various diagnostic positions of gaze, as well as those obtained with the head tilted to the right and to the left (Fig VI-6).

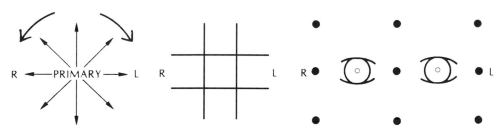

FIG VI-6—Three examples of methods for recording the results of ocular alignment testing.

A and V patterns should be noted at this point. An *A pattern* refers to an esotropia greatest in upgaze or an exotropia greatest in downgaze, while a *V pattern* denotes an esotropia greatest in downgaze or an exotropia greatest in upgaze. The patient should be observed carefully for any chin elevation or depression. See chapter X for a full discussion of A and V patterns.

Convergence

Alignment at near is usually measured at 13 inches (33 cm) directly in front of the patient in the horizontal plane. Comparison of the alignment in the primary position at both distance and near fixation helps assess the accommodative convergence (synkinetic near) reflex. The *near point of convergence* is determined by placing a fixation object at 40 cm in the midplane of the patient's head. As the subject fixates on the object, it is moved toward the subject until one eye loses fixation and turns out. The point at which this action occurs is the near point of convergence. The eye that is able to maintain fixation is considered to be the dominant eye. The normal near point of convergence is 8–10 cm or less.

AC/A ratio   The *accommodative convergence/accommodation (AC/A) ratio* is defined as the amount of convergence measured in prism diopters per unit (diopter) change in accommodation. There are two methods of clinical measurement.

□ The *gradient method* arrives at the AC/A ratio by the change in deviation in prism diopters divided by the change in lens power. An accommodative target must be used, and the working distance is held constant. Plus or minus lenses (+1, +2, −1, −2, etc) are used to vary the accommodative requirement. This method measures the *stimulus AC/A ratio,* which is not necessarily identical to the *response AC/A ratio.* The latter can be determined only with the use of an optometer that records the change in accommodation actually produced.

□ The *heterophoria method* employs the distance–near relationship, measuring the distance and near deviations. A similar alignment is normally present for distance and near fixation. If the patient is more exotropic or less esotropic at near, too little convergence, or a low AC/A ratio, is present; if more esotropic or less exotropic at near, a high AC/A ratio is present.

The AC/A ratio can be clinically manipulated either optically or pharmacologically. For example, plus spectacles for hyperopia reduce accommodation and therefore reduce accommodative convergence. This principle is the mainstay of the medical management of esotropia. Bifocals reduce or eliminate the need to accommodate for near fixation. This optical management is used for excess convergence at near, that is, an esodeviation greater at near. Underplussed or overminused spectacles create the need for greater-than-normal accommodation. This excess accommodation creates more accommodative convergence and is occasionally used to reduce an exodeviation.

Long-acting cholinesterase inhibitors (e.g., echothiophate iodide) can be used to decrease accommodative convergence. These drugs act directly on the ciliary body, facilitating transmission at the myoneural junction. They reduce the central demand for accommodative innervation and, thus, reduce the amount of convergence induced by accommodation.

Fusional Vergence

Vergences move the two eyes in opposite directions. Fusional vergences are motor responses used to eliminate horizontal, vertical, or torsional image disparity. They can be grouped by the following functions:

- *Fusional convergence* eliminates bitemporal retinal disparity and controls an exophoria.
- *Fusional divergence* eliminates binasal retinal disparity, and it controls an esophoria.
- *Vertical fusional vergence* controls a hyperphoria or hypophoria.
- *Torsional fusional vergence* controls intorsion or extorsion.

Fusional vergences can be measured by using a haploscopic device, a rotary prism, or a bar prism, increasing the prism power until diplopia occurs. Accommodation must be controlled during fusional vergence testing. Fusional vergences can be changed by a number of mechanisms:

- *Involuntary by patient:* As a tendency to deviate evolves, the patient gradually develops a larger-than-normal fusional vergence for that deviation. Very large fusional vergences are seen regularly in congenital vertical deviations and in exodeviations.
- *Visual acuity:* Improved acuity improves the fusional vergence mechanism. The treatment of reduced vision may change a symptomatic intermittent deviation to an asymptomatic phoria.
- *State of awareness:* Fatigue, illness, or hypoxia may decrease the fusional vergence mechanism, converting a phoria to a tropia.
- *Orthoptics:* The magnitude of the fusional vergence mechanism may be increased by exercises. This treatment works best for near fusional convergence, particularly for the relief of convergence insufficiency.
- *Optical stimulation of fusional vergence:* (1) In controlled accommodative esotropia, reducing the strength of the hyperopia correction induces an esophoria that will stimulate the fusional divergence. (2) Prisms to control diplopia may be gradually reduced to stimulate a compensatory fusional vergence.

Tests of Binocular Sensory Cooperation

Assessment of the vergence system indicates the extent to which the two eyes can be directed at the same object of regard. Sensory binocularity involves the use of both eyes together to form one perception. In general, normal sensory binocularity is dependent upon normal fusional vergence. Ideally, testing should therefore be performed before binocularity is disrupted by occlusion of either eye. Two classes of tests are commonly used to assess sensory binocularity: Worth four-dot testing (and its equivalents) and stereo acuity testing.

Worth four-dot testing The mechanics of Worth four-dot testing have been described in chapter III. Only patients who are using the two eyes together can appreciate all four lights being projected (Fig VI-7). If the right eye is suppressed, as often occurs if that eye is deviated, the patient will see only the two green and one white light and will report seeing three green lights since the white light appears green. If the left eye is suppressed, the patient will see two red lights since the white

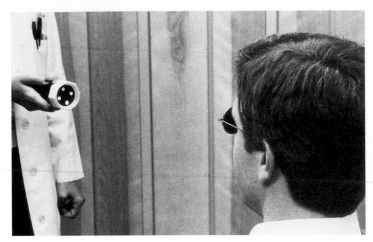

FIG VI-7—Worth four-dot test for near. The flashlight target, which illuminates the four dots, is held by the examiner. A larger, wall-mounted illuminated target with a similar distribution of the four lights is used for the distance test. The patient wears the same red-and-green glasses for both tests. (Reproduced with permission from Wilson FM II, ed. *Practical Ophthalmology: A Manual for Beginning Residents.* San Francisco: American Academy of Ophthalmology; 1996:111.)

light appears red. If alternate eyes are suppressed, the patient may see two red and three green lights alternating. Patients with diplopia may report seeing five lights simultaneously.

Use of the Worth four-dot test at distance illuminates a smaller, more central portion of the retina, while testing at closer distances illuminates a progressively larger, more peripheral portion. Distance testing can reveal small suppression scotomata that may be inapparent on testing at near. Results of testing should be reported as fusion or suppression of one eye at distance and at near. Many cases of small-angle strabismus, for example associated with monofixation syndrome, may combine fusion at near with suppression of one eye at distance.

Stereo acuity testing   While Worth four-dot testing is best at detecting suppression, stereo acuity testing assesses the use of the two eyes for binocular depth perception. Stereopsis occurs when the two retinal images, slightly disparate because of the normally different views provided by the horizontal separation of the two eyes, are cortically integrated. These views are more separated in individuals with larger interpupillary distances. Most tests of stereopsis use polarized glasses.

In the *Titmus stereo test* a card with superimposed images of a fly is shown to the patient. Ability to detect the elevation of the fly's wings above the plane of the card indicates stereopsis. Since the separation of the superimposed images is 3000 seconds of arc, this test is one of gross stereopsis. Other figures included on the same card contain less separated images. Thus, quantitation of stereo acuity down to as little as 20 seconds of arc may be possible in cooperative patients.

One system of stereo acuity testing, Wirt's stereo circles, is confounded by monocular clues. Random dot animals and Randot circles are therefore preferred by many examiners. As with Worth four-dot testing, stereopsis can also be measured at distance, using the AO Vectograph Project-O-Chart slide or the BVAT (Binocular Visual Acuity Test).

Special Motor Tests

Special motor tests include forced ductions, active force generation, and saccadic velocity. These are also discussed with illustrations in BCSC Section 5, *Neuro-Ophthalmology*.

□ *Forced ductions* are performed by using instruments to move the anesthetized eye mechanically into various positions, thus determining resistance to passive movement. This test is usually performed at the time of surgery but can sometimes be performed preoperatively in cooperative patients.

□ *Active force generation* assesses the relative strength of a muscle. The patient is asked to move the eye in a given direction while the observer fixates the eye with an instrument. If the muscle tested is paretic, the examiner will feel less than normal tension.

□ *Saccadic velocity* can be recorded using a special instrument that gives a graphic record of the speed and direction of eye movement. This test is useful to differentiate paralysis from restriction.

The limits of version movements, or field of binocular fixation, may be tested on either a Goldmann perimeter or a tangent screen. The subjective determination of diplopia is again more accurate and reliable than is the objective determination. A small white test object is followed by both eyes in the various cardinal positions throughout the visual field. When the patient comments that the test object is seen double, this point is plotted. The examiner then repeats the same procedure until the entire visual field has been plotted, noting the area in which the patient reported single vision and the area of double vision. The field of binocular fixation normally measures about 45°–50° from the fixation point except where it is restricted by the nose (Fig VI-8).

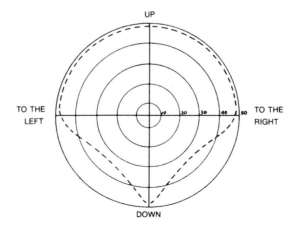

FIG VI-8—The normal binocular field of fixation as seen by the patient shows the limits of version movements.

Three-Step Test

Cyclovertical muscle palsies, especially involving the superior oblique muscles, are often responsible for hyperdeviations. The three-step test can be used to help identify the paretic muscle through a process of elimination. As helpful as this test is, it is not always diagnostic and can be misleading, especially in cases in which more than one muscle is paretic and in cases with restrictions.

The examiner must be familiar with the anatomy and motor physiology of the extraocular muscles in order to understand the test. Briefly, there are eight cyclovertically acting muscles; four work as depressors (two in each eye), and four as elevators (again, two in each eye). The two *depressors* of each eye are the *inferior rectus* and *superior oblique* muscles; the two *elevators* of each eye are the *superior rectus* and the *inferior oblique* muscles. The three-step test is performed in the following manner (Fig VI-9):

Step 1 Determine which eye is hypertropic by using the cover-uncover test. See Figure VI-1 and the discussion on p 59. Step 1 narrows the number of possibly underacting muscles from eight to four. In the example shown in Figure VI-9 the right eye has been found to be hypertropic. This means that the paresis will be found in either the depressors of the right eye (RIR, RSO) or the elevators of the left eye (LIO, LSR).

Step 2 Determine whether the vertical deviation is greater in right gaze or in left gaze. At the end of step 2, the two remaining possible muscles (one in each eye) are both intortors or extortors and both superior or inferior muscles (one rectus and one oblique). Note that in Figure VI-9, the increased left-gaze deviation eliminates two inferior muscles and implicates two superior muscles.

Step 3 Known as the *Bielschowsky head-tilt test,* the final step involves tilting the head to the right and then to the left. Head tilt to the right stimulates intorsion of the right eye (RSR, RSO) and extorsion of the left eye (LIR, LIO). Head tilt to the left stimulates extorsion of the right eye (RIR, RIO) and intorsion of the left eye (LSR, LSO). Normally, the two intortors and the two extortors of each eye have *opposite* vertical actions that cancel each other. If one intortor or one extortor is paretic, it cannot act vertically and the vertical action of the other ipsilateral torting muscle becomes manifest.

Figure VI-9 illustrates the results if step 2 above had demonstrated that the deviation was greater in left gaze and the RSO was the paretic muscle, as is commonly true. The dotted line indicates normal position, and the arrow shows abnormal movement.

Parks MM. Isolated cyclovertical muscle palsy. *Arch Ophthalmol.* 1958;60:1027–1035.

von Noorden GK. *Atlas of Strabismus.* 4th ed. St Louis: Mosby; 1983:149.

Cycloplegic Refraction

One of the most important tests in the evaluation of any patient with complaints pertinent to binocular vision and/or ocular motility is refraction with cycloplegic agents. *Cyclopentolate* (1.0%) is the preferred drug for routine use in children, especially when combined with phenylephrine, which has no cycloplegic effect itself. Use of

STEP 1

Possible paretic muscles: RSO, RIR, LSR, LIO

STEP 2

RIGHT GAZE
RIR and LIO
eliminated

LEFT GAZE
RSO or LSR
are possible paretic muscles

STEP 3

(for left-gaze
deviation only)

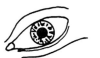

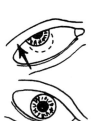

RSO is paretic

LSR not paretic

FIG VI-9—When an isolated cyclovertical muscle palsy is present, the three-step test can be used to identify the paretic muscle. *Step 1,* Cover-uncover test has been used to determine that patient has a *right hypertropia.* This step eliminates four of the cyclovertically acting muscles, in this case leaving right superior oblique (RSO), right inferior rectus (RIR), left superior rectus (LSR), and left inferior oblique (LIO) to be tested further. *Step 2,* Test shows no vertical deviation increase on right gaze, which could have implicated RIR and LIO as the possible paretic muscles. Deviation increases on left gaze; therefore either RSO or LSR is responsible. *Step 3,* Step 2 showed increased vertical deviation on *left gaze.* Head tilt to right followed by head tilt to left exposes muscle responsible for right hypertropia. *Top,* If RSO is paretic, deviation is larger on right head tilt (dotted line indicates normal position, and arrow shows abnormal movement). *Bottom,* If LSR were paretic, the deviation would have been larger on left head tilt. In this example, the three-step test result is consistent with an RSO palsy. (Illustration modified from von Noorden GK. *Atlas of Strabismus.* 4th ed. St Louis: Mosby; 1983:149.)

TABLE VI-2

ADMINISTRATION AND DURATION OF CYCLOPLEGICS

MEDICATION	ADMINISTRATION SCHEDULE	DURATION OF MYDRIATIC ACTION
Tropicamide	1 drop q 5 min × 2; wait 30 minutes	4–8 hours
Cyclopentolate	1 drop q 5 min × 2; wait 30 minutes	8–24 hours
Scopolamine	1 drop q 5 min × 2; wait 1 hour	1–3 days
Homatropine	1 drop q 5 min × 2; wait 1 hour	1–3 days
Atropine	1 drop tid × 3 days; then 1 drop morning of appointment	1–2 weeks

*Some physicians believe that atropine ointment is a safer vehicle for delivery of the drug, given q day × 3 days.

0.5% strength is suggested in infants, and the clinician should be aware that some adverse psychologic effects have been observed in children receiving cyclopentolate. *Homatropine* (5.0%) and *scopolamine* (0.25%) are occasionally used instead of cyclopentolate, but neither is as rapid acting or effective. *Tropicamide* (0.5% or 1.0%), which is used in conjunction with phenylephrine (2.5%) for routine dilation, is usually not strong enough for effective cycloplegia in children. Although *atropine* (0.5% or 1.0%, drops or ointment) is advocated by many, it may cause prolonged blurring and is often associated with toxic or allergic side effects (see below).

Table VI-2 shows the schedule of administration and duration of action for commonly used cycloplegics. The duration of action is highly variable, and the pupillary effect lasts longer than does the cycloplegic effect, so a dilated pupil does not necessarily indicate complete cycloplegia. For patients with accommodative esodeviations repeated cycloplegic examinations at frequent intervals are essential. Retinoscopic measurements should be made on the patient's visual axis.

Side effects   Adverse reactions to cycloplegic agents include allergic (or hypersensitivity) reaction with conjunctivitis, edematous eyelids, and/or dermatitis, seen more frequently with atropine than with any of the other agents. Hypnotic effect can be seen with scopolamine and occasionally with cyclopentolate or homatropine.

Systemic intoxication from atropine manifests in fever, dry mouth, flushing of the face, rapid pulse, nausea, dizziness, delirium, and erythema. Treatment is discontinuation of the medicine with supportive measures as necessary. If the reaction is severe, physostigmine may be given. Remember, one drop of 1.0% atropine = 0.5 mg of atropine.

Parks MM: *Ocular Motility and Strabismus.* Hagerstown, MD: Harper & Row; 1975.

Prism Adaptation Test

The prism adaptation test represents the formalization of a simple clinical practice that has been used for many years, especially in Europe. For a variety of reasons strabismus surgery in Europe is often delayed until the second half of the first decade of life. In the interim, in order to help the child obtain binocular fusion while awaiting surgical alignment of the eye, the patient is often fitted with prisms of sufficient magnitude to permit alignment of the visual axes. In many cases this step will provoke a restoration of sensory binocular cooperation in a form of fusion and even stereopsis. This technique then actually functions as a clinical trial of orthotropia, offering some predictive value of whether fusion may be restored when the patient is surgically aligned.

Some patients, however (especially those with acquired esotropia), respond to the placement of such prisms by increasing their deviation. In such cases anomalous retinal correspondence based on the objective angle may drive the eyes to maintain this adaptive alignment even with prismatic correction. After wearing such prisms, the patient will return with a greater angle of deviation corresponding to the addition of the prisms. The Prism Adaptation Study has concluded that these patients may require significantly more surgery than other patients in order to obtain correction of their deviation. In some cases patients who obtain fusion with this prism therapy may simply be weaned off the prisms if the angle of their deviation is not too large, and surgery may thereby be avoided. For patients in whom prism therapy results in an increase in the deviation rather than in fusion, some practitioners recommend successively increasing the prism until orthophoria with correction is obtained and then performing surgery for this maximal deviation rather than for the smaller deviation. This last concept of prism adaptation can be used to determine the target angle in cases of acquired esotropia.

Prism Adaptation Study Group. Efficacy of prism adaptation in the surgical management of acquired esotropia. *Arch Ophthalmol.* 1990;108:1248–1256.

CHAPTER VII

Esodeviations

The most common type of ocular misalignment, esodeviations represent more than 50% of ocular deviations in the pediatric population. An esodeviation is a latent or manifest convergent misalignment of the visual axes. Three commonly recognized forms of esodeviation are grouped according to variations in fusional capabilities:

□ *Esophoria* is a latent esodeviation that is controlled by fusional mechanisms so that the eyes remain properly aligned under normal binocular viewing conditions.

□ *Intermittent esotropia* is an esodeviation that is intermittently controlled by fusional mechanisms but spontaneously becomes manifest, particularly with fatigue or illness.

□ *Esotropia* is an esodeviation that is not controlled by fusional mechanisms, so the deviation is constantly manifest.

Esodeviations can occur as a result of innervational, anatomic, mechanical, refractive, genetic, and accommodative causes. Table VII-1 on p 76 lists the major types of esodeviation.

Pseudoesotropia

Infants often have a wide, flat nasal bridge with prominent medial epicanthal folds and a small interpupillary distance. Thus they may appear esotropic when in fact their eyes are straight. It is important to remember, however, that even though a child may indeed have a pseudoesodeviation as an infant, a bona fide esodeviation can also be present or appear later. A verbal report that one eye does not seem to "track" with the other eye should, therefore, not be taken lightly. In such a case, the child's alignment should be reexamined without delay.

Infantile (Congenital) Esotropia

Classic Congenital (Essential Infantile) Esotropia

Onset at birth is often the history of the esotropia given by the parents; however, the exact date is not precisely established in most cases. Documented presence of esotropia by 6 months of age has arbitrarily been accepted as the definition of congenital esotropia by most ophthalmologists. This criterion has been used in clinical studies.

A family history of esotropia or strabismus is often present, but well-defined genetic patterns are unusual. Other than their ocular misalignment, children with early-onset esotropia are usually normal. This type of esotropia is, however, seen quite frequently in children with cerebral palsy and hydrocephalus (up to 30%).

Equal visual acuity associated with alternation of fixation from one eye to the other is common in children with esotropia. Also frequent is cross-fixation, in which a large-angle esotropia is associated with the use of the adducted eye for fixation of

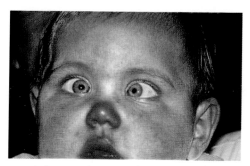

FIG VII-1—Classic congenital esotropia. (Reproduced from Archer SM. Esotropia. In: *Focal Points: Clinical Modules for Ophthalmologists.* San Francisco: American Academy of Ophthalmology; 1994;12:12.)

objects in the contralateral temporal field (Fig VII-1). Amblyopia may be present when a constant inturning of only one eye occurs with or without cross-fixation.

The misalignment is often quite apparent, characteristically larger than 30Δ. Abduction may be difficult to elicit. Associated vertical deviations, such as overaction of the inferior oblique muscles and/or dissociated vertical deviation (DVD), become common over time. Inferior oblique muscle overaction and DVD may occur in more than 50% of patients with congenital esotropia but are not commonly recognized until 1 year of age or older.

Asymmetry of monocular horizontal smooth pursuit is normal in infants up to 6 months of age, with nasal to temporal smooth pursuit less well developed than temporal to nasal smooth pursuit. Patients with congenital esotropia have persistent monocular smooth pursuit asymmetry that does not resolve.

Tychsen L, Lisberger SG. Maldevelopment of visual motion processing in humans who had strabismus with onset in infancy. *J Neurosci.* 1986;6:2495–2508.

Management Cycloplegic refraction characteristically reveals 1–2 D of hyperopia, which is the normal refractive error in young children. Significant astigmatism or myopia may be present and require correction. Repeat refractions are important because an accommodative component is sometimes discovered with follow-up of these children. Because accommodative esotropia can occur as early as 4 months of age and often responds to hyperopic correction, significant refractive errors (more than +2.00 D of sphere) are corrected by prescribing the full cycloplegic retinoscopy findings. An atropine refraction may be useful in some hyperopic patients with esotropia to ensure that all the hyperopia has been identified; this practice also ensures that esotropes who are surgical candidates receive a confirmation refraction prior to surgery.

Ocular alignment in the child with early-onset esotropia is rarely achieved without surgery. However, surgery should be undertaken only after correction of significant refractive errors and treatment of amblyopia, for failure to correct these problems will compromise a stable surgical alignment of the eyes. It is wise to repeat the measurement of the amount of esotropia shortly before surgery, because many infants will show a significant increase compared with their first evaluation.

TABLE VII-1

TYPES OF ESODEVIATION

Pseudoesotropia

Infantile (congenital) esotropia

    Classic congenital (essential infantile) esotropia

    Nystagmus and esotropia

        Ciancia syndrome

        Manifest latent nystagmus

        Nystagmus blockage syndrome

Accommodative esotropia

    Refractive (normal AC/A)

    Nonrefractive (high AC/A)

    Partially accommodative

Nonaccommodative acquired esotropia

    Basic

    Acute

    Cyclic

    Sensory deprivation

    Divergence insufficiency and divergence paralysis

    Spasm of the near synkinetic reflex

    Surgical (consecutive)

Incomitant esotropia

    Sixth nerve (abducens) paresis

    Medial rectus restriction

        Thyroid ophthalmopathy

        Medial orbital wall fracture

    Duane syndrome and Möbius syndrome

Most ophthalmologists agree that surgery should be undertaken early. The eyes should be aligned by 24 months of age to stimulate some form of sensory binocular cooperation or fusion. However, operation for congenital esotropia is frequently performed in healthy children at 6 months of age to try to maximize binocular visual function such as stereopsis, and surgery as early as 13 weeks of age has been advocated by some ophthalmologists to achieve a superior sensory outcome.

The child's development may improve and accelerate after the eyes are straightened. Psychological damage from cosmetic aspects of abnormal ocular alignment and from the surgical procedure itself is probably minimized by early correction. Although the risks of anesthesia are slightly greater in infants, improved anesthetic techniques have significantly minimized these risks and virtually eliminated such considerations in carrying out surgical treatment.

Many surgical approaches have been suggested for this common type of esotropia. The most commonly performed procedure for infantile esotropia is to recess both medial rectus muscles (BMR). Recession of a medial rectus muscle combined with resection of the ipsilateral lateral rectus muscle (R&R) is an acceptable alternative. Some surgeons operate on three or even four horizontal rectus muscles at the time of the initial surgery if the deviation is larger than 50Δ. Associated overaction of the inferior oblique muscles is often treated at the time of the initial surgery by inferior oblique muscle–weakening procedures. No single approach has been uniformly successful, and later operations for undercorrections, or less frequently for overcorrections, may be needed. Chapter XIII, Surgery of the Extraocular Muscles, discusses surgical procedures in greater detail.

Alignment within 8Δ of orthophoria has been suggested as an acceptable goal, because it frequently results in stable microstrabismus or monofixation with peripheral fusion, central suppression, and excellent appearance. Recent information, however, suggests that orthotropia and small-angle esotropia (≤8Δ) are superior outcomes to small-angle exotropia. Small-angle strabismus generally represents a stable functional surgical outcome even though bifoveal fusion is not achieved. Untreated patients do not improve spontaneously and may develop secondary contractures of the extraocular tissues.

Birch EE, Stager DR, Everett ME. Random dot stereo acuity following surgical correction of infantile esotropia. *J Pediatr Ophthalmol Strabismus.* 1995;32:231–235.

Kushner BJ, Fisher M. Is alignment within 8 prism diopters of orthotropia a successful outcome for infantile esotropia surgery? *Arch Ophthalmol.* 1996;114:176–180.

Wright KW, Edelman PM, McVey JH, et al. High-grade stereoacuity after early surgery for congenital esotropia. *Arch Ophthalmol.* 1995;112:913–919.

Nystagmus and Esotropia

Some patients with early-onset esotropia also have nystagmus. Three patterns of nystagmus and esotropia have been described. Patients with the *Ciancia syndrome* have a very large angle constant esotropia and often show a pattern of cross-fixation. Nystagmus is minimal with the fixing eye in adduction; however, nystagmus increases with attempted abduction of the fixing eye. Abduction is usually limited, and the nystagmus is similar to exaggerated end-position nystagmus on attempted abduction. Patients with Ciancia syndrome are often undercorrected after surgery and may require large bilateral medial rectus recessions.

Ciancia AO. On infantile esotropia with nystagmus in abduction. *J Pediatr Ophthalmol Strabismus.* 1995;32:280–288.

Patients with *latent nystagmus (LN)* show no nystagmus under binocular viewing conditions; with occlusion of one eye a jerk nystagmus develops in both eyes with the fast phase toward the viewing eye. If nystagmus is present when both eyes are open but only one eye is being used for vision (the other is suppressed), the patient is said to have *manifest latent nystagmus (MLN)*. This nystagmus is also jerk in type and may increase with monocular occlusion. Characteristic waveforms with quantitative eye movement recording distinguish LN and MLN from congenital nystagmus. Patients with LN and MLN frequently have an underlying esotropia but may also have other types of strabismus. In order to improve visual acuity the patient with MLN may adopt a face turn to place the fixing eye in adduction, where the amplitude of nystagmus is reduced.

Nystagmus blockage syndrome is a type of congenital nystagmus in which the angle of esotropia and the amplitude of nystagmus have an inverse relationship. The nystagmus intensity is greatest when the eyes are straight, and it is dampened or blocked by convergence of the eyes that leads to an esodeviation. The diagnosis is based on the appearance of nystagmus with attempted abduction of either eye, a head turn in the direction of the uncovered eye with occlusion of the fellow eye, and dampening of nystagmus with convergence of the eyes that results in an esodeviation.

Dell'Osso LF, Ellenberger C Jr, Abel LA, et al. The nystagmus blockage syndrome. Congenital nystagmus, manifest latent nystagmus, or both? *Invest Ophthalmol Vis Sci.* 1983;24:1580–1587.

Accommodative Esotropia

All accommodative esodeviations are acquired, with the following characteristics:

- Onset generally between 6 months and 7 years, averaging 2½ years of age (can be as early as 4 months of age)
- Usually intermittent at onset, becoming constant
- Often hereditary
- Sometimes precipitated by trauma or illness
- Amblyopia frequently associated
- Diplopia may occur early but usually disappears as patient develops facultative suppression scotoma in deviating eye

Types of accommodative esotropia are listed in Table VII-1 and discussed below.

Refractive Accommodative Esotropia

Two main mechanisms contribute to this type of esotropia: uncorrected hyperopia and insufficient fusional divergence. The uncorrected hyperopia forces the patient to accommodate to sharpen the retinal image, thus leading to increased convergence. If the patient's fusional divergence mechanism is insufficient to deal with the increased convergence tonus, esotropia results. The angle of esotropia is generally between 20Δ and 30Δ and approximately equal at distance and near fixation. The amount of hyperopia averages +4.00 D with a range of +3.00 to +10.00 D.

Treatment of refractive accommodative esotropia consists of amblyopia therapy if necessary and correction of the full amount of hyperopia as determined under cycloplegia with cyclopentolate or atropine. Bifocals may be required if the patient has excessive accommodative convergence. Significant delay in the initiation of treatment following the onset of esotropia increases the likelihood that a portion of the esodeviation will fail to respond to antiaccommodative therapy. A gradual reduction of hyperopic correction may be possible over time if the patient can maintain control of the ensuing esophoria. This reduction will stimulate the development of increased fusional divergence amplitudes, which in some patients may allow discontinuation of spectacle therapy in the future.

It is essential to emphasize to parents the importance of *full-time* wear of spectacle correction. A common cause of treatment failure or partial response to antiaccommodative management is inconsistent spectacle wear. Atropine 1.0% ointment applied to both eyes at bedtime may facilitate compliance.

Therapy with miotic agents (echothiophate iodide or isoflurophate) has been advocated as a substitute for glasses. However, because of potential ocular and systemic side effects from these medications, their use is usually confined to children who are uncooperative for wearing glasses at all or who spend long hours playing near the water in the summer.

Surgical correction may be required when a patient with refractive accommodative esotropia fails to regain fusion with glasses or subsequently develops a nonaccommodative component to the deviation. However, the ophthalmologist must be certain that there is no latent, uncorrected hyperopia before proceeding with surgery.

Nonrefractive Accommodative Esotropia

Patients with this form of esotropia have an abnormal relationship between accommodation and accommodative convergence, i.e., a high AC/A ratio. Excess convergence tonus results from accommodation, and esotropia develops in the setting of insufficient fusional divergence. Because more accommodation is required at near fixation than distance, the angle of esotropia is greater at near. It can be reduced by +3.00 D bifocal lenses. Measurement of the angle of esotropia with fixation targets that require appropriate accommodation is critical to making the diagnosis of this type of esotropia. The refractive error in these patients averages +2.25 D sphere but can range from myopic to highly hyperopic. Thus, patients with refractive and nonrefractive accommodative esotropia may show overlap in their amount of hyperopia.

Management No consensus exists on the best management of nonrefractive accommodative esotropia. Several options are available:

□ *Bifocals.* The most commonly used treatment option for nonrefractive accommodative esotropia is bifocal spectacles. If bifocals are employed, they should initially be prescribed in the executive or 35 mm flattop style with a power of +2.50 or +3.00 D. The top of the segment should cross the pupil and the vertical height of the bifocal should not exceed that of the distance portion of the lens. Detailed instructions concerning the bifocal should be given to the optician. Progressive bifocal lenses have been used successfully, but conventional bifocals are preferred. If progressive bifocals are used, they should be fitted higher than adult lenses (about 4 mm) and with maximum bifocal power (+3.50 D). An ideal response to bifocal glasses is restoration of normal binocular function (fusion and stereopsis) at both distance and near fixation. An acceptable response is fusion at distance with less than 10Δ of residual esotropia through the bifocal at near fixation.

□ *Long-acting cholinesterase inhibitors.* Ophthalmologists who use this form of treatment suggest starting with a maximum strength (0.125% echothiophate iodide drops) in both eyes once daily for 6 weeks. If effective, strength or frequency should be decreased to the minimum effective dose. Parents must be warned about the potentially serious side effects of these drugs, including deletion of pseudocholinesterase from the blood, which makes the patient very susceptible to depolarizing muscle relaxants such as succinylcholine.

□ *Surgery.* If a nonaccommodative esodeviation develops in the setting of full control of accommodation at distance and near, surgery may be indicated. Some ophthalmologists also advocate medial rectus muscle recessions for the near deviation so that the child, usually an adolescent, can discontinue bifocal wear and maintain control of the esodeviation with single-vision glasses or contact lenses. Despite recent controversy regarding surgery as an alternative to glasses for patients with fully accommodative esotropia, agreement is still strong among ophthalmologists that this is not a wise management option.

For the long-term management of both refractive and nonrefractive accommodative esotropia, it is important to remember that measured hyperopia usually increases until 5–7 years of age. Therefore, if esotropia with glasses increases, the cycloplegic refraction should be repeated and the full correction prescribed. After 5–7 years of age hyperopia may decrease, and the full cycloplegic refraction in place will thus blur vision. The ophthalmologist should seek the minimum hyperopic correction to provide optimal alignment and best visual acuity.

If glasses or drugs correct all or nearly all of the esotropia and some degree of sensory binocular cooperation or fusion is present, the clinician may begin to reduce the strength of glasses or drugs when the patient reaches 5 or 6 years of age to create a small esophoria. This reduction may stimulate the fusional divergence mechanism to redevelop normal magnitude. An increase in the fusional divergence combined with the natural decrease of both the hyperopia and the high AC/A ratio may enable the patient to maintain straight eyes without glasses, bifocals, or drugs. For example, in the case of a 5-year-old who has worn glasses since age 2 for esotropia and has a visual acuity of 20/25 in both eyes:

> Hyperopia +4.00 OU
> with +4.00 OU: orthophoria at distance and near
> after 6–12 months of spectacle wear: with +3.00 OU: $E = E' = 6\Delta$
> Prescribe +3.00 OU

Further reductions may be possible if the child maintains good visual acuity, has control of the esophoria, and does not have asthenopic symptoms.

Another example is an 8-year-old child who presented with new onset of esotropia at 3 years of age:

> Hyperopia +2.00 D
> with +2.00 D OU: $E = 4\Delta$; $E' = 24\Delta$
> +2.50 bifocals prescribed: $E = E' = 4\Delta$
> At age 6 hyperopia remains +2.00 D
> with +2.00 D add: $E = 4\Delta$; $E' = 8\Delta$
> with +1.50 D add: $E = 4\Delta$; $E(T)' = 12\Delta$
> Prescribe +2.00 D sphere OU with +2.00 D add

Further bifocal reductions may be possible as long as the child maintains an asymptomatic esophoria. If the amount of hyperopia increases and is prescribed in new glasses, the bifocal add can sometimes be reduced by the same amount that the hyperopia increased without affecting the resultant lens power through the bifocal. This change increases the chance that the child may eventually be able to discontinue bifocal use.

Partially Accommodative Esotropia

Patients with partially accommodative esodeviations show a reduction in the angle of esotropia with glasses but maintain a residual esotropia despite treatment of amblyopia and provision of full hyperopic therapy. In some instances partially accommodative esotropia is a result of decompensation of a fully accommodative esotropia, but in other instances the child may have had esotropia that subsequently developed an accommodative element. An interval of weeks to months between the onset of accommodative esotropia and the application of full cycloplegic refraction will often result in some residual esotropia even after the proper glasses are worn. Patients with pure refractive accommodative esotropia who have been made orthophoric with glasses are less likely to develop a nonaccommodative component to their esodeviation than patients with the high AC/A type of accommodative esotropia.

Treatment of partially accommodative esotropia consists of amblyopia management and prescription of the full hyperopic correction. Strabismus surgery may be warranted for the nonaccommodative portion. The amount of surgery should be conservative for hyperopes of +4.00 D or greater, because of an increased risk of developing a consecutive exotropia. It is important that the patient and parents understand before surgery that the purpose of surgery is to produce straight eyes *with* glasses— not to allow the child to discontinue wearing glasses altogether.

Nonaccommodative Acquired Esotropia

Basic (Acquired) Esotropia

Esotropia that develops after 6 months of age, but commonly before the end of childhood, is called *basic,* or *acquired, esotropia.* As with infantile esotropia, an accommodative factor is usually absent, the amount of hyperopia is not significant, and the near deviation is the same as the distance deviation. Although most children with this form of esotropia are otherwise healthy, central nervous system lesions must be considered. Therapy consists of amblyopia treatment and surgical correction as soon as possible after the onset of the deviation.

When planning surgery for patients with acquired esotropia, some ophthalmologists advocate prism adaptation. Prism adaptation is a process of prescribing the full hyperopic correction if indicated and adding press-on prisms to neutralize any residual esodeviation. The patient wears the glasses with the press-on prisms for 1 or 2 weeks and is then reexamined. If the esodeviation increases with the prisms, new prisms are prescribed to neutralize the deviation. In some patients the esodeviation will increase as the patient "eats up" the prism. Surgery is then planned for the full prism-adapted deviation. This process of prism adaptation reduces the relatively high undercorrection rate associated with acquired or decompensated accommodative esotropia, and it has been shown to produce a better motor outcome after surgery than that of the control group in a randomized clinical trial.

Repka MX, Connett JE, Scott WE. The one-year surgical outcome after prism adaptation for the management of acquired esotropia. *Ophthalmology.* 1996;103:922–928.

Acute Esotropia

Occasionally, an acquired esotropia is acute in onset. In such cases the patient immediately becomes aware of the deviation and frequently has diplopia. A careful motility evaluation is important to rule out an accommodative or paretic component. Artificial disruption of binocular vision, such as may follow treatment of an ocular injury or patching for amblyopia, is one of the known causes of acute esotropia. Physical and emotional stress, illness, and aging are other postulated causes. Because the onset of comitant esotropia in an older child may indicate an underlying neurologic disorder, neurologic evaluation may be indicated. Most patients with acute onset of esotropia have a history of normal binocular vision, and therefore the prognosis for restoration of single binocular vision with prisms and surgery is good. A period of observation during which prisms are employed may be indicated before surgery is performed.

Cyclic Esotropia

This type of esotropia is rare, with an estimated incidence of 1:3000–1:5000 strabismus cases. Onset occurs during the preschool years, although a congenital case and several adult cases have been reported. The esotropia is present intermittently, usually every other day (48-hour cycle). Variable cycles and 24-hour cycles have also been documented. Most patients with cyclic esotropia become constantly esotropic with time. In some ways cyclic esotropia resembles accommodative esotropia with a similar time of onset, moderate hyperopia, and a moderate angle of esotropia.

Amblyopia is occasionally present in cases of cyclic esotropia, and V-pattern esotropia is common (see chapter X). On the days when the cyclic esodeviation is not present, the individual has normal binocular vision and good stereo acuity.

Treatment of cyclic esotropia addresses the amblyopia and hyperopia. Some cases resolve with full hyperopic correction, while others continue the cyclic deviation and require surgery. Hyperopic correction and standard surgery for residual esotropia have resulted in functional cure. Phenobarbital and amphetamines have reportedly altered the frequency of the esotropic cycles in some patients.

Helveston EM. Cyclic strabismus. *Am Orthopt J.* 1973;23:48–51.

Sensory Deprivation Esodeviation

Monocular organic lesions such as cataract, corneal scarring, optic atrophy, or prolonged blurred or distorted retinal images may cause an esodeviation. Anisometropia with amblyopia is commonly seen in this type of esodeviation.

Obstacles preventing clear and focused retinal images and symmetrical visual stimulation must be identified and remedied as soon as possible. Animal and clinical data indicate that restoration of normal, symmetrical inputs must be accomplished at an early age if irreversible amblyopia is to be avoided. After all obstacles to balanced sensory inputs have been removed, any secondary amblyopia is treated. Surgery for residual esotropia may be indicated. The surgical management of these cases is similar to that of early-onset esotropia, except when good visual acuity cannot be restored as a result of irreversible amblyopia or organic defects. In such situations esotropia surgery should be done only on the abnormal eye.

Divergence Insufficiency

The characteristic finding of divergence insufficiency is an esodeviation greater at distance than at near. The deviation does not change with vertical or horizontal gaze, and fusional divergence is reduced. Most important, the clinician must rule out associated neurologic abnormalities. Treatment consists of base-out prisms and, rarely, surgery (lateral rectus resections).

Divergence Paralysis

The findings in divergence paralysis are the same as in divergence insufficiency, and differentiation from early, mild lateral rectus paresis may be extremely difficult. Divergence paralysis may be associated with pontine tumors, head trauma, and other neurologic conditions; consultation with a neuro-ophthalmologist is indicated.

Spasm of the Near Synkinetic Reflex

This term describes intermittent episodes of sustained convergence with accommodative spasm and miosis. Pseudomyopia may occur. The characteristic movement is the substitution of a convergence movement for a gaze movement on horizontal versions. Monocular abduction is normal in spite of marked abduction limitation on versions. Spasm of the near synkinetic reflex may occur in patients with conversion disorder, whose symptoms have no demonstrable physiological basis. It may also result from organic weakness of convergence as in myasthenia gravis. Occasionally, it may be a response to convergence/accommodative insufficiency of various causes.

Surgical (Consecutive) Esodeviation

Esodeviation following surgery for exodeviation frequently improves spontaneously. Treatment includes base-out prisms, plus lenses, miotics (if hyperopic), alternate occlusion, and, finally, surgery. Unless the deviation is very large, surgery should be postponed for several months because of the possibility of spontaneous improvement.

A completely detached or lost lateral rectus muscle will produce a large esotropia of the involved eye. A slipped lateral rectus muscle produces variable amounts of esotropia depending upon the amount of slippage. For lost muscles, surgical exploration and reattachment of the muscle to the globe is required. Transposition procedures may be necessary when lost muscles cannot be found. For slipped muscles, advancement of the muscle on the globe is required. (See Figures XIII-11 and XIII-12 and discussion in the text accompanying those illustrations.)

Incomitant Esodeviation

This term is used when esodeviation varies in different fields of gaze.

Sixth Nerve (Abducens) Palsy

Paresis of the lateral rectus muscle causes an incomitant esodeviation frequently associated with a head turn to maintain fusion. Spontaneous sixth nerve palsy in childhood occurs frequently. Older patients may complain of double vision and often have a head turn toward the side of the paretic sixth nerve. Approximately one third of these cases are associated with intracranial lesions and may have associated neurologic findings. Other cases may be related to infectious or immunologic processes that involve cranial nerve VI. Spontaneous benign lesions usually resolve over several months.

The vision in both eyes is equal unless other underlying errors of refraction or earlier strabismus are present. The esotropia increases in gaze toward the paretic lateral rectus muscle. Saccadic velocities show slowing of the affected lateral rectus muscle, and active force generation tests document the weakness of that muscle. Versions show limited or no abduction of the affected eye.

A careful history should be taken to define antecedent infections, head trauma, or other possible inciting factors for sixth nerve palsy. Neurologic evaluation with computed tomography (CT) or magnetic resonance imaging (MRI) is indicated when neurologic signs or symptoms are present.

Patching may be required to maintain vision in the esotropic eye, especially if the patient has no head turn to maintain binocular fusion. Fresnel press-on prisms are useful to correct the diplopia in primary position. Injection of botulinum toxin into the antagonist medial rectus muscle has successfully aligned the eye by temporarily paralyzing the medial rectus muscle. The botulinum treatment may be helpful in preventing contracture of the medial rectus muscle while the patient is observed for several months prior to surgical intervention. Spontaneous resolution of sixth nerve palsy sometimes occurs, making surgery unnecessary.

Surgery is indicated when spontaneous resolution does not take place after 6 months or more of follow-up and after exclusion of intracranial lesions. A large recession of the antagonist medial rectus muscle with resection of the lateral rectus muscle is often a successful first operation. If a mild paresis is present, the surgeon may consider weakening the contralateral medial rectus muscle with or without a posterior fixation procedure in addition to a recession and resection of the paretic eye. Adjustable sutures are helpful in paralytic strabismus if the patient is able to cooperate with this technique. In cases of total paralysis, muscle transposition procedures in conjunction with botulinum toxin injection into the ipsilateral medial rectus muscle may be required.

See additional discussions in chapter XI, Special Forms of Strabismus, and chapter XIV, Chemodenervation Treatment of Strabismus and Blepharospasm Using Botulinum Toxin. See also BCSC Section 5, *Neuro-Ophthalmology.*

Rosenbaum AL, Kushner BJ, Kirschen D. Vertical rectus transposition and botulinum toxin (Oculinum) to medial rectus for abducens palsy. *Arch Ophthalmol.* 1989;107:820–823.

Other Forms of Incomitant Esodeviation

Medial rectus muscle restriction   This restriction may result from thyroid myopathy, medial orbital wall fracture, or excessively resected medial rectus muscle (see chapter XIII).

Duane syndrome and Möbius syndrome   See discussions in chapter XI, Special Forms of Strabismus, and BCSC Section 5, *Neuro-Ophthalmology.*

Archer SM. Esotropia. In: *Focal Points: Clinical Modules for Ophthalmologists.* San Francisco: American Academy of Ophthalmology; 1994;12:12.

Preferred Practice Patterns Committee, Pediatric Panel. *Esotropia.* San Francisco: American Academy of Ophthalmology; 1997.

CHAPTER VIII

Exodeviations

An exodeviation is a divergent form of strabismus that can be latent (controlled by fusion) or manifest. While the exact cause of most exodeviations is unknown, proposed etiologies include anatomic and mechanical factors within the orbit as well as abnormalities of innervation such as excessive tonic divergence. A hereditary basis for exodeviation is apparent in some families.

Wilson ME. Exotropia. In: *Focal Points: Clinical Modules for Ophthalmologists*. San Francisco: American Academy of Ophthalmology; 1995;13:11.

Pseudoexotropia

The term *pseudoexotropia* refers to an appearance of exodeviation when in fact the eyes are properly aligned. Pseudoexotropia may occur as a result of the following:

□ Positive angle kappa without other ocular abnormalities

□ Wide interpupillary distance

□ Positive angle kappa together with ocular abnormalities such as temporal dragging of the macula in retinopathy of prematurity

Exophoria

Exophoria is a type of exodeviation controlled by fusion mechanisms under conditions of normal binocular vision. Exophorias are detected when binocular vision is interrupted, as during an alternate cover test. Exophoria may be asymptomatic if the angle of strabismus is small and fusional convergence amplitudes are adequate. Prolonged, detailed visual work or reading may bring about asthenopia. Treatment is usually not necessary unless an exophoria progresses to an intermittent exotropia.

Intermittent Exotropia

With the possible exception of exophoria at near, the most common type of exodeviation is intermittent exotropia, which is latent at some times and manifest at others (Fig VIII-1).

Clinical Characteristics

The onset of intermittent exotropia usually occurs early, before 5 years of age, but it may be detected for the first time much later in childhood. Since proper eye alignment in an intermittent exotropia requires that compensatory fusional factors be active, the deviation often becomes manifest during times of visual inattention, fatigue, or stress. Parents of affected children often report that exotropia occurs late in the day with fatigue or during illness, daydreaming, drowsiness upon awakening,

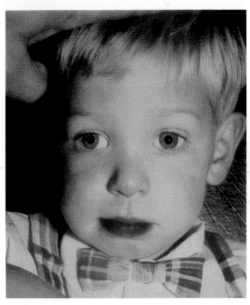

FIG VIII-1—This 3-year-old boy has been diagnosed with intermittent exotropia. (Reproduced with permission from Wilson ME. Exotropia. In: *Focal Points: Clinical Modules for Ophthalmologists.* San Francisco: American Academy of Ophthalmology; 1995;13:11.)

or when the child is being scolded. A reflex closure of one eye is often seen with exposure to bright lights.

In childhood deviation of the eyes is usually larger for distance viewing than for near, and exotropia manifests more frequently when the visual target is remote. In adults the near and distance exodeviation tend to be more equal in magnitude even if fusional control remains good. Intermittent exotropias can be associated with small hypertropias, A and V patterns, and oblique muscle dysfunction, all of which are discussed in the following two chapters. Inferior oblique muscle overaction can be detected in about one third of patients.

In many but not all patients untreated intermittent exotropia progresses toward constant exotropia. As exotropia progresses, tropic episodes occur at lower levels of fatigue and last longer than previously. Children younger than 10 years of age may develop sensory adaptations. Initial diplopia during manifest exotropia is often replaced by the cortical adaptations of suppression and abnormal retinal correspondence. However, normal retinal correspondence with high-grade or reduced stereoacuity remains when the eyes are straight. Amblyopia is uncommon unless progression to constant or nearly constant exotropia occurs.

Clinical Evaluation

The clinical evaluation begins with a detailed history to pinpoint as accurately as possible the age of onset of the strabismus and determine whether the exotropia is progressing toward constancy. The clinician records how often and under what specific circumstances the manifest exotropia occurs. Control of the exodeviation exhibited throughout the examination can be categorized as:

□ *Good control:* Exotropia is manifest only after cover testing, and patient resumes fusion rapidly without blinking or refixating.

□ *Fair control:* Exotropia is manifest after fusion is disrupted by cover testing, and the patient resumes fixation only after blinking or refixating.

□ *Poor control:* Exotropia is manifest spontaneously without disruption of fusion.

To bring out the maximum exodeviation, a far distance measurement is often made in addition to the standard measurements made at 20 feet and 14 inches. The patient can fixate a target 100–200 feet away at the end of a long hallway or out a window.

Classification   Intermittent exotropia has traditionally been classified into four groups, based on the difference between alternating prism and cover measurements at distance and at near and the change in near measurement produced by unilateral occlusion or +3.0 D lenses. *Basic* type exotropia is present when the exodeviation is approximately the same at distance and near fixation. *Divergence excess* type consists of an exodeviation that is greater at distance fixation than at near. *True divergence excess* type refers to those deviations that remain greater at distance than at near even after remeasurements at near either through a +3.00 D lens or after a period of uniocular occlusion. *Simulated divergence excess* type refers to a deviation that is initially greater at distance fixation than at near but that becomes about the same at both after one eye is occluded for 30–45 minutes (to remove binocular fusional impulses) or when +3.00 D sphere lenses are used (to suspend accommodation). The *convergence insufficiency* type is present when the near exodeviation is greater than the distance. This classification is different from isolated convergence insufficiency, which will be discussed later in this chapter.

This system of classification is still used by some surgeons for surgical planning. Recently, however, it has been recognized that differences between distance and near measurements are mostly the result of proximal vergence aftereffects, or *tenacious proximal fusion.* Furthermore, the gradient AC/A ratio in nearly all of these patients becomes normal after proximal vergence aftereffects are suspended by unilateral occlusion.

Sensory testing usually reveals excellent stereopsis with normal retinal correspondence when the exodeviation is latent and suppression with abnormal retinal correspondence when the exodeviation is manifest. However, if the deviation manifests very rarely, diplopia may persist during those manifestations. It is useful to measure stereopsis at 20 feet as well as at 14 inches, since reduced distance stereopsis may indicate poor control of a distance exodeviation.

Nonsurgical Management

Corrective lenses are prescribed for significant myopic, astigmatic, and hyperopic refractive errors. Correction of even mild myopia may improve control of the exodeviation. Mild to moderate degrees of hyperopia are not routinely corrected in children with intermittent exotropia, for fear of worsening the deviation. However, some patients with more than 4.0 D of hyperopia (or more than 1.5 D of hyperopic anisometropia) may actually gain better control of the exodeviation after optical correction. Children with severe hyperopia may be unable to sustain the necessary accommodation for a clear image, and the lack of accommodative effort produces a blurred retinal image and manifest exotropia. Optical correction may improve retinal image clarity and help control the exodeviation.

Iacobucci IL, Archer SM, Giles CL. Children with exotropia responsive to spectacle correction of hyperopia. *Am J Ophthalmol.* 1993;116:79–83.

Additional minus lens power, usually 2–4 D beyond refractive error correction, is used by some physicians to temporarily stimulate accommodative convergence to help control the exodeviation. This therapy may cause asthenopia in school-age children, but it can be very effective as a temporizing measure to promote fusion and avoid surgery during the most visually immature years when amblyopia and loss of stereopsis can occur in the event of a surgical overcorrection.

Caltrider N, Jampolsky A. Overcorrecting minus lens therapy for treatment of intermittent exotropia. *Ophthalmology.* 1983;90:1160–1165.

A rare but distinct group of intermittent exotropia patients have a true high AC/A ratio measured by the gradient method after fusional aftereffects have been eliminated with 30–60 minutes of unilateral patching. Conventional surgery may cause these patients to overcorrect to a high AC/A ratio accommodative esotropia. Minus lenses and bifocals may eliminate the need for surgery by effectively controlling the deviation in this small group of patients.

Part-time patching of the dominant (nondeviating) eye 4–6 hours per day, or alternate daily patching when no strong ocular preference is present, can be a very effective treatment for small to moderate-sized deviations, although the benefit produced is often temporary. The exact mechanism by which patching improves control of intermittent exotropia is not known; presumably it disrupts suppression in some manner and is characterized as a *passive orthoptic treatment.*

Freeman RS, Isenberg SJ. The use of part-time occlusion for early onset unilateral exotropia. *J Pediatr Ophthalmol Strabismus.* 1989;26:94–96.

Active orthoptic treatments that consist of antisuppression therapy/diplopia awareness and fusional convergence training can be used alone or in combination with patching, minus lenses, and/or surgery. For deviations of 20Δ or less, orthoptic treatment has been reported by some to have a long-term success rate comparable to surgery. Others have found no benefit and recommend surgery for any poorly controlled deviation.

Fusional convergence training works best for patients old enough to cooperate who have a remote near point of convergence or poor fusional amplitudes. Diplopia awareness and antisuppression therapy provide the patient with a sensory biofeedback mechanism (diplopia) that stimulates the fusional vergence system. These methods are more controversial but may still be appropriate when dense suppression is present, especially when the deviation is 20Δ or less and the patient is old enough to cooperate. Since conflicting data on the effectiveness of this latter orthoptic treatment are present in the literature, further study is needed to define which patients might benefit. In addition, the pre- and postoperative role of orthoptic treatment remains unclear.

The wearing of base-in prisms can be used to promote fusion in intermittent exotropia, but this treatment option is seldom chosen for long-term management because it can cause a reduction in fusional vergence amplitudes.

Surgical Treatment

Many patients with intermittent exotropia ultimately require surgery, which is customarily performed when progression toward constant exotropia is documented despite the use of appropriate nonsurgical treatments. No consensus exists, however, regarding specific indications. Some surgeons advocate very early surgery for any deviation of 15Δ or more that is intermittently manifest in hopes that realignment before suppression is firmly established will lead to long-term stability of proper alignment. Other surgeons prefer to be very conservative, reserving surgery for patients who have progressed to nearly constant exotropia. The conservative group often advises withholding surgery whenever possible in very young patients to avoid the amblyopia and loss of fine stereopsis that could result from an overcorrection. These risks are minimized with close postoperative follow-up, however.

Most strabismus surgeons today prefer to use lateral rectus muscle recessions bilaterally as the initial surgical procedure for all types of intermittent exotropia. Some surgeons perform unilateral medial rectus muscle resection combined with lateral rectus muscle recession for basic and simulated divergence excess types, bilateral lateral rectus muscle recessions for true divergence excess, and bilateral medial rectus muscle resections for the convergence insufficiency type. However, the benefit of this treatment scheme remains unproven. With little evidence to suggest that results differ according to the type of surgery used, the decision becomes one of the surgeon's choice.

Management of surgical overcorrection   A moderate temporary overcorrection is desirable after bilateral lateral rectus muscle recessions. Persistent overcorrection (beyond 3–4 weeks) may require treatment with base-out prisms (usually Fresnel Press-On prisms) or alternate patching to prevent amblyopia or relieve diplopia. Corrective lenses or miotics should be considered if a moderate amount of hyperopia is present. Bifocals can be used if a high AC/A ratio is present. Unless deficient ductions suggest a slipped or lost muscle, a delay of 4–6 months is recommended before reoperation since spontaneous improvement is common. Following a bilateral lateral rectus muscle recession, medial rectus muscle recessions can be performed provided the lateral rectus muscle ductions are normal. Unilateral lateral rectus muscle recession/medial rectus muscle resection surgery can be followed by medial rectus muscle recession/lateral rectus muscle resection surgery on the other eye.

Management of surgical undercorrection   Mild to moderate residual exodeviation is often treated by observation alone if fusional control is good. However, return of manifest exotropia is common with time. Therefore, some surgeons recommend aggressive base-in prism management for undercorrections with a gradual weaning of the prism dosage. Postoperative patching and orthoptic treatment using the same techniques listed under nonsurgical treatment can be applied to surgical undercorrections. Botulinum toxin injection, in small dosages, has also been used to treat surgical undercorrections, but data supporting its effectiveness are limited. Indications for reoperation in undercorrected patients are the same as for initial surgery. If lateral rectus muscle recessions have been performed bilaterally, medial rectus muscle resections are often chosen when reoperation is needed. Unilateral lateral rectus muscle recession/medial rectus muscle resection is often followed by a similar recess/resect procedure of the other eye. The surgical dose/response curve appears to be similar to the initial surgery. Therefore, surgical dosage can often be selected as though the surgery were a primary operation.

Constant Exotropia

Constant exotropia is encountered more often in older patients manifesting sensory exotropia or decompensated intermittent exotropia. Oblique muscle overaction is often present in a large-angle exotropia. This large-angle exotropia may be associated with an *X pattern,* possibly as a result of overaction of all four oblique muscles. The deviation in an X pattern increases in both upgaze and downgaze.

Surgical treatment for constant exotropia consists of appropriate recessions of lateral rectus muscles with or without tightening of the medial rectus muscles. Oblique muscle surgery may be required. In some cases the patient might have been aware of an enlarged field of peripheral vision because of rapid alternation of fixation and will miss it when the eyes are straight.

Congenital Exotropia

Congenital exotropia presents before 6 months of age with a large-angle constant exotropia, often in association with neurologic impairment or craniofacial disorders (Fig VIII-2). The potential for high-grade stereopsis and bifoveal fixation is poor. Early surgery may help establish peripheral fusion, but little verification of this potential is present in the literature. Late consecutive esotropia, recurrent exotropia, and dissociated vertical deviation are all common, even with early successful surgical alignment.

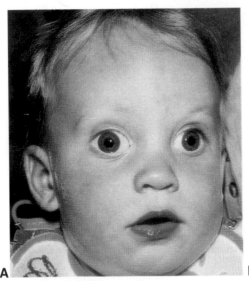 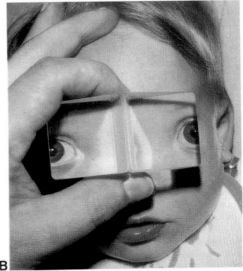

A   B

FIG VIII-2—*A,* This 10-month-old infant with congenital exotropia also shows moderate motor developmental delay. *B,* Krimsky testing uses two 45Δ prisms placed base-to-base in the frontal plane to measure 90Δ of exotropia. (Reprinted with permission from Wilson ME. Exotropia. In: *Focal Points: Clinical Modules for Ophthalmologists.* San Francisco: American Academy of Ophthalmology; 1995;13:11.)

Sensory Exotropia

Any condition that reduces visual acuity in one eye can cause sensory exotropia, a divergent strabismus in a poorly seeing eye. The causes include anisometropia, corneal or lens opacities, optic atrophy or hypoplasia, and macular lesions. It is not known why some individuals become esotropic after unilateral visual loss, while others become exotropic. Both sensory esotropia and sensory exotropia are common in children, but exotropia predominates in older children and adults.

If the eye with sensory exotropia can be visually rehabilitated, peripheral fusion may sometimes be reestablished after surgical realignment, provided the sensory exotropia has not been present for an extended period. Loss of fusional amplitudes, known as *central fusional disruption,* or *horror fusionis,* can lead to constant and permanent diplopia when adult-onset sensory exotropia has been present for more than 10 years prior to visual rehabilitation and realignment. In these patients intractable diplopia may persist, even with well-aligned eyes.

Consecutive Exotropia

Consecutive exotropia may follow previous strabismus surgery for esotropia.

Exotropic Duane (Retraction) Syndrome

Duane syndrome can present with exotropia, usually accompanied by a face turn away from the affected eye. Adduction is most often markedly deficient; other signs include eyelid narrowing, globe retraction, and characteristic upshoots and downshoots. See chapter XI for further discussion of Duane syndrome.

Neuromuscular Abnormalities

A constant exotropia may result from third nerve palsy, internuclear ophthalmoplegia, or myasthenia gravis. These conditions are all discussed in detail in BCSC Section 5, *Neuro-Ophthalmology.*

Dissociated Horizontal Deviation (DHD)

Dissociated strabismus may contain vertical, horizontal, and torsional components. When the dissociated abduction movement is prominent, it is referred to as *dissociated horizontal deviation.* While not a true exotropia, DHD can be confused with a constant or intermittent exotropia. DVD and latent nystagmus often coexist with DHD (Fig VIII-3).

Wilson ME, McClatchey SK. Dissociated horizontal deviation. *J Pediatr Ophthalmol Strabismus.* 1991;28:90–95.

Convergence Insufficiency

Characteristics of convergence insufficiency include asthenopia, blurred near vision, and reading problems in the presence of poor near fusional convergence amplitudes and a remote near point of convergence. The patient may have an exophoria for near but, by definition, should not have an exotropia. Rarely, accommodative spasms may occur if voluntary accommodation and convergence are stimulated in an effort

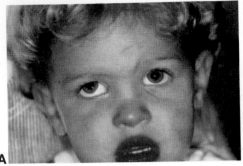 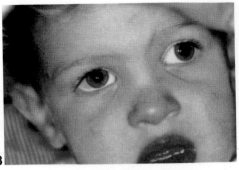

A   B

FIG VIII-3—Dissociated strabismus complex. *A,* When patient fixates with the left eye, a prominent dissociated vertical deviation (DVD) is shown in the right eye. *B,* However, when patient fixates with the right eye, a prominent dissociated horizontal deviation (DHD) is shown in the left eye. (Reproduced with permission from Wilson ME. Exotropia. In: *Focal Points: Clinical Modules for Ophthalmologists.* San Francisco: American Academy of Ophthalmology; 1995;13:11.)

to overcome the convergence insufficiency. Convergence insufficiency, as discussed here, should not be confused with the convergence insufficiency type of intermittent exotropia discussed on p 87.

Treatment of convergence insufficiency usually involves orthoptic exercises. Base-out prism reading can be used to stimulate fusional convergence. Stereograms, "pencil-pushups," and other near point exercises are often used. If these exercises fail, base-in prism reading glasses may be needed. Medial rectus muscle resection, unilaterally or bilaterally, has been used in rare cases when nonsurgical treatments have been unsatisfactory, but surgery carries a substantial risk for diplopia in distance viewing. Some patients with convergence insufficiency also have an accommodative insufficiency.

Convergence Paralysis

Convergence paralysis secondary to intracranial lesions is characterized by normal adduction and accommodation with exotropia and diplopia on attempted near fixation only. An organic intracranial lesion in the corpora quadrigemina or the nucleus of cranial nerve III is frequently associated with Parinaud syndrome.

Treatment is limited to providing base-in prisms at near to alleviate the diplopia. Occasionally, accommodation will also be weakened, particularly in a chronically ill patient, and plus lenses may also be required at near. These patients will have little if any fusional vergence amplitudes at near, and it may not be possible to restore them to comfortable single binocular vision. Occlusion of one eye at near is indicated in such cases, and eye muscle surgery is contraindicated.

Cooper J, Medow N. Major review: Intermittent exotropia; basic and divergence excess type. *Binocular Vision & Eye Muscle Surgery Quarterly.* 1993;8:185–216.

Kushner BJ. Exotropic deviations: a functional classification and approach to treatment. 18th Richard G. Scobee Memorial Lecture. *Am Orthoptic J.* 1988;38:81–93.

Repka MX, Arnoldi KA. Lateral incomitance in exotropia: fact or artifact? *J Pediatr Ophthalmol Strabismus.* 1991;28:125–130.

CHAPTER IX

Vertical Deviations

A vertical deviation is a vertical misalignment of the visual axes. Such a deviation may be comitant but is usually incomitant, or noncomitant. Either comitant or incomitant vertical deviations can occur alone or with a horizontal component (e.g., pure hypertropia or a hypertropia with esotropia or exotropia). A vertical deviation is named after the vertically deviating nonfixating eye. If the right eye is higher than the left and the left eye is fixating, this is called a *right hypertropia*. If the nonfixating right eye is lower than the fixating left eye, this is called a *right hypotropia*. If alternate fixation is present, the deviation is usually named for the hyperdeviating eye (e.g., right hypertropia rather than left hypotropia).

Types of Vertical Deviations

Comitant Vertical Deviations

Most comitant vertical deviations are small and frequently associated with comitant horizontal deviations. Although nearly every vertical paretic deviation starts out incomitant, a vertical misalignment may become comitant with time in the absence of any mechanical restrictions as might occur with a blowout fracture or thyroid ophthalmopathy. However, in most (some say all) vertical deviations, some difference in the magnitude of deviation is found if measurements are made in the diagnostic positions of gaze and with the head tilted.

Incomitant Vertical Deviations

The vast majority of vertical deviations are incomitant. They are produced by paresis or contracture of one or more cyclovertical muscles, or by mechanical restriction of vertical movement.

Differential Diagnosis and Management

Vertical deviations may be caused by innervational or restrictive (mechanical) factors. Combinations of these factors also occur.

Dissociated Vertical Deviation (DVD)

Dissociated vertical deviation is a common innervational disorder found in two thirds or more of patients with congenital esotropia. The etiology is unknown, but it appears to be associated with early disruption of binocular development. Either eye may spontaneously and slowly drift upward and outward with a simultaneous extorsion when an eye is occluded or during periods of visual inattention without occlusion (Fig IX-1). The vertical movement usually predominates and is referred to as

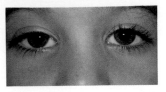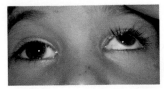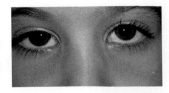

FIG IX-1—Dissociated vertical deviation, left eye. *Left,* Binocular gaze. *Center,* A large left hyperdeviation immediately after the eye is uncovered. *Right,* Left eye drifts back down toward horizontal.

DVD. When the dissociated abduction movements are prominent, the term *dissociated horizontal deviation (DHD)* is used. DHD is rarely seen without simultaneous DVD.

When the vertically deviated eye moves down toward horizontal, the fixating fellow eye makes no downward movement from the object of regard. Note that in hypertropia, when the hypertropic eye fixates a target, the other eye moves downward into a hypotropic position of equal magnitude. In contrast, eyes with DVD have no corresponding hypotropia of the fellow eye when the hypertropic eye fixates.

Hering's law of equal innervation does not apply to dissociated vertical deviation. The condition is usually bilateral, although frequently asymmetrical. It may occur spontaneously (manifest DVD) or only when one eye is occluded (latent DVD). In addition to DHD, latent nystagmus and horizontal strabismus are often associated with DVD. A prior history of congenital esotropia is particularly common. A superimposed vertical deviation, in which Hering's law of equal innervation does apply, can also be seen.

Measurement of DVD is difficult, and the results are variable. One method uses base-down prism in front of the deviating eye under an occluder. The occluder is then switched to the fixating eye. Base-down prism is added until no downward movement of the deviating eye is observed on switching occlusion. Each eye is tested separately in cases of bilateral DVD. Another method using a modified form of the Krimsky test is particularly useful in evaluating patients who cannot fixate with the deviating eye. The deviation can also simply be graded on a 1+ to 4+ scale, where 1+ = a slight deviation, 2+ = a small deviation, 3+ = a moderate deviation, and 4+ = a large deviation.

Treatment for DVD is indicated if the vertical deviation occurs spontaneously, is frequent, and is cosmetically significant. Nonsurgical treatment, which changes the fixation pattern by patching or by optical means, is most effective in unilateral or highly asymmetric bilateral DVD. Surgical treatment often improves the condition but rarely eliminates it (see chapter XIII). It is important to differentiate DVD from overaction of the inferior oblique muscles, since the surgical approach to these two conditions may be different.

Inferior Oblique Muscle Overaction

Primary overaction of the inferior oblique muscle is so named because it is not associated with superior oblique muscle paresis. This type of muscle overaction may be a result of mechanical or innervational causes or a combination of the two; its etiology is not well understood. Primary inferior oblique muscle overaction has been

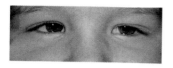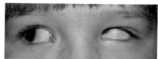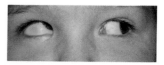

FIG IX-2—Small esotropia with marked overaction of both inferior oblique muscles. Note the elevation and slight abduction of the adducting eye.

reported to develop between ages 1 and 6 in approximately two thirds of patients with congenital esotropia. More rarely, it is seen in association with acquired esotropia or exotropia and even in patients with no other evidence of strabismus. It tends not to cause a primary gaze hypertropia even when asymmetric or unilateral. *Secondary overaction* of the inferior oblique muscle is caused by a paresis or paralysis of its antagonist superior oblique muscle.

Clinical characteristics include overelevation of the eye in adduction (Fig IX-2). With the eyes in lateral gaze and the abducting eye fixating, the adducted eye is overelevated as a result of overaction of the inferior oblique muscle. When the eyes are in lateral gaze and the adducting eye is fixating, the abducted eye will be depressed and manifest a hypotropia on alternate cover testing. By contrast, in DVD the nonfixating abducting eye in lateral gaze does *not* manifest a hypotropia. In addition, the hyperdeviation in DVD can be demonstrated not only in adduction but also in abduction and primary position. Finally, primary position extorsion of the fundus on indirect ophthalmoscopy and V pattern are present with overacting inferior oblique muscles but not with DVD.

When hyperdeviation of the adducted eye becomes clinically significant, a weakening procedure on the inferior oblique muscle is indicated. Many ophthalmologists prefer inferior oblique muscle recession; some prefer inferior oblique myectomy (see chapter XIII). Anteriorization of the recessed inferior oblique muscle is a procedure that has been used to correct both marked overaction of the inferior oblique muscles and DVD when both are present simultaneously.

Kratz RE, Rogers GL, Bremer DL, et al. Anterior tendon displacement of the inferior oblique for DVD. *J Pediatr Ophthalmol Strabismus.* 1989;26:212–217.

Superior Oblique Muscle Overaction (Fig IX-3)

Unlike inferior oblique muscle overaction, superior oblique muscle overaction is usually not divided into primary and secondary forms, because pareses of the inferior rectus and inferior oblique muscles are uncommon. Therefore, almost all bilateral superior oblique muscle overaction can be considered primary.

Also in contrast to primary inferior oblique muscle overaction, a vertical deviation often occurs in primary position with unilateral or asymmetric bilateral overaction of the superior oblique muscles. The hypotropia is on the side of the unilaterally overacting superior oblique muscle. An associated horizontal deviation, most often exotropia, may be present, and the overacting superior oblique muscle also causes depression with resulting hypotropia on adduction.

In a patient with clinically significant ocular deviation or A pattern secondary to bilateral superior oblique overaction, a bilateral superior oblique weakening

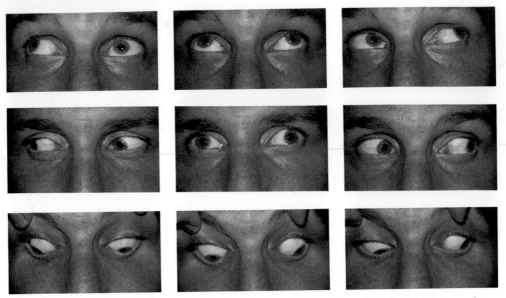

FIG IX-3—Exotropia with A pattern, marked overaction of superior obliques OU, and moderate underaction of inferior obliques OU. Note depression of adducting eye in lateral gaze and depression and abduction of the adducting eye in gaze to the side and down. Note slight limitation of elevation of the adducting eye in gaze to the side and up.

procedure is indicated. This surgery may consist of a superior oblique tenotomy or a superior oblique lengthening by insertion of a silicone expander or nonabsorbable suture. Both procedures are clinically effective in patients who have reduced binocularity (monofixation or suppression). However, many surgeons are reluctant to perform superior oblique tenotomies in patients with bifixation and normal stereopsis in whom the uncontrolled torsional and sometimes asymmetric vertical effect obtained with this surgery can result in torsional diplopia or symptoms of secondary superior oblique palsy with head tilt.

> Wright KW, Ryan SJ. *Color Atlas of Ophthalmic Surgery: Strabismus.* Philadelphia: Lippincott; 1991:210–216. (An excellent illustrated description of the technique for weakening the superior oblique by insertion of a silicone tendon expander.)

Superior Oblique Muscle Paresis (Fourth Cranial Nerve Palsy)

The most common isolated cyclovertical muscle palsy encountered by the ophthalmologist is the fourth, or trochlear, nerve palsy. The palsy may be congenital, resulting from a defect in the nucleus or the motor portion of cranial nerve IV, or it may be acquired, most commonly as a result of closed head trauma or, rarely, from central nervous system vascular problems, diabetes, or brain tumors. The palsy may be unilateral or bilateral. Markedly asymmetric bilateral palsies that initially appear to be unilateral have prompted the term *masked bilateral.* The examiner should maintain a high index of suspicion for possible bilaterality when evaluating patients with superior oblique muscle palsy.

To differentiate congenital from acquired palsies it is helpful to examine old family photographs to detect an appropriate head tilt extending back to childhood. Facial asymmetry from long-standing childhood head tilting and large vertical fusional amplitudes also indicate chronicity. In addition, patients with a congenital palsy will more frequently demonstrate a long, redundant, or "floppy" superior oblique tendon at the time of surgery.

The patient may present fixating with the unaffected eye and showing a hypertropia of the involved eye. Or the patient may present fixating with the paretic eye and a hypotropia of the unaffected eye, sometimes called *fallen eye syndrome.* Abnormal head positions are common, usually a head tilt toward the shoulder opposite the side of the paresis. Amblyopia is uncommon in acquired pareses but may be present in congenital ones. Extorsion and a complaint of apparent tilting of objects are common in acquired cases. Congenital cases are usually unilateral, and acquired cases are more often bilateral.

The possibility of bilaterality should always be considered. To differentiate bilateral from unilateral superior oblique paresis the following criteria are used:

□ *Bilateral cases.* Bilateral cases usually have a V-pattern esotropia in downgaze (see chapter X, A and V Patterns). Torsion, when measured by the double Maddox rod test, is usually greater than 10° excycloduction. The Bielschowsky head-tilt test (see chapter VI) is positive to each side; i.e., right head tilt shows a right hypertropia and left head tilt a left hypertropia. The ductions of the superior oblique muscles are usually diminished in bilateral cases. Signs of bilaterality in cases initially thought to be unilateral include bilateral objective fundus extorsion, esotropia in downgaze, and even the mildest degree of inferior oblique overaction on the presumed uninvolved side.

□ *Unilateral cases.* Unilateral cases usually show little esotropia in downgaze; torsion, measured by the double Maddox rod test, shows less than 10° excycloduction; the head tilt test is positive for the involved side only; and the actions of the superior oblique muscle may be normal or diminished.

The diagnosis of superior oblique muscle palsy is supported by results of the three-step test, double Maddox rod testing to measure torsion, and a careful analysis of the ductions and versions. The three-step test does not provide a diagnosis or rule out bilaterality; it merely identifies the paretic muscle when an isolated cyclovertical muscle palsy is known to occur. The test can be misleading in cases of dissociated vertical deviation, restrictive muscle disorders that may occur with orbital blowout fracture, or other innervational disorders such as skew deviation. Diplopic fields are also important, as in all cases of acquired strabismus. Documentation of deviation using the Hess screen or Lancaster red-green test is used by some ophthalmologists to follow patients with superior oblique muscle palsy.

Measurement of ocular deviation in all nine diagnostic gaze positions, as well as with right and left head tilt, is important in diagnosing and planning treatment for superior oblique muscle palsy (Fig IX-4). For example, in a right superior oblique muscle paresis the deviations in gaze left and up and left and down give important information to the clinician planning surgery. The versions should be examined, with attention paid to the actions of the involved superior oblique muscle, the antagonist inferior oblique muscle, the inferior rectus muscle in the involved eye (because contracture of the ipsilateral superior rectus muscle may occur with subsequent

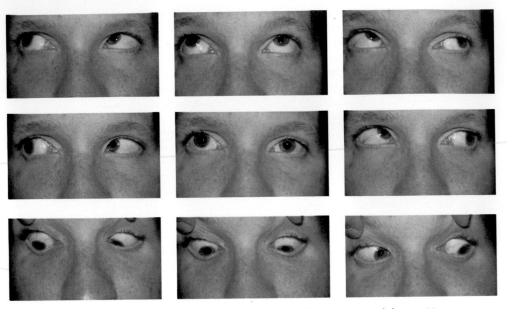

FIG IX-4—Right superior oblique palsy with a right hypertropia that increases on left gaze. Note accompanying overaction of right inferior oblique.

limitation of depression by the ipsilateral inferior rectus muscle), and the superior rectus muscle in the involved eye.

Indications for treatment are abnormal head position, significant vertical deviation, or diplopia. Prisms may be used to overcome diplopia in small, symptomatic, comitant, or nearly comitant deviations that do not have a symptomatic torsional component. If this treatment alleviates the symptoms, surgery is not warranted.

Surgical management The surgical principles that apply to the treatment of vertical deviations are followed. To plan a surgical treatment for superior oblique muscle paresis the clinician must undertake an analysis of both the versions and the diagnostic gaze position measurements. Common surgical strategies are discussed below and in chapter XIII.

When the antagonist inferior oblique muscle is overacting and the deviation in primary position is no greater than 15Δ, the inferior oblique muscle should be weakened. The amount of deviation in primary position that is corrected is proportional to the amount of overaction of the inferior oblique muscle.

If the deviation is greater than 15Δ with an overacting antagonist inferior oblique muscle, the inferior oblique muscle and the yoke contralateral inferior rectus muscle should be weakened. Again, the amount of primary gaze correction achieved by the inferior oblique muscle weakening will depend more on the amount of overaction present preoperatively than on the specific inferior oblique muscle–weakening technique used. Correcting mild overaction may yield only 5–8Δ of primary gaze correction. Operating on a moderate to severely overacting muscle can often achieve 10–15Δ of correction. The remainder of the primary gaze deviation is then corrected by a recession of the contralateral inferior rectus muscle. A basic guideline: Each millimeter of recession of a vertical rectus muscle will result in approximately 3Δ of vertical correction.

Some surgeons prefer to tuck the ipsilateral superior oblique tendon rather than perform a recession of the contralateral inferior rectus muscle. The ability to titrate the quantity of a superior oblique tendon tuck comes with experience. An attempt should be made to tuck the tendon until a positive forced traction test is created for elevation in adduction just as the inferior limbus crosses an imaginary line drawn between the medial and lateral canthus. In adults inferior rectus muscle recession has the advantage of facilitating use of an adjustable suture. If the antagonist inferior oblique muscle is not overacting, either the yoke contralateral inferior rectus muscle should be recessed or the ipsilateral superior oblique tendon should be tucked.

The surgical plan may need to include recession of the ipsilateral superior rectus muscle if a forced duction test shows limited depression on the side of the deviation. This finding is more common when the paresis is long-standing. In fact, much of the "spread of comitance" that occurs over time in superior oblique muscle paresis is a result of ipsilateral superior rectus muscle contracture. For example, with a right superior oblique muscle weakness, the hypertropia is usually greatest in left gaze. In cases with contracture of the ipsilateral superior rectus muscle the deviation in right gaze will be more like the deviation in primary position and left gaze. Thus, the superior rectus muscle would need to be recessed (often only a small amount) as part of the surgical strategy in these cases.

Ipsilateral superior rectus muscle contracture can also produce a depression deficiency in abduction. On version testing this deficiency may appear to represent superior oblique muscle *overaction* in the normal eye. If the surgeon is misled by this appearance and performs a superior oblique tenotomy on the normal eye, iatrogenically converting a unilateral superior oblique paresis to a bilateral one, disabling torsional diplopia can result.

If the deviation is greater than 35Δ in primary position, three-muscle surgery may be required. This treatment might include recession of the overacting antagonist inferior oblique muscle, superior oblique tendon tuck, or vertical rectus muscle surgery as necessary.

The superior oblique tendon tuck is often used in cases of acquired bilateral superior oblique muscle paresis or weakness. Many surgeons also recommend a superior oblique tendon tuck to reduce or eliminate the head tilt in a congenital superior oblique muscle palsy that presents in early childhood and is accompanied by a loose, floppy tendon at the time of surgery.

An alternative to tucking the superior oblique tendons in bilateral paretic cases with predominantly torsional complaints is anterior temporal displacement of the anterior halves of the superior oblique muscle tendons (sometimes called the *Harada-Ito procedure*). This procedure corrects the extorsion and abducting weakness of the superior oblique muscle in downgaze. It does not correct any vertical deviation in primary position.

Harada M, Ito Y. Surgical correction of cyclotropia. *Jpn J Ophthalmol.* 1964;8:88–96.

Mitchell PR, Parks MM. Surgery for bilateral superior oblique palsy. *Ophthalmology.* 1982;89:484–488.

Saunders RA. Superior oblique muscle surgery. In: Tasman W, Jaeger EA, eds. *Duane's Clinical Ophthalmology.* Philadelphia: Lippincott; 1997, vol 6, chap 86, 1–20.

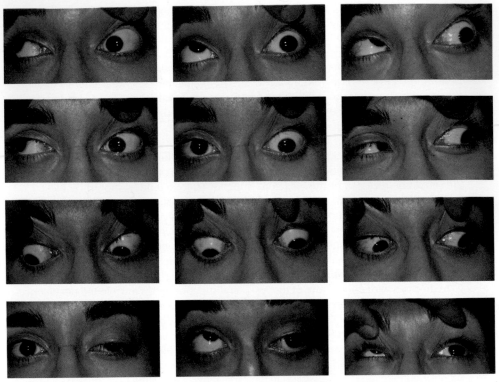

FIG IX-5—*Top three rows,* Monocular elevation deficiency of the left eye, with no voluntary elevation of the left eye above horizontal in nine diagnostic positions. *Bottom left,* Ptosis of the left upper eyelid when fixing with the right eye persists when fixing with the left eye (*bottom center*). The bottom center photograph also shows the marked secondary deviation of elevation in the right eye when fixing with the left eye. *Bottom right,* A partially intact Bell's phenomenon with the left eye elevating above the horizontal on forced eyelid closure.

Monocular Elevation Deficiency (Double Elevator Palsy)

The term *double elevator palsy* implies a paresis of both the inferior oblique and superior rectus muscles. However, double elevator palsy has become an umbrella term for any strabismus manifesting deficit elevation in all positions of gaze. Since this motility pattern is well known to be caused by inferior rectus muscle restriction as well as paresis of one or both elevator muscles, double elevator muscle palsy is a misleading name and has been replaced by *monocular elevation deficiency* (Fig IX-5). Three types of monocular elevation deficiency are found:

With inferior rectus restriction. These deficiencies are diagnosed by:

□ Positive forced ductions to elevation

□ Normal force generations (no muscle paralysis)

□ Normal saccades of the superior rectus muscle

With elevator weakness. These deficiencies are diagnosed by:

□ Free forced ductions

□ Reduced force generations of elevators (evidence of paralysis)

□ Reduced saccadic velocities in upgaze movements of affected eye (often with Bell's phenomenon preserved, indicating a supranuclear etiology)

Combination. These deficiencies have inferior rectus restriction and also weak elevators. They are diagnosed by:

□ Positive forced ductions in elevation

□ Reduced force generations of elevators of involved eye

□ Reduced upward vertical saccadic velocities in involved eye

Characteristics Clinical characteristics of all three types described above include

□ Limitation of elevation; elevation in adduction as well as abduction, both on versions and ductions (elevation in abduction often more reduced than in primary gaze and improving somewhat in adduction—in contrast to Brown syndrome)

□ Hypotropia of involved eye that increases in upgaze

□ Chin-up position with fusion in downgaze or straight head with amblyopia in the hypotropic eye

□ Ptosis or pseudoptosis often present in primary position (an element of true ptosis present in 50% of patients—among monocular elevation deficiency patients with ptosis, up to one third will also show Marcus Gunn jaw-winking phenomenon)

□ Inferior rectus muscle restriction

Patients with inferior rectus muscle restriction often have an extra or deeper lower eyelid fold on the affected side. Bell's phenomenon is usually asymmetric. The eye with the inferior rectus muscle restriction has a very poor or absent Bell's, as compared to the eye without the inferior rectus muscle restriction.

Metz HS. Double elevator palsy. *Arch Ophthalmol.* 1979;97:901–903.

Management Indications for treatment include large vertical deviation in primary position, with or without ptosis, and abnormal head position, usually chin up. If inferior rectus muscle restriction is present, the muscle should be recessed. If there is no restriction, the medial rectus and the lateral rectus muscles should be transposed toward the superior rectus muscle *(Knapp procedure).*

Brown Syndrome (Superior Oblique Tendon Sheath Syndrome)

The motility disorder described by Brown in 1950 and originally named *superior oblique tendon sheath syndrome* is now known simply as *Brown syndrome.* The characteristic restriction of elevation in adduction was originally thought to be caused by secondary shortening of the anterior sheath of the superior oblique tendon from congenital palsy of the ipsilateral inferior oblique muscle. Brown later abandoned this theory, which has subsequently been disproven and dismissed.

Brown syndrome occurs in congenital, acquired, constant, and intermittent forms. Restriction of free passage of the superior oblique tendon through the trochlear pulley is central to all forms of Brown syndrome even when related to trauma or systemic inflammatory (rheumatological) conditions. Acquired Brown

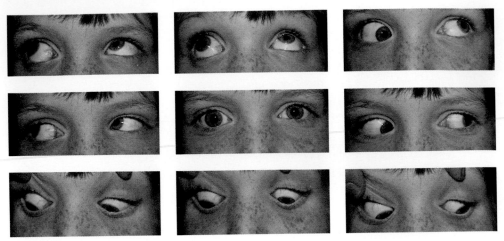

FIG IX-6—Brown syndrome, right eye. There is no elevation of the right eye when adducted; in this patient, the right eye is depressed when adducted.

syndrome is more likely to be intermittent and to spontaneously resolve than congenital Brown syndrome, which is more likely to be constant and less likely to resolve. However, exceptions occur. Even congenital constant Brown syndrome may spontaneously resolve over many years, sometimes becoming intermittent before resolving completely. Brown syndrome is bilateral in approximately 10% of cases.

Well-recognized features of Brown syndrome include a deficiency of active and passive elevation in adduction (Fig IX-6). With rotation of the eye out of the field of vertical action of the superior oblique muscle, elevation improves so that restriction is reduced in midline, and minimal or no elevation deficit is present in abduction. Divergence is usually seen with midline elevation. In adduction the palpebral fissure widens and a downshoot of the eye is often seen. Version testing reveals minimal or no ipsilateral superior oblique muscle overaction. This finding along with positive forced duction testing differentiates Brown syndrome from inferior oblique muscle palsy (discussed below).

Brown syndrome can be graded as mild, moderate, or severe. In the mild form no hypotropia is present in primary position and no downshoot of the eye occurs in adduction. Moderate cases have a downshoot in adduction but still no primary gaze hypotropia. Severe Brown syndrome cases have both a downshoot in adduction and a primary gaze hypotropia often accompanied by abnormal head posturing. A chin-up head posture is most commonly seen, although a face turn away from the affected eye may be present. Occasionally, patients present with a manifest hypotropia and no compensatory head posturing. These patients often have associated horizontal strabismus and are at greater risk for amblyopia. Mild and moderate forms make up about two thirds of all Brown syndrome cases. These cases do not have strabismus in primary position, and they are most often left untreated.

An unequivocally positive forced duction test demonstrating restricted passive elevation in adduction is essential for the diagnosis of Brown syndrome. Forced retroplacement of the globe during forced duction testing places the superior oblique muscle on stretch and accentuates the restriction in Brown syndrome. When inferior rectus muscle fibrosis or inferior orbital blowout fracture produces a restrictive elevation deficiency, the limitation to passive elevation will be accentuated by proptosing the eye rather than retroplacing it. In addition, the elevation deficiency produced by inferior rectus fibrosis or blowout fracture is usually more marked in abduction rather than adduction.

Treatment Observation alone remains the most common management for all forms of Brown syndrome. Range-of-motion eye exercises, oral corticosteroids, and corticosteroids injected near the trochlea have each produced improvement in selected patients. When Brown syndrome occurs in association with adult rheumatoid arthritis, juvenile rheumatoid arthritis, or other systemic inflammatory diseases, resolution may occur as systemic treatment brings the underlying disease into remission. Sinusitis has also led to Brown syndrome, and it has been suggested that patients presenting with acute-onset Brown syndrome of undetermined cause undergo CT scans of the orbits and paranasal sinuses.

Surgical treatment is indicated when a primary position hypotropia and/or anomalous head posture is present and spontaneous resolution seems unlikely. Brown's sheathectomy surgery has been abandoned in favor of more effective procedures. Ipsilateral superior oblique tenotomy is effective in improving elevation in adduction. However, iatrogenic superior oblique muscle palsy may occur postoperatively. Although the incidence has been reported to be 44%–82%, careful preservation of intermuscular septum during tenotomy can reduce this complication to approximately 20%. This modified tenotomy often produces an early undercorrection that gradually improves with time.

To further reduce the incidence of superior oblique muscle palsy after tenotomy some surgeons perform a simultaneous ipsilateral inferior oblique muscle recession or myectomy. More recently, a guarded tenotomy has been performed by some surgeons using an inert spacer formed from a solid silicone retinal band sewn to the cut ends of the superior oblique tendon at tenotomy. This procedure eliminates the need for simultaneous inferior oblique muscle weakening but has resulted in a downgaze deficiency from adhesions to the nasal border of the superior rectus muscle in some cases. Care must be taken to place the silicone spacer nasal to the superior rectus muscle and to avoid direct contact of the spacer with sclera by preserving the intermuscular septum.

Crawford JS. Surgical treatment of true Brown's syndrome. *Am J Ophthalmol.* 1976; 81:289–295.

Parks MM, Eustis HS. Simultaneous superior oblique tenotomy and inferior oblique recession in Brown's syndrome. *Ophthalmology.* 1987;94:1043–1048.

Parks MM, Mitchell PR. Ophthalmoplegic syndromes and trauma. In: Tasman W, Jaeger EA, eds. *Duane's Clinical Ophthalmology.* Philadelphia: Lippincott; 1997; vol 1, chap 20, 5–7.

Wilson ME, Eustis HS Jr, Parks MM. Brown's syndrome. *Surv Ophthalmol.* 1989; 34:153–172.

Wright KW. Superior oblique silicone expander for Brown syndrome and superior oblique overaction. *J Pediatr Ophthalmol Strabismus.* 1991;28:101–107.

Inferior Oblique Muscle Paresis

Damage to the inferior division of cranial nerve III (oculomotor) and especially to the branch that supplies the inferior oblique muscle has been proposed as a possible etiology of inferior oblique muscle paresis. However, the exact cause is unknown. The condition is rare, controversial, and has not been reported to be associated with any other neurologic abnormalities.

Onset is not well documented. Underaction of the inferior oblique muscle is demonstrated by deficiency of elevation from an adducted position. An A pattern is usually present, and the superior oblique muscle usually overacts. The diagnosis of inferior oblique muscle paresis is supported by findings of the three-step test. However, many cases thought to be inferior oblique muscle paresis may in fact represent asymmetric or unilateral primary superior oblique muscle overaction with secondary underaction of the inferior oblique muscle and subsequent A pattern. Forced ductions are free when elevating the eye in an adducted position.

Although Brown syndrome and inferior oblique muscle paresis may both present with deficient elevation in adduction, they are easily distinguished by other clinical characteristics as listed in Table IX-1.

Indications for treatment of inferior oblique muscle palsy are abnormal head position, vertical deviation in primary gaze, and diplopia. Management is usually superior oblique tenotomy. Contralateral superior rectus muscle recession is used in those rare cases when ipsilateral superior oblique muscle overaction is not present.

TABLE IX-1

COMPARISON OF INFERIOR OBLIQUE MUSCLE PALSY
WITH BROWN SYNDROME

	INFERIOR OBLIQUE MUSCLE PALSY	BROWN SYNDROME
Forced ductions	Negative	Positive
Strabismus pattern	A pattern	V pattern
Superior oblique muscle overaction	Usually present	None or minimal

Orbital Floor Fractures (Blowout Fractures) (Fig IX-7)

Blunt facial trauma is the usual cause of orbital floor fractures; auto accidents account for the majority. Clinical characteristics include:

☐ Ecchymosis of the involved eye

☐ Diplopia in some or all positions of gaze immediately following injury; it may persist in upgaze or downgaze

☐ Paresthesia or hypoesthesia of the infraorbital area, secondary to damage of the infraorbital nerve

☐ Enophthalmos, either early or late

□ Entrapment of the inferior rectus muscle, inferior oblique muscle, or surrounding tissue

□ Hypotropia in the primary position that increases with upgaze and may decrease or become a hypertropia in downgaze, suggesting combined mechanical restriction to elevation and inferior rectus paresis or pseudoparesis to depression

□ Medial orbital wall fractures, resulting in entrapment of the medial rectus muscle

In the presence of a limitation of elevation or depression, forced duction testing will rule out restriction. Saccadic eye movement testing is sometimes helpful to determine whether the eye is limited in movement because of a restrictive or a paretic process. CT scans or MRIs are more sensitive than plain-film radiograms and have largely replaced them. Consultation with other specialists who have experience with orbital fractures may be quite helpful in determining the extent of damage to the orbit and surrounding tissues and in planning appropriate management. Intraocular damage is frequently associated, requiring a complete eye examination.

Surgical management of orbital floor fractures is controversial. Some clinicians advocate immediate exploration once the diagnosis is made, while others recommend waiting for orbital edema and hematoma to subside, which usually takes 5–10 days, before considering surgery. Some ophthalmologists wait 6 weeks before surgical intervention, and others wait 3–6 months before exploration if the hypotropia persists. Residual strabismus can generally be corrected by using standard eye muscle surgical techniques (recession or resection) without the necessity of exploring or repairing the orbital floor. A posterior fixation suture is sometimes used on the inferior rectus muscle of the uninjured eye to limit downgaze and match a duction deficiency in the injured eye. This approach is particularly useful when diplopia occurs in the reading position but no deviation is present in primary position. See also BCSC Section 7, *Orbit, Eyelids, and Lacrimal System.*

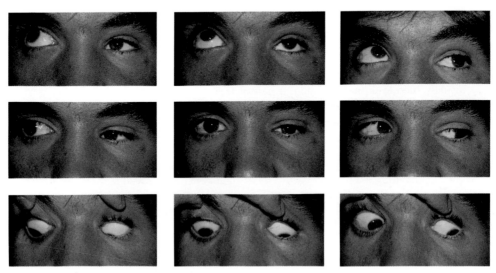

FIG IX-7—Orbital fracture OS with inferior rectus entrapment. Note ptosis from enophthalmos and limitation of elevation OS.

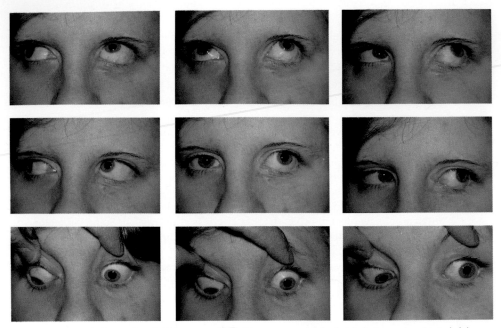

FIG IX-8—Traumatic laceration, left lower eyelid, with severance of the left inferior rectus. Note left hypertropia with limitation of depression of left eye.

Inferior Rectus Muscle Paresis

This condition is a result of trauma to the nerve or to the inferior rectus muscle and can occur either at the time of injury or at the time of the repair of an orbital floor fracture (Fig IX-8). Care must be taken to make an accurate diagnosis before attempting repair.

If inferior rectus muscle paresis is present without entrapment, a hypertropia is usually seen in primary position. If paresis is present with entrapment, the patient may have very little deviation or even a slight hypotropia in primary position, which decreases in downgaze.

The management of inferior rectus muscle paresis is observation, as it may recover with time. If recovery does not take place within 6 months of the injury, muscle surgery may be indicated. For partial inferior rectus muscle paresis a resection of the affected muscle combined with a recession of the ipsilateral superior rectus muscle can be performed. Alternatively, a recession of the contralateral inferior rectus muscle with or without the addition of a posterior fixation suture can be used. Transposition of the ipsilateral medial and lateral rectus muscles to the inferior rectus muscle (inverse Knapp procedure) can be performed for complete inferior rectus muscle paralysis.

CHAPTER X

A and V Patterns

Horizontal deviations that change in magnitude with upgaze and downgaze, A patterns and V patterns, are incomitant subtypes of horizontal strabismus. According to the traditional (and somewhat arbitrary) definition, an A pattern is not considered clinically significant unless it measures 10Δ or more difference between gaze up 25° and down 25°. A V pattern is not considered clinically significant unless it measures 15Δ or more difference between gaze up 25° and down 25°.

An *A pattern* is present when a vertically incomitant horizontal deviation shows increasing convergence (decreasing divergence) in upgaze and increasing divergence in downgaze. *V pattern* designates a vertically incomitant horizontal deviation with increasing convergence (decreasing divergence) in downgaze and increasing divergence in upgaze. Other, less common, variations include Y, λ, ◇, and X patterns.

Between 15% and 25% of all strabismus cases have an associated A or V pattern. They are more commonly seen when measured in extreme positions of gaze. Common patterns found in clinical practice are V-pattern esotropia (Fig X-1), V-pattern exotropia (Fig X-2), A-pattern exotropia (Fig X-3), and A-pattern esotropia (Fig X-4).

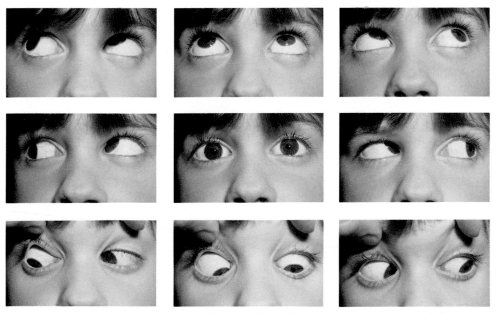

FIG X-1—V-pattern esotropia. Note overelevation of the adducted eye from overaction of the inferior obliques. Note also limitation of depression of the adducted eye from underaction of the superior obliques.

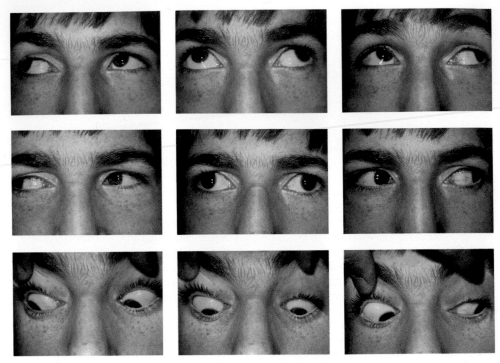

FIG X-2—V-pattern exotropia with moderate overaction of inferior oblique muscles OU. Note large exotropia in upgaze and small esotropia in downgaze.

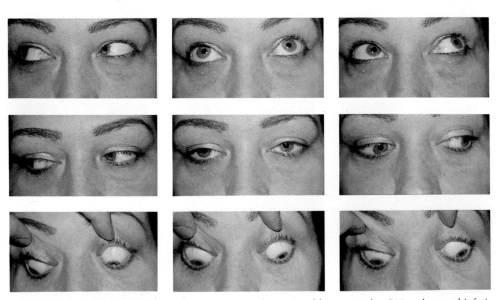

FIG X-3—A-pattern exotropia with marked overaction of superior oblique muscles OU and normal inferior oblique muscles OU. Note the depression of the adducted eye and abduction of the adducted eye in contralateral downgaze.

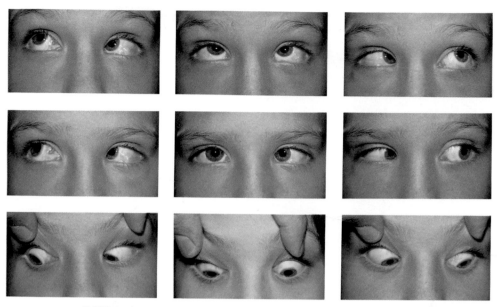

FIG X-4—A-pattern esotropia with minimal oblique muscle dysfunction.

Each of the following conditions has been firmly documented as a cause of A and V patterns. The ophthalmologist should pay careful attention to these anatomic or innervational anomalies before making any decisions about surgery.

□ *Oblique muscle dysfunction.* Inferior oblique muscle overaction is associated with V patterns, and superior oblique muscle overaction is associated with A patterns. Oblique muscle dysfunction is commonly found with clinically significant patterns.

□ *Horizontal rectus muscle dysfunction.* For example, increased lateral rectus muscle innervation in upgaze produces a V pattern.

□ *Vertical rectus muscle dysfunction.* If the superior rectus muscles are primarily underacting, for example, their adducting effect in upgaze will decrease, and a V pattern will result.

Patients with upward- or downward-slanting palpebral fissures may also show A and V patterns. Diagnosis of A and V patterns is made by measuring the patient's alignment while he or she is fixating an accommodative target at distance. Measurements are done in extreme positions of gaze, using the proper refractive correction, and prism cover tests are also employed. Underactions and overactions of the oblique muscles are noted with versions. Any compensatory head position such as chin up, chin down, or head turn is noted.

Patients with Apert syndrome or Crouzon syndrome (see craniosynostosis, p 350) frequently show a V-pattern exotropia or esotropia with marked elevation of the adducting eye, which resembles the pattern caused by overacting inferior oblique muscles. The etiology of this unusual motility disorder may be a combination of mechanical factors (e.g., extorsion of the entire bony orbit) and structural abnormalities (abnormal size, number, or insertion of muscles). Surgical correction can be difficult. In addition, facial surgery for these conditions may produce a large eye alignment shift, usually in an esotropic direction.

Surgical Considerations

Clinically significant patterns are typically treated surgically. Definitions of clinical significance for A and V patterns appear on p 107.

Principles of Treatment

The following are guidelines to help the clinician plan surgical correction of A- and V-pattern deviations:

- Primary and reading positions are functionally the most important positions of gaze.
- Surgery to eliminate horizontal deviation in primary position should be independently selected.
- Most patients with large A or V patterns will also have significant oblique muscle dysfunction.
- Most surgeons use "oblique dysfunction" to determine their surgical approach, referring to the vertical deviations in adduction. (For example they say there is right inferior oblique overaction if the right eye elevates in adduction. If the eye does not elevate in adduction they would say there is no oblique dysfunction.)
- Most surgeons feel horizontal rectus muscle transpositions are indicated when there is no oblique dysfunction but are not a substitute for oblique muscle surgery when oblique muscle overaction is present.
- Weakening the inferior oblique muscles or tucking the superior oblique muscles corrects up to $15-25\Delta$ of V pattern, but the tuck procedure is somewhat unpredictable for many surgeons.
- Inferior oblique muscle weakening tends to be self-adjusting, correcting all the V pattern present without overcorrection.
- Bilateral superior oblique tenotomies correct up to $35-45\Delta$ of A pattern; i.e., they produce $35-45\Delta$ of eso shift in downgaze.

Horizontal Rectus Muscle Transpositions

Horizontal rectus muscles can be vertically transposed to correct A- or V-pattern strabismus not caused by oblique muscle dysfunction, as shown in Figure X-5. The *medial rectus muscles* are always moved toward the direction of vertical gaze where the *convergence* is greater, i.e., upward in A patterns and downward in V patterns. The *lateral rectus muscles* are moved toward the direction of vertical gaze where the *divergence* is greater, i.e., upward in V patterns and downward in A patterns.

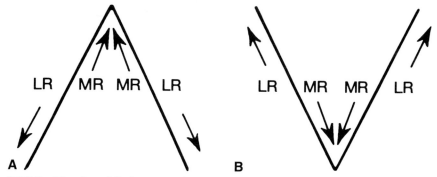

FIG X-5—Direction of displacement of medial and lateral rectus muscles in weakening operations to treat A-pattern deviations *(A)* and V-pattern deviations *(B)*. (Reprinted from von Noorden GK. *von Noorden–Maumenee's Atlas of Strabismus.* 3rd ed. St Louis: Mosby; 1977.)

When recess-resect surgery is indicated in an A pattern, a half- or full-tendon-width transposition of the medial rectus muscle up and the lateral rectus muscle down will have no net vertical effect in primary position. But in upgaze the medial rectus muscle will be relaxed and the lateral rectus will be tightened, thereby decreasing the A pattern. Similarly, for V patterns, the medial rectus muscle is transposed a half- or full-tendon-width down and the lateral rectus muscle is transposed a half- or full-tendon-width up. In downgaze the medial rectus muscle will be relaxed and the lateral rectus muscle will be tightened, thereby decreasing the V pattern.

A useful mnemonic for these procedures is MALE: *M*edial recti to the *A*pex, *L*ateral recti to the *E*mpty space. Other surgeons remember the association *L*ateral rectus moves toward the *L*eg of the deviation, and the *M*edial rectus moves to the *M*iddle of the deviation. Others, thinking of the muscle mechanics, remember that the surgeon moves the muscle in the direction where its horizontal effect is to be weakened (e.g., medials down in V pattern).

Horizontal transposition of the vertical recti has been proposed as an alternative treatment. The superior recti are moved temporally and the inferior recti moved nasally for an A pattern and the opposite for a V pattern. While this procedure is theoretically appealing, it is rarely used today because horizontal deviations, and therefore horizontal muscle surgery, are more common.

Sample Treatment Plans for the Various Patterns

Treatment of V-Pattern Esotropia

Inferior oblique muscle function should be assessed. If inferior oblique muscle overaction is present, the inferior oblique muscles should be weakened, and the deviation in primary position should be corrected with either bilateral medial rectus muscle recessions or a recess-resect operation.

If significant inferior oblique muscle overaction is not present, the procedure of choice is bilateral medial rectus muscle recessions with downward transposition or a recess-resect operation moving the medial rectus muscle down and the lateral rectus muscle up.

Treatment of V-Pattern Exotropia

Again, inferior oblique muscle function should be assessed. If inferior oblique muscle overaction is present, the inferior oblique muscles should be weakened, and each lateral rectus muscle should be recessed to correct the amount of deviation measured in primary position. Alternatively, a recess-resect operation may be performed to correct the deviation in primary position.

If inferior oblique muscle overaction is not present, the treatment of choice is bilateral lateral rectus muscle recessions with upward displacement or a recess-resect operation for the deviation in primary position. In this case the recessed lateral rectus muscle is moved upward, and the resected medial rectus muscle is moved downward.

Treatment of A-Pattern Esotropia

Superior oblique muscle function should be assessed. If superior oblique muscle overaction is present, the superior oblique muscles should be weakened with bilateral superior oblique tenotomies or tendon-lengthening procedures. Superior oblique muscle–weakening procedures are self-adjusting in A-pattern strabismus, correcting up to 40–45Δ of excess divergence in downgaze, if present.

Some controversy persists concerning the effect of bilateral superior oblique tenotomies on primary position horizontal alignment. Some surgeons feel that the loss of abducting forces resulting from bilateral superior oblique tenotomy increases convergence in primary position by 10–15Δ. These surgeons suggest adjusting horizontal surgery to compensate for this expected change. Others feel that superior oblique tenotomies have no significant effect on primary position alignment, and therefore, no adjustment of horizontal surgery is warranted. With this issue in mind, the ophthalmologist must plan appropriate surgery, either bilateral medial rectus recession or a recess-resect procedure to correct for horizontal position misalignment. Since the amount of horizontal surgery required is difficult to predict when superior oblique tenotomies are completed, adjustable sutures on the horizontal muscles may be helpful.

> Diamond GR, Parks MM. The effect of superior oblique weakening procedures on primary position horizontal alignment. *J Pediatr Ophthalmol Strabismus.* 1981; 18:35–38.

If superior oblique overaction is not present, the treatment of choice is bilateral medial rectus recession with upward displacement or a bilateral resection of the lateral rectus with downward displacement. Alternatively, a recession of the medial rectus muscle and a resection of the lateral rectus muscle can be performed, moving the medial rectus superiorly and the lateral rectus inferiorly.

Treatment of A-Pattern Exotropia

Again, superior oblique muscle function should be assessed. If superior oblique muscle overaction is present, weakening procedures should be performed. Bearing in mind the controversy discussed above, the ophthalmologist should plan horizontal rectus muscle surgery to correct the horizontal misalignment in primary position with either a bilateral lateral rectus recession or a recess-resect procedure. As mentioned above, adjustable sutures on the horizontal muscles may be helpful.

If superior oblique muscle overaction is not remarkable, bilateral lateral rectus recession with downward displacement or recession of the lateral rectus with downward displacement and resection of the medial rectus with upward displacement should be planned.

CHAPTER XI

Special Forms of Strabismus

Congenital Sixth Nerve (Abducens) Palsy

Palsies of cranial nerve VI (abducens) occurring shortly after birth have been reported. They are thought to be caused by the increased intracranial pressure associated with labor and delivery and usually resolve spontaneously. Permanent sixth nerve damage with resultant esodeviation can also be noted in the early neonatal period; see discussion under Incomitant Esodeviations, pp 83–84.

Duane Syndrome

Duane syndrome includes a spectrum of motility disturbances, which all feature retraction of the globe in adduction. Often some limitation of horizontal movement is also present. Vertical deviations are common, with a marked upshoot or downshoot (leash phenomenon) of the affected eye in adduction.

A defect in development in the fourth week of gestation appears to be the etiology of Duane syndrome, according to studies of patients exposed to thalidomide prenatally. While most affected patients have Duane syndrome alone, many associated systemic defects have been observed, including Goldenhar syndrome (hemifacial microsomia, ocular dermoids, ear anomalies, preauricular skin tags, and upper eyelid colobomas), and Wildervanck syndrome (sensorineural hearing loss, Klippel-Fiel anomaly with fused cervical vertebrae), which is limited to girls. Most cases of Duane syndrome are sporadic, but about 5%–10% show autosomal dominant inheritance. An interesting prevalence in girls has been observed in most reported series of patients. Discordance in monozygotic twins raises the possibility that intrauterine environment may have an important contribution. The many nonfamilial cases and the predilection for occurring in the left eye also point to nongenetic factors.

In the few anatomic studies performed the nucleus of the sixth nerve has been absent and an aberrant branch of the third nerve has innervated the lateral rectus muscle. Electromyographic studies have shown paradoxical innervation of the lateral rectus muscle, including innervation on attempted adduction and reduced innervation on attempted abduction. Anomalous synergistic innervation of the medial, inferior, and superior rectus muscles and the oblique muscles has been demonstrated as well.

> Hotchkiss MG, Miller NR, Clark AW, et al. Bilateral Duane's retraction syndrome. A clinical-pathologic case report. Arch Ophthalmol. 1980;98:870–874.

Many attempts to classify Duane syndrome patients have been made. Huber devised the most commonly used system: type I having poor abduction, type II having poor adduction, and type III having both poor abduction and adduction. Since many patients do not fit into these simple categories, other researchers have chosen to emphasize instead the direction of the strabismus in primary gaze.

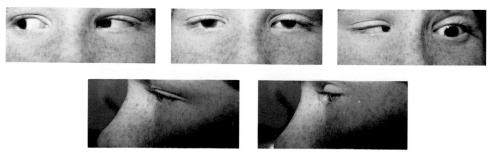

FIG XI-1—Duane syndrome with esotropia, left eye. Limitation of abduction. Retraction of globe in adduction becomes more obvious in side view.

Kraft SP. A surgical approach to Duane syndrome. *J Pediatr Ophthalmol Strabismus.* 1988;25:119–130.

Many Duane syndrome patients have some position of gaze in which the eyes are aligned, and they thus develop binocular vision. Amblyopia and refractive errors occur but less often than originally reported. Surgery is reserved primarily for those with deviated eyes in primary position or an abnormal head position and could be considered for those with marked globe retraction on adduction or a large upshoot or downshoot in adduction.

Duane syndrome with esotropia and deficient abduction is the most common form (50%–80% of series). Careful observation for globe retraction on adduction, particularly viewing from the side of the patient (Fig XI-1), will save the patient a neurologic work-up for a sixth nerve palsy. This retraction can be very hard to appreciate in an infant.

Parents often present complaining about the normal eye turning in, not realizing that the involved eye is not abducting. Recession of the medial rectus on the involved side has been most often used to correct the esotropia in primary position and eliminate the head turn. Abduction is not improved, but overcorrection is rare. Adding recession of the opposite medial rectus is recommended for deviations over 20Δ in primary position. Resection of the lateral rectus is not favored because of the likelihood that globe retraction will worsen. Transposition of the vertical rectus muscles with botulinum injection of the medial rectus has been used in cases of severe abduction deficit.

Duane syndrome with exotropia and deficient adduction (Fig XI-2) is the next most common type (2%–33%). The recommended surgery is comparable to that for esotropic Duane syndrome: recession of the lateral rectus on the involved side for small deviations and of both lateral recti for large deviations, with avoidance of resection of the medial rectus.

Duane syndrome patients with both poor abduction and poor adduction often have straight eyes in primary position. No surgery will improve the globe excursion. If the globe retraction is severe, it may be helped by recessing both the medial and lateral rectus muscles. For severe leash phenomenon that causes an upshoot in adduction, splitting the lateral rectus muscle in a Y configuration or performing a posterior fixation procedure on the lateral rectus muscle may be helpful (Fig XI-3).

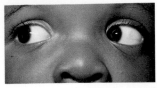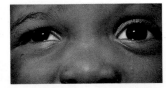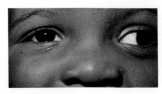

FIG XI-2—Duane syndrome with exotropia, right eye. Limitation of adduction.

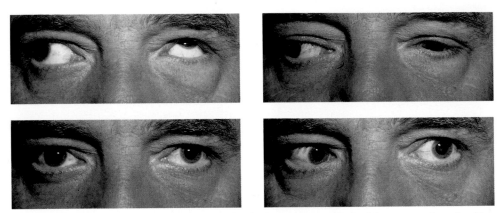

FIG XI-3—Duane syndrome, left eye, showing leash phenomenon with the left eye sometimes leashing up and other times leashing down in attempted adduction (*top left and right*). Also note primary position (*lower left*) and limitation of abduction in attempted left gaze (*lower right*).

Del Monte MA, Archer SM. Surgery to correct Duane syndrome and Brown syndrome. In: Tasman W, Jaeger EA, eds. *Duane's Clinical Ophthalmology*. Philadelphia: Lippincott; 1993; vol 6, chap 96, 1–20.

DeRespinis PA, Caputo AR, Wagner RS, et al. Duane's retraction syndrome. *Surv Ophthalmol.* 1993;38:257–288.

Molarte AB, Rosenbaum AL. Vertical rectus muscle transposition surgery for Duane's syndrome. *J Pediatr Ophthalmol Strabismus.* 1990;27:171–177.

Möbius Syndrome

Möbius syndrome is characterized by the association of both sixth and seventh nerve palsies, the latter causing masklike facies. These patients may also manifest gaze palsies that cannot be explained by a single cranial nerve involvement but can be attributed to abnormalities in the pontine paramedian reticular formation (see BCSC Section 5, *Neuro-Ophthalmology,* for discussion of the PPRF). Many patients also show limb, chest, and tongue defects, and some geneticists feel that Möbius syndrome is one of a family of syndromes in which hypoplastic limb anomalies are associated with orofacial and cranial nerve defects. Poland syndrome (absent pectoralis muscle) is seen in some patients with Möbius syndrome.

Motility disturbances reported in Möbius syndrome are frequently more complex than the limitation of abduction expected in sixth nerve palsy. Adduction may also be limited; at times adduction will be better with convergence than with versions, similar to a gaze paresis. Some patients appear to have palpebral fissure changes on adduction, and a few have vertical muscle involvement.

The patient may have an esotropia or straight eyes in primary position. If a significant deviation is present, medial rectus recession has been advocated, but in the presence of a significant limitation of adduction, a conservative approach is frequently indicated.

Third Nerve (Oculomotor) Palsy

Exodeviation may occur in third nerve palsy, whether congenital or acquired. The exotropia in this setting is generally associated with a hypotropia of the paretic eye, since the remaining unopposed muscles include the lateral rectus (abductor) and the superior oblique (depressor).

The causes of third nerve palsy in children include congenital (40%–50%), traumatic, inflammatory, and, infrequently, neoplastic lesions. It can also occur after viral infection and migraine. Because the visual system is still developing in children, amblyopia is commonly associated with third nerve palsy in pediatric patients, and it must be sought and treated aggressively. In addition, the clinical findings and treatment may be complicated in congenital and traumatic cases by aberrant regeneration (misdirection) of cranial nerve III. Anomalous eyelid, pupillary, and horizontal or vertical movements of the eye, such as eyelid elevation, pupil constriction, or depression of the globe on attempted adduction can result from aberrant regeneration (see BCSC Section 5, *Neuro-Ophthalmology*, for further discussion and extensive illustration).

In adults third nerve palsy may be caused by aneurysm, diabetes, neuritis, trauma, infection, or, rarely, tumor. Many patients with aneurysm are poor surgical candidates and therefore not referred for surgery. Diabetic third nerve palsy generally resolves spontaneously within 3–4 months. Therefore, the majority of adults referred for surgical treatment have third nerve palsy of traumatic origin.

Third nerve palsies present particular surgical therapeutic challenges, since multiple extraocular muscles as well as levator, iris, and ciliary muscle may be involved. Replacing the many lost vector forces on the globe with the remaining two active muscles is impossible; therefore, the goals of surgery must be thoroughly discussed with patients so that their expectations concerning treatment are realistic. Frequently, adequate alignment for binocular function in primary position and slight downgaze for reading may be all that can be expected. Before any surgical correction is planned, it is advisable to wait 6–12 months to observe for spontaneous recovery.

Although good motor alignment can be achieved in most patients, surgery should be undertaken cautiously in patients with complete palsy and good binocular visual function, since elevation of the eyelid and incomplete realignment without useful single binocular fields may produce incapacitating diplopia. Patients with at least partial recovery of their nerve function or incomplete paralysis are much better candidates for good functional as well as cosmetic results. Prism adaptation testing has shown that patients who can achieve single binocular vision with prisms

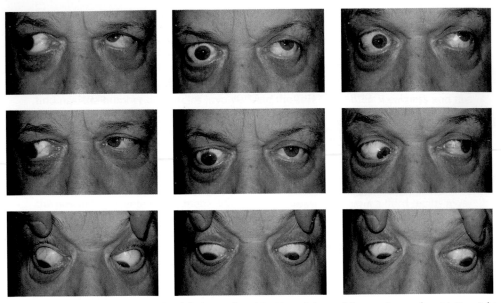

FIG XI-4—Graves disease (thyroid ophthalmopathy) OD. Note right eyelid retraction and restrictive right hypotropia with no elevation of the right eye above the midline.

It is usually preferable to postpone strabismus surgery until orbital decompression has been completed, as diplopia can occur after orbital decompression, particularly in patients with muscle restriction.

Eyelid surgery is usually deferred until after strabismus surgery because upper eyelid retraction may be quite improved when the patient does not have to strain as hard to elevate the eye. Additionally, large recessions of very tight inferior rectus muscles can cause lower eyelid retraction severe enough to need eyelid surgery later despite extensive dissection around the muscle. Some success at preventing lower eyelid retraction has been reported with separate treatment of the lower eyelid retractors at the time of the strabismus surgery.

Recession of the affected muscles is the primary surgical treatment. Strengthening procedures are performed rarely as worse restriction can be induced. Extraocular muscle surgery may eliminate diplopia in primary gaze but rarely restores normal motility because of the restrictive myopathy, the need to do very large recessions to allow the eye to be in primary position, and the replacement of muscle tissue by fibrous scar. Limited depression of the eyes after large inferior rectus recessions can prevent bifocal use by patients after surgery. Proptosis can become worse after muscle recessions.

Adjustable strabismus sutures may improve the alignment and rotations in these difficult cases. Since late overcorrection frequently occurs, especially with large inferior rectus recessions, slight undercorrection (fusion with a slight chin-up position) is desirable at the time of surgery or suture adjustment.

Chronic Progressive External Ophthalmoplegia (CPEO)

Chronic progressive external ophthalmoplegia (CPEO) usually begins in childhood with ptosis and slowly progresses to total paralysis of the eyelids and extraocular muscles. CPEO may be sporadic or familial. Although a true pigmentary dystrophy like retinitis pigmentosa is usually not present, constricted fields and electrodiagnostic abnormalities can occur. Defects in mitochondrial DNA have been found in some patients. The triad of retinal pigmentary changes, CPEO, and cardiomyopathy (especially heart block) is called *Kearns-Sayre syndrome.* BCSC Section 2, *Fundamentals and Principles of Ophthalmology,* discusses this in greater detail.

Myasthenia Gravis

Onset of myasthenia gravis may occur at any age, although it is uncommon in children. The disease may be purely ocular with ptosis and extraocular muscle weakness, or it may occur as part of a systemic disorder with other skeletal muscles involved as well. The strabismus that occurs is usually variable. BCSC Section 5, *Neuro-Ophthalmology,* discusses both the ocular and the systemic aspects of myasthenia gravis in depth.

Diagnosis involves several tests. Marked variability of motility measurements should suggest the presence of the disease. Affected muscles fatigue rapidly with the *muscle fatigue test,* which involves having the patient look up for 30 seconds and observing for worsening of ptosis. In the *sleep test* if the ptosis has resolved after 20–30 minutes with the eyelids closed in a dark room, a definite diagnosis of myasthenia gravis can be made. The presence of *Cogan's twitch,* an overshoot of the eyelid when the patient looks straight ahead after looking down for several minutes, is also diagnostic.

In a *Tensilon test* for an adult a test dose of 0.2 cc edrophonium chloride is injected intravenously. The patient's eyelids and eye movements are observed for improvement in function (Fig XI-5). If improvement occurs, no additional dosing is needed. If no adverse reaction or improvement occurs, 0.2 cc increments are injected IV up to 0.8 additional dose to avoid severe cholinergic reactions. Measurements of deviations can also be used. Atropine for IV administration is kept available as an antidote should an adverse reaction occur. A similar test using neostigmine (Prostigmin) administered intramuscularly following pretreatment with atropine has been described for use in children, since the neostigmine effect is prolonged, allowing more time for measurement. *Increased saccadic velocity* of affected muscles following the administration of edrophonium or neostigmine may be recorded.

Electromyography shows decreased electrical activity of involved muscles after prolonged voluntary innervation, and increased activity after the administration of Tensilon. Documentation of abnormalities in single-fiber electromyography or the presence of circulating anti–acetylcholine receptor antibodies is necessary in difficult cases.

Ocular myasthenia gravis is frequently resistant to the usual systemic myasthenia treatment. If and when ocular deviation has stabilized (i.e., the condition has become inactive), standard eye muscle surgery can be helpful in restoring binocular function in at least some gaze positions.

that overshoots the target, followed by a rotation of the head back in the opposite direction once fixation is established. The initial thrust serves to break fixation and may be associated with a blink that serves the same purpose. Vertical saccades and random eye movements are intact, but vestibular and optokinetic nystagmus are impaired. Reading can be difficult. Symptoms may improve over time.

The pathogenesis of this disorder is not known. It has been associated with premature birth, and developmental delay, especially motor milestones, may be present. Central nervous system abnormalities, including agenesis of the corpus callosum and hydrocephalus, have also been associated. Several case reports have identified mass lesions of the cerebellum that compressed the rostral part of the brain stem in infants presenting with ocular motor apraxia. Assessment of children with ocular motor apraxia by neuroimaging of the skull as well as with a complete systemic and developmental evaluation is therefore prudent.

Acquired ocular motor apraxia has been associated with bilateral lesions of the frontoparietal cortex. The differential diagnosis of acquired ocular motor apraxia subsumes conditions that affect the generation of voluntary saccades, including metabolic and degenerative diseases such as Huntington's chorea.

Cogan DG. Congenital ocular motor apraxia. *Can J Ophthalmol.* 1966;1:253–260.

Harris CM, Shawkat F, Russell-Eggitt I, et al. Intermittent horizontal saccade failure ('ocular motor apraxia') in children. *Br J Ophthalmol.* 1996;80:151–158.

CHAPTER XII

Childhood Nystagmus

The child who presents with nystagmus represents a difficult diagnostic challenge. The concern is to ensure that the nystagmus is not a sign of a significant neurologic abnormality, which would necessitate immediate intervention (Table XII-1). BCSC Section 5, *Neuro-Ophthalmology,* discusses the neurologic implications of nystagmus, and Section 4, *Ophthalmic Pathology and Intraocular Tumors,* covers some of the tumors mentioned in Table XII-1.

> Lavery MA, O'Neill JF, Chu FC, et al. Acquired nystagmus in early childhood: a presenting sign of intracranial tumor. *Ophthalmology.* 1984;91:425–435.

> Newman NM. Discussion of acquired nystagmus in early childhood: a presenting sign of intracranial tumor. *Ophthalmology.* 1984;91:435.

Many children with nystagmus have an ophthalmic etiology that can be elicited with simple examination techniques. Certain types of nystagmus do not necessitate further intervention, and these are usually readily identifiable.

TABLE XII-1

COMMON INTRACRANIAL TUMORS IN CHILDHOOD

TYPE	LOCATION
Glial tumors	
Astrocytoma	Cerebellum Brain stem Hypothalamus Optic nerve/chiasm
Ependymoma	Fourth ventricle
Neural tumors	
Medulloblastoma	Cerebellum
Neuroblastoma	
Congenital tumors	
Germinomas	
Craniopharyngioma	Suprasellar, chiasmal
Arachnoid cysts	

TABLE XII-4

CONDITIONS ASSOCIATED WITH DECREASED VISION AND
MINIMAL FUNDUS CHANGES

Leber congenital amaurosis

Rod monochromacy

Blue-cone monochromacy

Hereditary optic atrophy

Optic nerve hypoplasia

Ocular albinism

Congenital stationary night blindness

Childhood Nystagmus Types

Congenital Nystagmus

Congenital motor nystagmus (CN) This form is a binocular conjugate nystagmus that is usually uniplanar and horizontal, and it commonly remains horizontal on up- and downgaze. It can be pendular, jerk, circular, or elliptical, and more than one type may exist in the same individual. The characteristic waveform of congenital motor nystagmus is a slow phase with an exponential increase in velocity. CN is dampened by convergence and therefore often associated with an esotropia. A *null point,* or *neutral zone,* may be present where the intensity of oscillations is diminished and the visual acuity improves. If the null point is not in primary position, anomalous head postures may be assumed to dampen the nystagmus and provide the best visual acuity. Oscillopsia is usually not present.

Approximately two thirds of patients with congenital motor nystagmus with a jerk waveform exhibit a paradoxical inversion of the optokinetic nystagmus (OKN) response. Normally, if a patient with a right jerk nystagmus views an OKN drum rotating to the patient's left (eliciting a pursuit left, jerk right response), the patient will have an increased right jerk nystagmus. However, patients with congenital motor nystagmus exhibit either a damped right jerk nystagmus or possibly even a left jerk nystagmus. This paradoxical response of left jerk instead of right jerk nystagmus is seen only in CN.

Some cases of congenital motor nystagmus may be inherited as an autosomal dominant, recessive, or X-linked trait. Purely congenital nystagmus is not associated with other central nervous system abnormalities.

Sensory defect nystagmus This type of congenital nystagmus is secondary to an abnormality in the afferent visual pathway. Inadequate image formation results in failure of development of the normal fixation reflex. If visual loss is present at birth, the resulting nystagmus begins in the first 3 months of life. The severity of the nystagmus usually depends on the severity of the visual loss. All waveforms may be present, but pendular nystagmus occurs most frequently. On lateral gaze the nystagmus may become jerk. Searching, slow, wandering, or conjugate eye movements may also be observed.

Periodic alternating nystagmus   Periodic alternating nystagmus is an unusual form of congenital motor jerk nystagmus that periodically changes direction with a certain frequency that usually lasts between 60 and 120 seconds. Typically, the patient starts with a jerk nystagmus in one direction that lasts for 60–90 seconds and then slowly begins to dampen. A period of no nystagmus lasts anywhere from 10 to 20 seconds, and then the nystagmus begins to jerk in the opposite direction. The nystagmus continues to jerk in the opposite direction for 60–90 seconds, and then the process repeats itself. Some children adopt an alternative head position to take advantage of the changing null position. The etiology of congenital periodic alternating nystagmus is unknown, but it has been associated with oculocutaneous albinism.

Latent nystagmus   Latent nystagmus is a congenital conjugate horizontal jerk nystagmus that occurs under conditions of monocular fixation. When one eye is occluded, a jerk nystagmus develops in both eyes with the fast phase directed toward the uncovered eye. Thus, a left jerk nystagmus of both eyes occurs when the right eye is covered. When the left eye is covered, there is a right jerk nystagmus of both eyes. This nystagmus is the only form that reverses with a change in fixation. Asymmetries in amplitude, frequency, and velocity of the nystagmus can also be noted, depending on which eye is covered.

Latent nystagmus is often noted in early childhood, especially in patients with congenital esotropia and dissociated vertical deviation. The etiology is unknown. Because a nystagmus is induced when an eye is covered, binocular visual acuity is better than monocular, and occlusion must be avoided when testing the vision monocularly. Use of polarizing lenses and polarized chart, blurring of the nontested eye with a +5.00 D sphere, or repositioning of the occluder several inches in front of the eye not being tested are methods that can be effective.

A latent nystagmus may become manifest *(manifest latent nystagmus)* when both eyes are open but only one eye is being used for vision (i.e., the other eye is suppressed or amblyopic). Just as with latent nystagmus, occlusion of the preferred eye will result in a change in the direction of the jerk nystagmus. Electronystagmographic evaluation of latent and manifest latent nystagmus reveals a similar waveform with an exponential decrease in velocity of the slow phase. This pattern is the opposite of congenital motor nystagmus, which shows an exponential increase in velocity of the slow phase (Fig XII-1). Latent nystagmus may be superimposed on congenital motor nystagmus.

Dell'Osso LF, Schmidt D, Daroff RB: Latent, manifest latent, and congenital nystagmus. *Arch Ophthalmol.* 1979;97:1877–1885.

Acquired Nystagmus

Spasmus nutans   Spasmus nutans is an acquired nystagmus that occurs in children from ages 3 to 15 months. It is usually associated with a triad of findings including nystagmus, head nodding, and torticollis. The nystagmus is generally bilateral; however, it can be asymmetric, monocular, and variable in different gaze positions. It is a small-amplitude, high-frequency nystagmus (shimmering) and often difficult to see. It can be horizontal, vertical, or rotary and is occasionally intermittent. In most cases spasmus nutans is a benign disorder, but a nystagmus form very characteristic of spasmus nutans has been associated with chiasmal or suprachiasmal tumors in children who have also had other central nervous system findings. When doubt persists

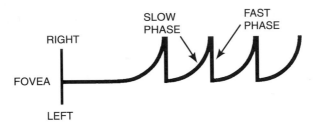

Congenital Motor Nystagmus

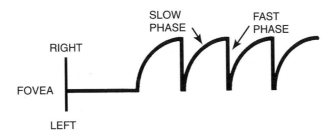

Manifest Latent Nystagmus

FIG XII-1—Left jerk nystagmus. *Top,* Electronystagmographic evaluation of congenital motor nystagmus shows exponential increase in velocity of the slow phase. *Bottom,* Manifest latent nystagmus shows a waveform with an exponential decrease in velocity of the slow phase.

about the etiology of presumed spasmus nutans, neuroradiologic investigation should be employed. Spasmus nutans can occasionally be familial and has been present in monozygotic twins. It usually disappears by age 3–4 years.

Arnoldi KA, Tychsen L. Prevalence of intracranial lesions in children initially diagnosed with disconjugate nystagmus (spasmus nutans). *J Pediatr Ophthalmol Strabismus.* 1995;32:296–301.

Garty BZ, Weitz R, Mimouni M, et al. Spasmus nutans as a presenting sign of diencephalic syndrome. Correspondence. *J Pediatr.* 1985;107:484.

Koenig SB, Naidich TP, Zaparackas Z. Optic glioma masquerading as spasmus nutans. *J Pediatr Ophthalmol Strabismus.* 1982;19:20–24.

Norton EWD, Cogan DG. Spasmus nutans: a clinical study of twenty cases followed two years or more since onset. *Arch Ophthalmol.* 1954;52:442–446.

See-saw nystagmus An unusual but quite dramatic type of nystagmus, see-saw nystagmus has both vertical and torsional components. The name comes from the action of the playground device. If the eyes were placed on a seesaw, one at either end, they would "roll down the plank" as the seesaw rose, with the high eye intorting and the low eye extorting. As the direction of the seesaw changed, so would the eye movement. Thus the eyes make alternating movements of elevation and intorsion followed by depression and extorsion.

This type of nystagmus is often associated with a lesion in the rostral midbrain or the suprasellar area. In children the most likely intracranial tumor is a craniopharyngioma. Confrontation visual fields may elicit a bitemporal visual field defect. Neuroradiologic evaluation is necessary. The treatment for see-saw nystagmus is to remove the inciting etiology.

Daroff RB. See saw nystagmus. *Neurology.* 1963;13:306–311.

Nystagmus retractorius (dorsal midbrain syndrome) *Convergence-retraction nystagmus* is a part of a dorsal midbrain syndrome associated with paralysis of upward gaze, defective convergence, and light–near dissociation. Unlike other types of childhood nystagmus, this form may be noticed only under particular circumstances. It is best elicited on attempted fast upgaze, when co-contraction of all the horizontal extraocular muscles occurs and the eyes are pulled into the orbit (hence the term *retractorius*). The eyes will often converge as well on attempted upgaze. Voluntary convergence, however, is minimal. There is an associated pupillary abnormality with marked light–near dissociation. In the pediatric age group convergence-retraction nystagmus is most commonly secondary to congenital aqueductal stenosis or a pinealoma.

Opsoclonus Opsoclonus is an extremely rare eye movement disorder that is not a true nystagmus but a bizarre ocular oscillation. It is rapid, involuntary, and multivectorial. It can be present intermittently and often has a very high frequency, low-amplitude movement. The movements are so fast and chaotic that they are not easily confused with other forms of infantile nystagmus. Probably the most common cause of opsoclonus is an acute cerebellar ataxia of childhood. The child presents with "dancing eyes and dancing feet." Opsoclonus can be a sign of occult neuroblastoma, a consequence of epidemic encephalitis of viral origin, or associated with hydrocephalus.

Vertical nystagmus (upbeat, downbeat) Vertical nystagmus is usually a jerk nystagmus with a fast phase either up or down. Children most commonly have a downbeat nystagmus that is associated with an Arnold-Chiari malformation or spinal cerebellar degeneration.

Schulman JA, Shults WT, Jones JM Jr. Monocular vertical nystagmus as an initial sign of chiasmal glioma. *Am J Ophthalmol.* 1979;87:87–90.

Monocular nystagmus Monocular nystagmus has been reported to occur in severely amblyopic and blind eyes. The oscillations are pendular, chiefly vertical, slow, small in amplitude, and irregular in frequency. Monocular nystagmus is often difficult to detect, and it may be rare in infants and small children.

Farmer J, Hoyt CS. Monocular nystagmus in infancy and early childhood. *Am J Ophthalmol.* 1984;98:504–509.

Yee RD, Jelks GW, Baloh RW, et al. Uniocular nystagmus in monocular visual loss. *Ophthalmology.* 1979;86:511–522.

Dissociated nystagmus   Dissociated nystagmus, referring to nystagmus in the abducting eye, occurs in several instances. The nystagmus seen with internuclear ophthalmoplegia is most common. Surgical weakening of the medial rectus muscle has also been reported to cause a nystagmus of the contralateral abducting eye similar to that seen with internuclear ophthalmoplegia. With INO, however, a slowing of saccades in the adducting eye also occurs that is not seen with pseudo–internuclear ophthalmoplegia after surgical paresis of the medial rectus muscle. Myasthenia gravis may also simulate an internuclear ophthalmoplegia with nystagmus of the abducting eye.

Cogan DG. Dissociated nystagmus with lesions in the posterior fossa. *Arch Ophthalmol.* 1963;70:361–368.

von Noorden GK, Tredici TD, Ruttum M. Pseudo–internuclear ophthalmoplegia after surgical paresis of the medial rectus muscle. *Am J Ophthalmol.* 1984;98:602–608.

Differential Diagnosis

The flowchart in Figure XII-2 lists the signs and symptoms of various forms of horizontal nystagmus in children along with guidelines for testing and systemic associations.

Treatment

Providing the patient with the best acuity achieved with the least effort may require treatment of associated problems. Although refraction can be difficult when nystagmus is present, significant refractive errors should be corrected. Therapy for amblyopia should be prescribed if needed. If latent nystagmus is present, patching may still be an option, but optical degradation may have to be substituted (see chapter IV, Amblyopia).

A trial of prisms may be advisable prior to considering surgery for a face turn. Fresnel prisms may be successful in eliminating a face turn. Each prism is mounted with the base opposite to the direction of the null zone. For example, with a left face turn and a null zone in dextroversion, prism before the right eye would be oriented base in, and prism before the left eye would be oriented base out.

Base-out prism spectacles have been prescribed to stimulate fusional convergence and dampen the nystagmus. If a face turn remains after a Kestenbaum-Anderson procedure performed for congenital nystagmus, spectacles with prisms oriented with the bases opposite to the side of the null zone may be given in order to abolish the torticollis often seen with nystagmus (the Kestenbaum-Anderson procedure is described below). Prisms have also been used to reestablish fusion when a heterotropia has occurred postoperatively.

Surgery

Surgery for nystagmus is indicated to correct a head turn or improve visual function. By shifting the null point to primary position, surgery can obtain the best vision without the need for a head turn. Both horizontal face turns and the less common vertical torticollis may be ameliorated by the appropriate procedure. Surgery has been reported to decrease nystagmus intensity, broaden the null zone, and, in some cases, improve visual acuity.

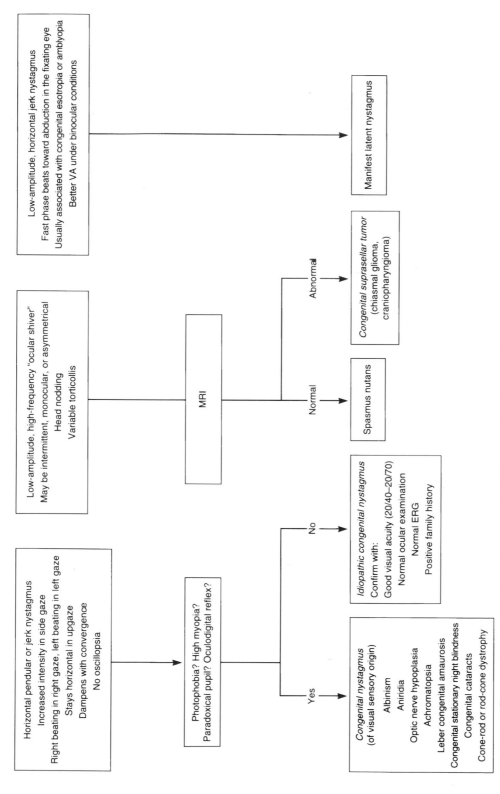

FIG XII-2—Differential diagnosis of horizontal nystagmus in children. (Modified from Brodsky MC, Baker RS, Hamed LM. *Pediatric Neuro-Ophthalmology.* New York: Springer-Verlag; 1995:339.)

Dell'Osso LF, Flynn JT. Congenital nystagmus surgery: a quantitative evaluation of the effects. *Arch Ophthalmol.* 1979;97:462–469.

Flynn JT, Dell'Osso LF. The effects of congenital nystagmus surgery. *Ophthalmology.* 1979;86:1414–1425.

Kestenbaum A. Nouvelle opération du nystagmus. *Bull Soc Ophtalmol Fr.* 1953; 6:599–602.

Surgery for congenital nystagmus usually involves a recess-resect procedure, often performed on both eyes. This surgery may be referred to as a *Kestenbaum* or *Kestenbaum-Anderson procedure.* The eyes are surgically rotated in the direction of the head turn, that is, away from the null zone, or preferred position of gaze. If surgery is to be performed on four rectus muscles, *recession* of the yoked rectus muscles on the side *opposite* the head turn is accompanied by *resection* of the yoked rectus muscles on the side *ipsilateral* to the head turn. For example, if a patient with congenital nystagmus has a left face turn and a null zone in dextroversion, the eyes are surgically rotated to the left by recession of the right lateral and left medial rectus muscles and resection of the right medial and left lateral rectus muscles.

The Kestenbaum procedure has been modified in an attempt to achieve better long-term results, quantitate the surgery to the amount of head turn present, and assist in preoperative planning when a strabismus coexists. Table XII-5 shows the original Kestenbaum procedure for horizontal rectus muscle surgery to both eyes with two different modifications. Each eye receives a recess-resect procedure to move the eyes in the appropriate direction. Note that the total numbers of millimeters of surgery for the two eyes are equal in order to rotate each globe an equal amount. The two modifications in Table XII-5 are based on the amount of surgery proposed by Parks. Each of the modifications recommends greater amounts of surgery by increasing Parks's original figures by 40% or 60%. Measurements are rounded off to the nearest 0.5 mm at surgery. For head turns of 30° the 40% augmented procedure is recommended; the 60% augmentation procedure is used with face turns of 45°. The augmented procedures may cause restriction of motility.

Calhoun JH, Harley RD. Surgery for abnormal head position in congenital nystagmus. *Trans Am Ophthalmol Soc.* 1973;71:70—83.

TABLE XII-5

KESTENBAUM PROCEDURE AND MODIFICATIONS

PROCEDURE	KESTENBAUM	40% AUGMENTED	60% AUGMENTED
Recess medial rectus	5.0 mm	7.0 mm	8.0 mm
Resect medial rectus	6.0 mm	8.4 mm	9.6 mm
Recess lateral rectus	7.0 mm	9.8 mm	11.2 mm
Resect lateral rectus	8.0 mm	11.2 mm	12.8 mm
Total Surgery	13.0 mm	18.2 mm	20.8 mm
R + R	(5+8) = (6+7)	(7+11.2) = (8.4+9.8)	(8+12.8) = (9.6+11.2)

Nelson LB, Ervin-Mulvey LD, Calhoun JH, et al. Surgical management for abnormal head position in nystagmus: The augmented modified Kestenbaum procedure. *Br J Ophthalmol.* 1984;68:796–800.

Roberts EL, Saunders RA, Wilson ME. Surgery for vertical head position in null point nystagmus. *J Pediatr Ophthalmol Strabismus.* 1996;33:219–224.

Zubcov AA, Stark N, Weber A, et al. Improvement of visual acuity after surgery for nystagmus. *Ophthalmology.* 1993;100:1488–1497.

If vertical torticollis is present with congenital nystagmus, the chin-up or -down posturing may be ameliorated by surgery on the vertical rectus muscles. The eyes are rotated away from the null point. When operating on the vertical rectus muscles, the possibility of creating cyclovertical deviations must be taken into consideration.

Surgery is also modified if strabismus is associated with congenital nystagmus. The dominant eye used for fixation is moved according to the prescribed amount of surgery. Then the amount of surgery performed on the nondominant eye is adjusted to correct the heterotropia. Alternatively, surgery on the nondominant eye may be performed secondarily, so that the effects of the Kestenbaum procedure on the heterotropia can be evaluated. An alternative to the standard Kestenbaum procedure is to recess all the horizontal rectus muscles posterior to the equator. This process usually requires a recession of both medial rectus muscles of 8–10 mm and both lateral rectus muscles of 10–12 mm. This approach may be beneficial in improving visual function even in cases where head position is not a problem.

Surgery for nystagmus blockage syndrome often involves recession of the medial rectus muscles, sometimes combined with a posterior fixation suture.

Helveston EM, Ellis FD, Plager DA. Large recession of the horizontal recti for the treatment of nystagmus. *Ophthalmology.* 1991;98:1302–1305.

Shuckett EP, Hiles DA, Biglan AW, et al. Posterior fixation suture operation (fadenoperation). *Ophthalmic Surg.* 1981;12:578–585.

von Noorden GK. Indications of the posterior fixation operation in strabismus. *Ophthalmology.* 1978;85:512–520.

von Noorden GK, Springer DT. Large rectus muscle recessions for the treatment of congenital nystagmus. *Arch Ophthalmol.* 1991;109:221–224.

CHAPTER XIII

Surgery of the Extraocular Muscles

Both the experienced and the beginning strabismus surgeon will benefit by becoming familiar with the basic references and surgical atlases listed below. While specific references to these texts are not made in the following discussion, the reader should refer to them when additional information is needed. See also chapters I and II of this volume.

Calhoun JH, Nelson LB, Harley RD. *Atlas of Pediatric Ophthalmic Surgery.* Philadelphia: Saunders; 1987.

Del Monte MA, Archer SM. *Atlas of Pediatric Ophthalmology and Strabismus Surgery.* New York: Churchill Livingstone; 1993.

Helveston EM. *Atlas of Strabismus Surgery.* 4th ed. St Louis: Mosby; 1993.

von Noorden GK. *Burian–von Noorden's Binocular Vision and Ocular Motility: Theory and Management of Strabismus.* 5th ed. St Louis: Mosby; 1996.

Wright KW. *Color Atlas of Ophthalmic Surgery: Strabismus.* Philadelphia: Lippincott; 1992.

A thorough knowledge of the anatomy of the extraocular muscles and surrounding fascia, along with an understanding of their motor physiology, is essential to planning and executing strabismus surgery. Lifelong problems for the patient can be avoided by the use of appropriate surgical technique guided by knowledge of the anatomy of the extraocular muscles and surrounding fascia. The references mentioned above are excellent resources for this understanding.

Similarly, the surgeon should become familiar with the appropriate types of surgical instruments, sutures, and needles for strabismus surgery. The surgeon must also be knowledgeable about operating room procedures in order to perform the surgery in an efficacious and controlled manner. The classic references listed below address these issues in greater detail.

Helveston EM. Sutures and needles for strabismus surgery. *Int Ophthalmol Clin.* 1976;16:39–45.

Parks MM. The role of the fascia in muscle surgery. *Int Ophthalmol Clin.* 1976; 16:17–37.

White RH Jr, Parks MM. Polyglycolic acid sutures in ophthalmic surgery. *Trans Am Acad Ophthalmol Otolaryngol.* 1974;78:632–636.

The history and a detailed motility evaluation (often repeated at a subsequent visit to corroborate the initial findings) in conjunction with a complete ocular examination will provide the surgeon the information necessary to plan the correct surgery. This evaluation may include sensory testing, forced duction testing, active force generation testing, saccadic velocities, and diplopia visual fields. Preoperative planning must address the patient's and/or family's expectations for the outcome as well as those of the surgeon, and risks and complications must be discussed. Such communication is the basis for informed patient consent.

Indications for Surgery

Surgery is performed to improve function or to improve the patient's appearance and well-being. The indications for surgery may be subtle or more obvious. *Asthenopia,* a vague but real sense of ocular fatigue, is frequently found in patients with phorias or intermittent tropias. Occasionally, there may be subconjunctival scar tissue from prior muscle surgery that may warrant additional surgical revision to improve appearance or to relieve mechanical restriction.

Double vision in one or all fields of gaze is often the complaint of patients with adult-onset strabismus, and eliminating diplopia is one of the goals of strabismus surgery. If some degree of fusion can be achieved, it will help the patient maintain ocular alignment postsurgically. Alignment of the visual axes can restore stereopsis in some patients or produce a certain amount of stereopsis in others, especially if the preoperative deviation is intermittent or of recent onset.

An abnormal head position is assumed by some patients to relieve diplopia (e.g., with superior oblique or lateral rectus muscle weakness) or to improve vision (e.g., with nystagmus and an eccentric null point). Surgical treatment may not only increase the field of useful vision but also reduce the habitual head posturing. Correcting an abnormal head position or eliminating an ocular deviation can, in turn, improve the patient's self-image and sense of well-being. Society does not consider strabismus to be a variation of normal and, therefore, correcting it should be considered reconstructive rather than cosmetic surgery, even if a fusional result is not feasible.

Surgical Techniques for the Muscles and Tendons

Weakening Procedures

Table XIII-1 defines the various weakening procedures and describes when each would be used. Combinations of techniques are also listed.

Del Monte MA, Parks MM. Denervation and extirpation of the inferior oblique. An improved weakening procedure for marked overaction. *Ophthalmology.* 1983; 90:1178–1185.

Guyton DL. The posterior fixation procedure: mechanism and indications. *Int Ophthalmol Clin.* 1985;25:79–88.

Hardesty HH. Superior oblique tenotomy. *Arch Ophthalmol.* 1972;88:181–184.

Helveston EM. Indications for marginal myotomy and technique. *Am J Ophthalmol.* 1970;70:574–578.

Parks MM. The weakening surgical procedures for eliminating overaction of the inferior oblique muscle. *Am J Ophthalmol.* 1972;73:107–122.

Wright KW. Superior oblique silicone expander for Brown syndrome and superior oblique overaction. *J Pediatr Ophthalmol Strabismus.* 1991;28:101–107.

TABLE XIII-1

WEAKENING PROCEDURES USED IN STRABISMUS SURGERY

PROCEDURE	USED FOR
Myotomy: cutting across a muscle *Myectomy:* removing a portion of muscle	Used by some surgeons to weaken the inferior oblique muscles
Marginal myotomy: cutting partway across a muscle, usually following a maximal recession	To weaken a rectus muscle further
Tenotomy: cutting across a tendon *Tenectomy:* removing a portion of tendon	Both used routinely to weaken the superior oblique muscle; recently, silicone spacers have been interposed by some surgeons to control the weakening effect
Recession: removal and reattachment of a muscle (rectus or oblique) so that its insertion is closer to its origin	The standard weakening procedure for rectus muscles
Denervation and extirpation: the ablation of the entire portion of the muscle, along with its nerve supply, within Tenon's capsule	Used only on severely or recurrently overacting inferior oblique muscles
Recession and anteriorization: Movement of the muscle's insertion anterior to its original position	Also used only on the inferior oblique muscle, to change its action from elevation to depression; particularly useful when an inferior oblique muscle overaction and dissociated vertical deviation (DVD) both exist
Posterior fixation suture (fadenoperation): Attachment of a rectus muscle to the sclera 11–18 mm posterior to the insertion using a nonabsorbable suture; this procedure is difficult to perform	Used to weaken a muscle in its field of action by decreasing its mechanical advantage; often used in conjunction with recession; sometimes used in DVD, nystagmus, high AC/A esotropia, and noncomitant strabismus

Strengthening Procedures

To strengthen or enhance the effect of a muscle or tendon, surgeons most frequently use the *resection technique:*

▫ Absorbable sutures are placed at a predetermined distance posterior to the muscle insertion

▫ The muscle anterior to the position of the sutures is excised (resected)

▫ The shortened muscle is reattached to the globe at or near the original insertion

This technique is commonly used on any of the rectus muscles and rarely used to strengthen either of the oblique muscles. For detailed descriptions of the techniques, see the basic references listed on p 136.

A muscle's function can also be augmented by *advancing the insertion* nearer the limbus. The technique is commonly used for rectus muscles if the muscle has been previously recessed. Advancement of a muscle to a position anterior to its original anatomical insertion is rarely performed, because the muscle may become visible under the conjunctiva. The anterior half of the superior oblique tendon may be advanced temporally and toward the limbus, as described by Harada and Ito, to reduce excycloduction in patients with superior oblique muscle paresis.

The *tucking procedure* can be performed on the superior oblique tendon to enhance its effect, especially for superior oblique muscle paresis. However, tucking the superior oblique tendon may produce an iatrogenic Brown syndrome. For step-by-step techniques, see the basic references listed on p 136.

Harada M, Ito Y. Surgical correction of cyclotropia. *Jpn J Ophthalmol.* 1964;8:88–96.

Helveston EM. Surgery of the superior oblique muscle. In: Helveston EM. *Symposium on Strabismus.* St Louis: Mosby; 1978:150–153.

Adjustable Suture Techniques

Adjustable strabismus sutures have been used for many years in one form or another to improve the outcome of strabismus surgery. The purpose of adjustable strabismus sutures is to increase the likelihood of reaching the desired surgical alignment with one operation, thereby decreasing the need for staged operations and reoperations. Adjustable suture techniques do not solve the problem of long-term alignment (or permanence of the surgical results), which depends on fusional potentials, focused symmetrical retinal images, and tonic and innervational forces acting on the extraocular muscles.

Improved synthetic suture materials, refined surgical techniques, and the continued unpredictability of strabismus surgery have all stimulated increased use of adjustable suture techniques. Various types of adjustable suture techniques have been described; some are included below.

Postoperative adjustable (two-stage) techniques   The strabismus surgery is completed in the operating room using externalized sutures and knots so that the position of the muscle can be altered during the postoperative period as needed to obtain alignment.

Nelson LB, Wagner RS, Calhoun JH. The adjustable suture technique in strabismus surgery. *Int Ophthalmol Clin.* 1985;25:89–105.

Wright KW. Adjustable suture technique. In: Wright KW. *Color Atlas of Ophthalmic Surgery: Strabismus.* Philadelphia: Lippincott; 1992:87–124.

Operation/reoperation techniques The strabismus surgery is completed using only short-acting or reversible anesthetic agents and externalized sutures and knots. The patient is examined a short time after surgery and reanesthetized for the final tying or adjustment of the sutures as indicated by the postoperative evaluation. This method has been used successfully in children, but since a second general anesthesia is required, it offers little advantage over standard nonadjustable surgery with possible reoperation.

Topical anesthesia techniques The strabismus surgery is completed with the patient awake. Drugs that might affect ocular motility are avoided, and the patient's dynamic ocular motility and ocular alignment are observed and adjusted at the time of surgery. This technique requires a cooperative patient and is not appropriate for most patients who have significant scarring and need a reoperation, individuals with thyroid ophthalmopathy, and almost all children. (Anesthesia is discussed on p 147.)

Thorson JC, Jampolsky A, Scott AB. Topical anesthesia for strabismus surgery. *Trans Am Acad Ophthalmol Otolaryngol.* 1966;70:968–972.

Pull-over (stay) sutures A temporary suture is attached to the limbus and secured to periocular skin to fix the eye in a selected position during postoperative healing. This technique is particularly useful in cases with severely restricted rotations.

Transposition Procedures

Transposition procedures involve moving the extraocular muscles out of their original planes of action. They are generally reserved for treatment of paralytic strabismus, small vertical and horizontal deviations, and A and V patterns. The usual situations in which transposition procedures are used include paralysis of cranial nerves III and VI as well as monocular elevation deficiency. See the basic references on p 136 for detailed descriptions of these techniques.

Harley RD. Complete tendon transplantation for ocular muscle paralysis. *Ann Ophthalmol.* 1971;3:459–463.

Helveston EM. Muscle transposition procedures. *Surv Ophthalmol.* 1971;16:92–97.

Jensen CD. Rectus muscle union: A new operation for paralysis of the rectus muscles. *Trans Pac Coast Otoophthalmol Soc.* 1964;45:359–384.

Considerations in Planning Surgery for Strabismus

Incomitance

Deviations that vary according to positions of gaze require special variations in technique to make the postoperative alignment more nearly comitant.

Vertical incomitance If a horizontal deviation in the primary position is significantly different in upgaze and downgaze, an A or a V pattern is present (see chapter X). Surgical treatment may include surgery on the oblique muscles or offsetting up or down of the horizontal rectus muscles.

Horizontal incomitance   If the deviation in left and right gaze is significantly different from the deviation in primary gaze, a paresis or restriction may be present. If the restriction is stable, surgical correction as illustrated in the following example might be considered:

XT = 20Δ	XT = 30Δ	XT = 40Δ
right gaze	primary position	left gaze

The surgeon might do one of the following:

☐ Perform a recession of each lateral rectus muscle, the left more than the right, to achieve greater reduction of the exotropia in the field of action of the left lateral rectus, i.e., left gaze.

☐ Perform a greater recession of the left lateral rectus muscle and lesser resection of the left medial rectus muscle than the standard amount in order to achieve greater effect in left gaze.

Lateral incomitance   Standard amounts of surgery for intermittent exotropia may result in overcorrection if measurements in side gaze are substantially less than in primary position, for example:

XT = 15Δ	XT = 30Δ	XT = 15Δ
right gaze	primary position	left gaze

Some surgeons recommend reducing the amount of recession of each lateral rectus slightly in these patients.

> Moore S. The prognostic value of lateral gaze measurements in intermittent exotropia. *Am Orthopt J.* 1969;19:69–71.

Prior Surgery

It is technically easier and therefore preferable to operate on muscles that have not had prior surgery. However, each case must be considered individually. In cases of mechanical restriction from excessive resection/scarring or weakness from excessive recession, these problems must be relieved by reoperation on the involved muscle to obtain optimal surgical results. Previous operative reports may be helpful in surgical planning. If retinal detachment surgery has been performed in the past, consultation with the retinal surgeon is advisable.

Cyclovertical Strabismus

In many patients with vertical strabismus the vertical deviation is different in right and left gaze. In some patients the vertical deviation is different between upgaze to one side and downgaze to that side. In general, surgery should be performed on those muscles whose field of action is in the same field as the greatest vertical deviation. For example, in a patient with a right hypertropia that is greatest down and to the patient's left, the surgeon should strongly consider either strengthening the right superior oblique muscle or weakening the left inferior rectus muscle. If the right hypertropia is the same in left upgaze, straight left, and left downgaze, then any of the four muscles whose greatest vertical action is in left gaze may be chosen for surgery. In this example the left superior rectus muscle or right superior oblique muscle could be strengthened, or the left inferior rectus muscle or right inferior oblique muscle could be weakened.

Visual Acuity

Surgery is normally delayed until the vision has been made equal or nearly so by whatever means are appropriate, including spectacles and amblyopia therapy.

Guidelines for Strabismus Surgery

These guidelines should be considered general approximations only. It is essential to recognize that each individual case must be evaluated from all standpoints. Among the factors to be considered are

- Amblyopia
- Restriction
- A or V patterns
- Incomitance
- Previous surgery
- Unequal distance and near deviations
- Predictability of postoperative diplopia

The surgical decision is therefore based on many clinical findings, not just on measurement of the primary position deviation.

Two surgeons are unlikely to perform a specific surgical procedure in exactly the same fashion. Thus, the amount of dissection, the suturing technique and placement in the muscle and sclera, the number of sutures used, and the nature of the incision will vary slightly between surgeons, even when both are following the same surgical table. Nonetheless, these guidelines are useful as a starting point for routine strabismus surgery when performed by the beginning surgeon.

Each surgeon must standardize his or her own approach by continually reviewing the results and adjusting the amount of surgery to achieve the best possible outcomes. Thus, the surgery should be planned based on the surgeon's own ocular motility measurements and judgment.

Esodeviation

Symmetrical surgery   In addition to the guidelines listed in Table XIII-2, some surgeons would also advocate medial rectus muscle recessions of 6.5–7.0 mm for 60–80Δ of esotropia, while other surgeons avoid these very large recessions and favor operating three or four muscles initially.

Monocular recess-resect procedures   The same figures given in Table XIII-2 may be used, selecting the appropriate number of millimeters for each muscle as shown in Table XIII-3. For example, for an esotropia of 30Δ the surgeon would recess the medial rectus muscle 4.5 mm and resect the lateral rectus muscle 7.0 mm.

Exodeviation

Symmetrical surgery   The guidelines for exodeviation listed in Table XIII-4 are designed to give an initial overcorrection. Some surgeons advocate bilateral rectus muscle recessions of 9.0 mm or greater for deviations larger than 45Δ.

TABLE XIII-2

SYMMETRICAL SURGERY FOR ESODEVIATION

ANGLE OF ESOTROPIA	RECESS MR OU	OR	RESECT LR OU
15Δ	3.0 mm		4.0 mm
20Δ	3.5 mm		5.0 mm
25Δ	4.0 mm		6.0 mm
30Δ	4.5 mm		7.0 mm
35Δ	5.0 mm		8.0 mm
40Δ	5.5 mm		9.0 mm
50Δ	6.0 mm		9.0 mm

TABLE XIII-3

MONOCULAR RECESS-RESECT PROCEDURES FOR ESODEVIATION

ANGLE OF ESOTROPIA	RECESS MR	AND	RESECT LR
15Δ	3.0 mm		4.0 mm
20Δ	3.5 mm		5.0 mm
25Δ	4.0 mm		6.0 mm
30Δ	4.5 mm		7.0 mm
35Δ	5.0 mm		8.0 mm
40Δ	5.5 mm		9.0 mm
50Δ	6.0 mm		9.0 mm

TABLE XIII-4

SYMMETRICAL SURGERY FOR EXODEVIATION

ANGLE OF EXOTROPIA	RECESS LR OU	OR	RESECT MR OU
15Δ	4.0 mm		3.0 mm
20Δ	5.0 mm		4.0 mm
25Δ	6.0 mm		5.0 mm
30Δ	7.0 mm		6.0 mm
40Δ	8.0 mm		6.0 mm

TABLE XIII-5

MONOCULAR RECESS-RESECT PROCEDURES FOR EXODEVIATION

ANGLE OF EXOTROPIA	RECESS LR	AND	RESECT MR
15Δ	4.0 mm		3.0 mm
20Δ	5.0 mm		4.0 mm
25Δ	6.0 mm		5.0 mm
30Δ	7.0 mm		6.0 mm
40Δ	8.0 mm		6.0 mm
50Δ	9.0 mm		7.0 mm
60Δ	10.0 mm		8.0 mm
70Δ	10.0 mm		9.0 mm
80Δ	10.0 mm		10.0 mm

Monocular recess-resect procedures As with esodeviations, the surgical table can be used for monocular procedures as well as for symmetrical surgery, reading across according to the angle of deviation (Table XIII-5). For example, for an exodeviation of 15Δ the surgeon would recess the lateral rectus muscle 4.0 mm and resect the antagonist medial rectus muscle 3.0 mm. Monocular surgery of large-angle exotropia is likely to result in a limitation of abduction postoperatively.

Value of Immediate Overcorrection in Exodeviation

The surgical dosages listed in Table XIII-4 for bilateral lateral rectus recessions tend to produce a small overcorrection of exotropia in the early postoperative period. Available evidence suggests a small, temporary esotropia during the first few days or weeks after surgery may yield the most favorable long-term result. Many patients will have diplopia during the time they are esotropic, and they should be advised of this possibility.

> Raab EL, Parks MM. Recession of the lateral recti. Early and late postoperative alignment. *Arch Ophthalmol.* 1969;82:203–208.

> Scott WE, Keech R, Mash AJ. The postoperative results and stability of exodeviations. *Arch Ophthalmol.* 1981;99:1814–1818.

Oblique Muscle–Weakening Procedures

Weakening the inferior oblique muscle In cases that show a marked asymmetry of the overactions of the inferior oblique muscles with no superior oblique muscle paresis, unilateral surgery on the muscle with the most marked overaction will often be followed by a significant degree of overaction in the unoperated eye. Therefore, bilateral inferior oblique–weakening procedures, which can be graded if recessions are performed, are indicated for bilateral overaction, even if asymmetrical. A good symmetrical result is the rule, and overcorrections are rare. Inferior oblique muscles that are not overacting should not have a surgical weakening procedure.

Secondary overaction of the inferior oblique muscle occurs in some patients who have superior oblique muscle paresis. In this situation the greatest vertical deviation appears in the field of action of the ipsilateral inferior oblique muscle. A weakening of that inferior oblique muscle could be expected to correct up to 15Δ of vertical deviation in primary position. The amount of vertical correction is roughly proportional to the degree of preoperative overaction (see chapter IX).

Weakening each inferior oblique muscle has little to no effect on horizontal alignment in primary position. Frequently, a weakening procedure is performed on each inferior oblique muscle for V-pattern strabismus. That surgery can be expected to cause 15Δ or more of eso shift in upgaze (decrease of an exodeviation or increase of an esodeviation), but it has almost no effect in primary position or downgaze.

Stager DR, Parks MM. Inferior oblique weakening procedures. Effect on primary position horizontal alignment. *Arch Ophthalmol.* 1973;90:15–16.

Weakening the superior oblique muscle *Unilateral weakening* of a superior oblique muscle is not commonly performed except as part of the treatment for Brown syndrome (see also pp 101–103). It may also be performed for an isolated inferior oblique muscle weakness, which is rare.

Crawford JS, Orton RB, Labow-Daily L. Late results of superior oblique muscle tenotomy in true Brown's syndrome. *Am J Ophthalmol.* 1980;89:824–829.

Del Monte MA, Archer SM. Surgery to correct Duane syndrome and Brown syndrome. In: Tasman W, Jaeger EA, eds. *Duane's Clinical Ophthalmology.* Philadelphia: Lippincott; 1993; vol 6, chap 96, 1–20.

Scott WE, Nankin SJ. Isolated inferior oblique paresis. *Arch Ophthalmol.* 1977; 95:1586–1593.

Bilateral weakening of the superior oblique muscle is often performed with or without horizontal muscle surgery for A-pattern deviations. This surgery can be expected to cause an eso shift of up to 30–40Δ in downgaze, little change in primary position, and almost no effect in upgaze. In surgery on patients with normal binocularity, the possibility of creating diplopia from vertical or torsional strabismus must be considered.

Fierson WM, Boger WP 3rd, Diorio PC, et al. The effect of bilateral superior oblique tenotomy on horizontal deviation in A-pattern strabismus. *J Pediatr Ophthalmol Strabismus.* 1980;17:364–371.

Scott WE, Jampolsky AJ, Redmond MR. Superior oblique tenotomy: indications and complications. *Int Ophthalmol Clin.* 1976;16:151–159.

Vertical Rectus Muscle Surgery for Hypotropia and Hypertropia

Because vertical deviations have many causes (e.g., cyclovertical muscle palsy, mechanical restriction, etc.), no single approach for surgical correction can be recommended for all situations. Surgical planning must be individualized based on suspected etiology and size of deviation. However, for small, largely comitant vertical deviations, recession or resection of vertical rectus muscles is frequently advocated. The atlases by Calhoun, Del Monte, and Wright cited on p 136 offer more specific guidance concerning selection of muscles and determination of the size of the recession or resection.

Dissociated vertical deviation (DVD)   When treatment of DVD is indicated, one of several surgical methods can be used. A recession of the superior rectus muscle, possibly on a "hang-back" suture, of 6–10 mm is considered effective. Bilateral superior rectus muscle recession may be indicated whenever either eye can fixate. If only one eye can fixate, then unilateral surgery is possible. Resection of the inferior rectus muscle for DVD ranges from 4 mm for small deviations to 8 mm for large angles. This technique may advance the lower eyelid, especially if careful dissection is not performed.

Anchoring the superior rectus muscle to the globe with a nonabsorbable suture 12–15 mm posterior to the insertion is another technique for managing DVD. This posterior fixation suture (fadenoperation) is usually combined with a recession of the superior rectus muscle.

Recession of the inferior oblique muscle with anteriorization of its insertion to a point temporal to the lateral border of the inferior rectus has been found effective in reducing or eliminating DVD; the mechanical tethering/depressing effect is important. This procedure is especially useful in cases when both DVD and a component of inferior oblique overaction occur in the same patient.

Kratz RE, Rogers GL, Bremer DL, et al. Anterior tendon displacement of the inferior oblique for DVD. *J Pediatr Ophthalmol Strabismus.* 1989;26:212–217.

Magoon E, Cruciger M, Jampolsky A. Dissociated vertical deviation: an asymmetric condition treated with large bilateral superior rectus recession. *J Pediatr Ophthalmol Strabismus.* 1982;19:152–156.

Sprague JB, Moore S, Eggers H, et al. Dissociated vertical deviation. Treatment with the faden operation of Cüppers. *Arch Ophthalmol.* 1980;98:465–468.

Other Rectus Muscle Surgery

Vertical displacement of the horizontal rectus muscles for A and V patterns
Vertical displacement of the horizontal rectus muscles one-half-tendon width will produce about 15Δ of additional weakening of that muscle in the direction of gaze the muscle is displaced. The muscle should thus be displaced in the direction of the desired additional weakening effect. The medial rectus muscle should be moved toward the apex of the A or V pattern (up in A pattern, down in V pattern). The lateral rectus muscle should be moved toward the open end of the A (down) or V (up). This guideline applies whether surgery is performed on one or both eyes.

Knapp P. A and V patterns. In: Burian HM. *Symposium on Strabismus.* St Louis: Mosby; 1971:242–254.

Metz HS, Schwartz L. The treatment of A and V patterns by monocular surgery. *Arch Ophthalmol.* 1977:95:251–253.

Lateral rectus muscle paralysis   The treatment of lateral rectus muscle paralysis varies with the degree of weakness of the lateral rectus muscle and the degree of contracture of the antagonist, ipsilateral medial rectus muscle. Apart from the use of botulinum toxin, there are basically two treatment options:

□ Resection of the lateral rectus muscle with recession of the ipsilateral medial rectus muscle

□ Recession of the ipsilateral medial rectus muscle combined with a transposition procedure

Cline RA, Scott WE. Long-term follow-up of Jensen procedures. *J Pediatr Ophthalmol Strabismus.* 1988;25:264–269.

Frueh BR, Henderson JW. Rectus muscle union in sixth nerve paralysis. *Arch Ophthalmol.* 1971;85:191–196.

Scott AB. Active force tests in lateral rectus paralysis. *Arch Ophthalmol.* 1971; 85:397–404.

Anesthesia for Extraocular Muscle Surgery

Topical anesthetic drops alone (e.g., tetracaine 0.5%, proparacaine 0.5%, cocaine 4%) can be used effectively in cooperative patients for certain procedures. Lid blocks are not necessary if the eyelid speculum is not spread to the point of causing pain. Topical anesthesia is effective for making incisions in the conjunctiva and Tenon's capsule, placing sutures into the muscle, and disinserting the muscle from the globe. It is not effective in controlling the pain produced by pulling on or against a muscle. Topical anesthesia is effective for simple recession procedures but not for resection procedures or for recession procedures involving restricted muscles where exposure is difficult.

Both *local infiltration* and *retrobulbar anesthesia* produce freedom from pain for most extraocular muscle procedures. Their use should be considered in those adults for whom general anesthesia may pose an undue hazard. The administration of a short-acting hypnotic by an anesthesiologist just before retrobulbar injection greatly improves patient comfort.

General anesthesia is necessary for children and is frequently used for adults as well, particularly those requiring bilateral ocular manipulation or surgery. Neuromuscular blocking agents such as succinylcholine, which are often administered to facilitate intubation for general anesthesia, can temporarily affect the results of a traction test.

France NK, France TD, Woodburn JD Jr, et al. Succinylcholine alteration of the forced duction test. *Ophthalmology.* 1980;87:1282–1287.

Conjunctival Incisions

Fornix Incision

This conjunctival incision is made in either the superior or the inferior cul-de-sac, usually in the inferior. It is located on bulbar conjunctiva, not actually in the fornix, 1–2 mm to the limbal side of the cul-de-sac. The incision is parallel to the fornix, approximately 8 mm in length. For surgery on the medial rectus muscle, the incision terminates just temporal to the semilunar fold. For lateral rectus surgery, the incision extends temporally from an imaginary line dropped into the cul-de-sac that divides the lateral and middle thirds of the cornea. Bare sclera is exposed by incising Tenon's capsule perpendicular to the conjunctival incision in its midportion. The muscle is engaged from this bare scleral exposure. The conjunctival incision is pulled or stretched over the point of the hook that has passed under the muscle belly.

When properly placed, the two-plane incision can be self-closed by gently massaging the conjunctiva into the fornix. Some surgeons prefer to close the incision with conjunctival sutures.

Del Monte MA. Conjunctival incisions. In: Del Monte MA, Archer SM. *Atlas of Pediatric Ophthalmology and Strabismus Surgery.* New York: Churchill Livingstone; 1993.

Parks MM. Fornix incision for horizontal rectus muscle surgery. *Am J Ophthalmol.* 1968;65:907–915.

Limbal or Peritomy Incision

The initial incision through conjunctiva and Tenon's capsule to the sclera is made in an oblique quadrant, close to and radial to the limbus, on the side of the eye nearest the muscle. The combined layer of conjunctiva and Tenon's capsule is then cleanly severed from the limbus with scissors. A second radial incision is made in the other quadrant so that the combined conjunctiva–Tenon's capsule flap can be retracted to expose the muscle for surgery. At the completion of surgery, the flap is reattached to its original position with a single suture in each corner.

von Noorden GK. The limbal approach to surgery of the rectus muscles. *Arch Ophthalmol.* 1968;80:94–97.

Complications of Strabismus Surgery

Unsatisfactory Alignment

The most common complication of surgery for strabismus is an unsatisfactory alignment. Undercorrections are more common with the above guidelines than overcorrections. In some cases it is apparent to both the patient and the surgeon in the immediate postoperative period that the alignment is not satisfactory. The development of the adjustable suture technique has provided an opportunity to improve the immediate postoperative alignment in cooperative patients (see pp 139–140).

A satisfactory alignment obtained in the immediate postoperative period may not be permanent for a variety of reasons. Some of these reasons are poor fusion, poor vision, altered accommodation, and contracture of scar tissue, but in many patients the cause for the unstable alignment is unknown. Reoperations may be necessary.

Refractive Changes

Changes in refractive error are most common when strabismus surgery is performed on two rectus muscles of one eye. An induced with-the-rule astigmatism of low magnitude usually resolves within several months.

Thompson WE, Reinecke RD. The changes in refractive status following routine strabismus surgery. *J Pediatr Ophthalmol Strabismus.* 1980;17:372–374.

Diplopia

Diplopia is common following strabismus surgery in older children and especially in adults. The surgery can move the image of the object of regard in the deviating eye out of a suppression scotoma. In the hours to several months following surgery, various responses can occur:

□ A new suppression scotoma may form, which corresponds to the new angle of alignment

□ Fusion of the two images can occur, obviating the need for a suppression scotoma

□ The diplopia may persist

If the initial strabismus was acquired before age 10, the ability to suppress is generally well developed, even if unused during many years of fusion, and prolonged postoperative diplopia is uncommon unless the patient's strabismus is overcorrected. If strabismus was first acquired in adulthood, however, the diplopia that was symptomatic before surgery will persist unless fusion is regained. Prisms may be helpful in assessing fusional potential and the risk of bothersome postoperative diplopia.

Further treatment is indicated for those patients, mainly adults, whose symptomatic diplopia persists more than 3–4 weeks following surgery. Patients with unequal acuities can frequently be taught to ignore the dimmer, fuzzier, nondominant image by closing the nondominant eye intermittently. If vision is equal or nearly so, press-on prisms should be tried, generally with the full correction in a single prism over the nonpreferred eye, tilted to correct both vertical and horizontal deviation. If diplopia is eliminated, then attempted weaning or later replacement with permanent ground-in prism split between both eyes may provide long-term relief. If this approach fails, additional surgery or botulinum toxin injection may be needed (see chapter XIV).

Perforation of the Sclera

A needle may perforate into the suprachoroidal space or through the choroid and retina. In most cases this perforation creates no problem other than a chorioretinal scar. However, perforation can lead to vitreous hemorrhage, retinal detachment, or endophthalmitis (Fig XIII-1). Presumably, inadvertent perforation of the sclera with a suture pass provides access for infection within the globe. Some surgeons advocate laser or cryotherapy over the site of the perforation. Funduscopy with observation is advised, with further treatment as indicated. Preoperative antibiotics are generally used.

Basmadjian G, Labelle P, Dumas J. Retinal detachment after strabismus surgery. *Am J Ophthalmol.* 1975;79:305–309.

Gottlieb F, Castro JL. Perforation of the globe during strabismus surgery. *Arch Ophthalmol.* 1970;84:151–157.

Simon JW, Lininger LL, Scherage JL. Recognized scleral perforation during eye muscle surgery: incidence and sequelae. *J Pediatr Ophthalmol Strabismus.* 1992;29: 273–275.

Postoperative Infections

Serious infection is uncommon following strabismus surgery. Some patients develop mild conjunctivitis, which may be caused by allergy to suture material or postoperative medications as well as by infectious agents. Preseptal or orbital cellulitis with proptosis, eyelid swelling, chemosis, and fever are also rare complications of strabismus surgery (Fig XIII-2). These conditions usually develop 2–3 days after surgery

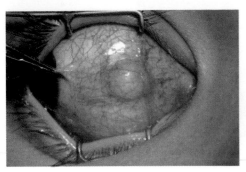

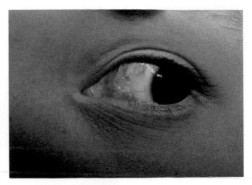

FIG XIII-5—Postoperative conjunctival epithelial inclusion cyst following right medial rectus recession using fornix incision technique.

FIG XIII-6—Involvement of plica semilunaris in incision.

□ *Advancement of the plica semilunaris onto bulbar conjunctiva.* Sometimes in surgery on the medial rectus muscle using the limbal approach, the surgeon may mistake the plica semilunaris for a conjunctival edge and incorporate it or a portion of it into the closure. Although not strictly a conjunctival scar, the plica semilunaris, now pulled forward over bulbar conjunctiva, will retain its normal fleshy color long after the remainder of the conjunctiva has returned to its normal color (Fig XIII-6). A restrictive esotropia is also likely.

Adherence Syndrome

Violation of Tenon's capsule with prolapse of orbital fat into the sub-Tenon's space can cause formation of a pink fibrofatty scar to the operated muscle and globe, which may produce restriction of motility. This complication may occur after surgery of any extraocular muscles, and when it occurs after inferior oblique muscle surgery, hypotropia can result. If an inadvertent rent in Tenon's capsule is recognized at the time of surgery, the prolapsed part can be excised and the rent closed with absorbable sutures. Otherwise, further surgery, including the use of sleeves and caps, may be needed, and the response to such surgery is usually poor. Meticulous surgical technique will usually prevent this serious complication.

Dunlap EA. Use of plastics and adhesives in strabismus surgery. In: Burian HM. *Symposium on Strabismus.* St Louis: Mosby; 1971:268–280.

Parks MM. The overacting inferior oblique muscle. The XXXVI DeSchweinitz Lecture. *Am J Ophthalmol.* 1974;77:787–797.

Dellen

The term *dellen* (*delle,* singular), derived from the German word for "dents," refers to shallow depressions or corneal thinning just anterior to the limbus. They occur when raised abnormal tissue on the bulbar conjunctiva prevents the eyelid from adequately bathing the cornea during blinking (Fig XIII-7). Fluorescein pools in these

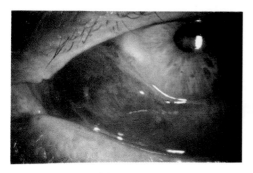

FIG XIII-7—Corneal delle subsequent to postoperative subconjunctival hemorrhage.

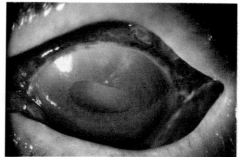

FIG XIII-8—Superotemporal segmental anterior segment ischemia after simultaneous superior rectus muscle and lateral rectus muscle surgery following scleral buckling procedure.

depressions but does not stain the stroma. Dellen are seen occasionally when the limbal approach to muscle surgery is used. They should be followed carefully, and artificial tears or lubricants may be needed until the chemosis and conjunctival hemorrhage subside. Patching of the eye may be helpful.

Anterior Segment Ischemia

Most of the blood supply to the anterior segment of the eye comes through the anterior ciliary arteries that travel in the four rectus muscles. Simultaneous surgery on three of these rectus muscles, or even two of them in patients with poor blood flow, may lead to anterior segment ischemia. This complication is characterized by corneal epithelial edema, folds in Descemet's membrane, and other signs of an anterior uveitis (Fig XIII-8). If severe, it may lead to phthisis bulbi. Treatment is directed at the anterior uveitis, which often responds to frequent administration of topical, subconjunctival, or systemic steroids.

It may be possible to recess or resect a rectus muscle while sparing its anterior ciliary vessels by using an operating microscope and vitrectomy microinstruments. Although difficult and time-consuming, this technique may be indicated in high-risk cases.

McKeown CA, Lambert HM, Shore JW. Preservation of the anterior ciliary vessels during extraocular muscle surgery. *Ophthalmology.* 1989;96:498–506.

Saunders RA, Bluestein EC, Wilson ME, et al. Anterior segment ischemia after strabismus surgery. *Surv Ophthalmol.* 1994;38:456–466.

Change in Eyelid Position

Change in the position of the eyelids is most likely to occur with surgery on the vertical rectus muscles. Pulling the inferior rectus muscle forward, as in a resection, will pull the lower eyelid up, over the lower limbus; recessing the muscle will pull the

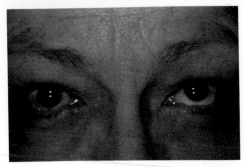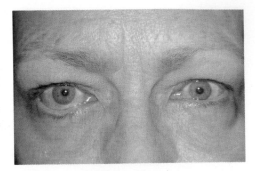

FIG XIII-9—*Left,* Preoperative photograph of patient who had recession of the right inferior rectus muscle, which pulled the right lower eyelid down, and a resection of the left inferior rectus muscle, which pulled the left lower eyelid up, causing postoperative asymmetry. *Right,* Postoperative photograph.

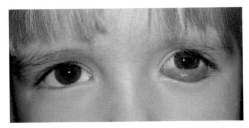

FIG XIII-10—One year after resection of left inferior rectus muscle, with down-pulled left lower eyelid and conjunctival prolapse.

lower eyelid down, exposing bare sclera below the lower limbus (Figs XIII-9 and XIII-10). Surgery on the superior rectus muscle is less likely to affect the upper eyelid position when proper dissection is performed.

Eyelid position changes can be obviated somewhat by careful dissection. In general, all intermuscular septum and fascial connections between the eyelid and associated vertical rectus muscle must be severed at least 12–15 mm posterior to the muscle insertion (to the point at which the muscle disappears through Tenon's capsule). Some surgeons have advocated release of the lower eyelid retractors or advancement of the capsulopalpebral head to prevent lower eyelid retraction after inferior rectus muscle recession.

Kushner BJ. A surgical procedure to minimize lower-eyelid retraction with inferior rectus recession. *Arch Ophthalmol.* 1992;110:1011–1014.

Meyer DR, Simon JW, Kansora M. Primary infratarsal eyelid retractor lysis to prevent eyelid retraction after inferior rectus muscle recession. *Am J Ophthalmol.* 1996; 122:331–339.

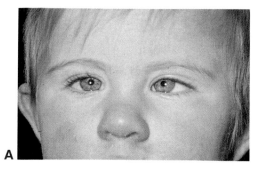

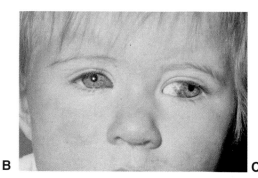

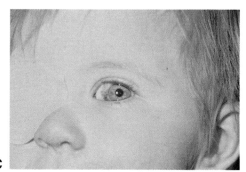

FIG XIII-11—Lost left medial rectus muscle. *A,* Preoperative congenital (essential infantile) esotropia. *B,* Postoperative day 2. Patient shows inability to adduct left eye to midline. *C,* Patient uses right head turn to keep left eye in abduction as a result of inability to adduct left eye.

Lost Muscle

Sometimes after a muscle is freed from its insertion, it can slip out of the sutures or surgical instruments and be lost posteriorly in the orbit (Fig XIII-11). The surgeon should immediately make every attempt to find the lost muscle, which retracts into its sleeve of Tenon's capsule. It is important to realize that a lost or retracted muscle will usually not remain next to the globe posterior to the equator but will instead retract into Tenon's capsule along the orbital wall. Generally, pulling Tenon's capsule forward in a "hand over hand" fashion will bring the muscle into view. Malleable retractors and a headlight may be helpful. Care must be taken not to violate Tenon's capsule, in which case fibrofatty proliferation can occur (see p 152).

When the diagnosis is made in the immediate postoperative period, the patient should be promptly returned to surgery for exploration and attempted retrieval of the lost muscle by a surgeon experienced with this potentially complex surgery. Muscle transposition surgery may be required if the lost muscle is not found.

Slipped Muscle

It is uncommon for a muscle to become detached from the sclera or to "slip" posteriorly within the muscle capsule during the postoperative period. Clinically, the patient manifests a weakness of that muscle with limited rotations and decreased saccades in the field of action. The muscle capsule may be found attached at the previous surgical site, but the muscle fibers within it have slipped posteriorly in the

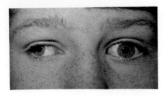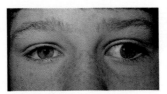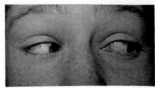

FIG XIII-12—Slipped left medial rectus muscle. *Left,* Gaze right shows widening of palpebral fissure of left eye and inability to adduct. *Middle,* Exotropia in primary position with widened palpebral fissure. *Right,* Gaze left shows full abduction with normal width of fissure.

capsule. Surgery should be performed as soon as possible in order to replace the slipped muscle before further retraction and contracture take place. This problem can be prevented by adequately securing the muscle prior to tenotomy with full-thickness lock bites to include muscle tissue and not just capsule (Fig XIII-12).

Bloom JN, Parks MM. The etiology, treatment and prevention of the "slipped muscle." *J Pediatr Ophthalmol Strabismus.* 1981;18:6–11.

Postoperative Nausea and Vomiting

Nausea and vomiting are common following eye muscle surgery. The incidence and severity can be reduced using newer anesthetic agents and antiemetics.

Oculocardiac Reflex

The oculocardiac reflex is a slowing of the heart rate that is caused by traction on the extraocular muscles. In its most severe form it can produce asystole. The surgeon should be aware of the possibility of inducing the oculocardiac reflex when manipulating a muscle and should be prepared to release tension if the heart rate drops excessively. Intravenous atropine can protect against the oculocardiac reflex.

Malignant Hyperthermia

Malignant hyperthermia (MH) is an acute metabolic disorder that can be fatal if diagnosis and treatment are delayed. In its fully developed form it is characterized by extreme heat production. MH is often triggered by the potent inhalation anesthetics halothane, enflurane, and isoflurane and the muscle relaxant succinylcholine. Local anesthetics of the amide type have also been implicated.

MH is a disorder of calcium binding by the sarcoplasmic reticulum of skeletal muscle. In the presence of an anesthetic triggering agent, unbound intracellular calcium increases, stimulating muscle contracture. As this increased metabolism outstrips oxygen delivery, anaerobic metabolism develops with lactate production and massive acidosis. Hyperthermia occurs as a result of the hypermetabolic state. As cells are depleted of adenosine triphosphate (ATP), cell breakdown occurs with loss of potassium and myoglobin.

MH can occur as an isolated case or as a dominantly inherited disorder with incomplete penetrance. Other disorders associated with MH include strabismus, myopathies, ptosis, and other musculoskeletal abnormalities. The incidence is variously reported as between 1:6000 and 1:60,000 and is thought to be higher in children. It occurs in all age groups. Although the mortality rate used to be as high as 70%, it is probably lower than 10% now.

Diagnosis   The diagnosis of MH is made on the basis of clinical signs and may be confirmed by laboratory studies. Muscle biopsy with in vitro halothane and caffeine contraction testing is the most specific test to confirm the clinical diagnosis. Patients who have an unconfirmed diagnosis, but also have a suspicious history or a relative with MH, may undergo testing to see if they are susceptible. If testing is not available, nontriggering anesthetic agents should be used and the patient treated as if MH is a possibility.

Clinical picture   Frequently, the earliest sign of MH is a tachycardia that is greater than expected for the patient's anesthetic and surgical status. Other arrhythmias may also occur, as well as unstable blood pressure. Other early signs include tachypnea, sweating, muscle rigidity, blotchy discoloration of skin, cyanosis, and dark urine. Onset may be manifested during the induction of anesthesia by trismus caused by masseter muscle spasm, although the significance of masseter spasm is controversial. Most of these patients do not develop MH, but they should be observed closely. If the patient is being monitored with capnography, an elevated end-tidal carbon dioxide may be the presenting sign.

A later sign is a rise in temperature, which may reach extremely high levels. Other later signs include respiratory and metabolic acidosis, hyperkalemia, hypercalcemia, myoglobinuria and renal failure, skeletal muscle swelling, heart failure, disseminated intravascular coagulation, and cardiac arrest. Ideally, MH should be diagnosed and treated before a marked rise in temperature occurs. Survival is greatly improved when treatment begins early.

Treatment   Early treatment of unexpected cases of MH cannot be overemphasized. Table XIII-6 gives the protocol for treatment of malignant hyperthermia. Once the condition is recognized, anesthetic agents should be discontinued, hyperventilation with oxygen started, and treatment with intravenous dantrolene begun. Dantrolene works to prevent release of calcium from the sarcoplasmic reticulum, preventing the excessive contractile response of muscle. Surgery should be terminated as soon as possible, even if incomplete. Temperature monitoring should be established along with an intra-arterial catheter for the monitoring of blood pressure and arterial blood gases. Electrolytes, ECG, urine output, PT, PTT, fibrinogen, and pulse oximetry should also be monitored. Central venous or pulmonary artery pressure may be monitored if indicated by the patient's condition.

TABLE XIII-6

MALIGNANT HYPERTHERMIA PROTOCOL

1. Stop the triggering agents immediately and conclude surgery as soon as possible.

2. Hyperventilate with 100% oxygen at high flow rates.

3. Administer

a. Dantrolene: 2–3 mg/kg initial bolus with increments up to 10 mg/kg total. Continue to administer dantrolene until symptoms are controlled. Occasionally, a dose greater than 10 mg/kg may be needed.

b. Sodium bicarbonate: 1–2 mEq/kg increments guided by arterial pH and pCO_2. Bicarbonate will combat hyperkalemia by driving potassium into cells.

4. Actively cool patient:

a. If needed, IV iced saline (not Ringer's lactate) 15 ml/kg q 10 minutes × 3. Monitor closely.

b. Lavage stomach, bladder, rectum, and peritoneal and thoracic cavities with iced saline.

c. Surface cool with ice and hypothermia blanket.

5. Maintain urine output. If needed, administer mannitol 0.25 gm/kg IV, furosemide 1 mg/kg IV (up to 4 doses each). Urine output greater than 2 ml/kg/hr may help prevent subsequent renal failure.

6. Calcium channel blockers *should not* be given when dantrolene is administered, as hyperkalemia and myocardial depression may occur.

7. Insulin for hyperkalemia: Add 10 units of regular insulin to 50 ml of 50% glucose and titrate to control hyperkalemia. Monitor blood glucose and potassium levels.

8. Postoperatively: Continue dantrolene 1 mg/kg IV q 6 hours × 72 hours to prevent recurrence. Lethal recurrences of MH may occur. Observe in an intensive care unit.

9. For expert medical advice and further medical evaluation, call the MHaus MH hotline consultant at (800) 644-9737. For nonemergency professional or patient information, call (800) 986-4287. E-mail address is mhaus@norwich.net.

CHAPTER XIV

Chemodenervation Treatment of Strabismus and Blepharospasm Using Botulinum Toxin

Pharmacology and Mechanism of Action

Botox, formerly called *Oculinum* (purified botulinum toxin A), is a protein drug produced from the bacterium *Clostridium botulinum.* The toxin is injected directly into the orbicularis muscle or into selected extraocular muscles localized with a portable electromyographic device. Following injection, botulinum toxin is bound and internalized in 24–48 hours within local motor nerve terminals, where it remains for many weeks to interfere with the release of acetylcholine. Paralysis of the injected muscle begins within 2–4 days after injection and lasts clinically for at least 5–8 weeks in the extraocular muscle and for 3 or more months in the orbicularis muscle. An extraocular muscle lengthens while it is paralyzed by botulinum, and its antagonist contracts. These changes may produce long-term improvement in the alignment of the eyes. Botox was approved by the Food and Drug Administration for use in strabismus and blepharospasm in 1990.

Indications, Techniques, and Results

Strabismus Correction

Clinical trials have shown botulinum to be most effective when used in the following conditions:

□ Small- to moderate-angle esotropia and exotropia (less than 40Δ)

□ Postoperative residual strabismus (2–8 weeks following surgery or later)

□ Weakening of an antagonist muscle in acute paralytic strabismus (especially sixth nerve palsy) to block its contracture while the agonist recovers

□ Cyclic esotropia

□ Active thyroid ophthalmopathy (Graves disease) or inflamed or prephthisical eyes, when surgery is inappropriate

Studies have shown this treatment to be disappointing in patients with large deviations, restrictive or mechanical strabismus (trauma or multiple reoperations), or secondary strabismus where a muscle has been over-recessed. Injection is ineffective in A and V patterns, dissociated vertical deviations (DVD), oblique muscle disorders, and chronic paralytic strabismus. Multiple injections are frequently required for maximal benefit. As with surgical treatment, best results occur when there is fusion to stabilize the alignment.

Results of treatment The percentage of patients achieving a deviation of 10Δ or less at least 6 months after the last injection has ranged from 33% for large-angle exotropia to 72% for small-angle esotropia. Overcorrections are rare, and adults and children have had similar responses.

Eyelid Disorders

Botulinum toxin has proven effective in the treatment of essential blepharospasm and hemifacial spasm. Although relief from these eyelid disorders is only temporary, requiring repeated injections into the orbicularis muscle for maintenance, the lack of other reliable effective drugs has made botulinum the medical treatment of choice. Orbicularis extirpation for blepharospasm or nerve decompression for hemifacial spasm are effective surgical treatments.

Complications

The most common side effects have been temporary ptosis lasting from 3 weeks to 3 months (16% of adults and 25% of children) and induced secondary vertical strabismus (17% of all patients). Rarely, these effects have persisted beyond 6 months (0.16% with slight residual ptosis and 2% with residual vertical strabismus of 2Δ or more). Other reported rare complications include scleral perforation (0.13%), retrobulbar hemorrhage (0.2%), pupillary dilation (0.6%), and permanent diplopia in one patient as a result of loss of suppression. Thus far in clinical use, no toxic systemic effects or loss of vision have been reported.

Biglan AW, Burnstine RA, Rogers GL, et al. Management of strabismus with botulinum A toxin. *Ophthalmology.* 1989;96:935–943.

Cohen DA, Savino PJ, Stern MB, et al. Botulinum injection therapy for blepharospasm: a review and report of 75 patients. *Clin Neuropharmacol.* 1986;9:415–429.

Gammon JA, Gemmill M, Tigges J, et al. Botulinum chemodenervation treatment of strabismus. *J Pediatr Ophthalmol Strabismus.* 1985;22:221–226.

Metz HS, Mazow M. Botulinum toxin treatment of acute sixth and third nerve palsy. *Graefes Arch Clin Exp Ophthalmol.* 1988;226:141–144.

Scott AB. Botulinum toxin: treatment of strabismus. In: *Focal Points: Clinical Modules for Ophthalmologists.* San Francisco: American Academy of Ophthalmology; 1989;7:12.

Scott AB, Magoon EH, NcNeer KW, et al. Botulinum treatment of strabismus in children. *Trans Am Ophthalmol Soc.* 1989;87:174–184.

PART 2

PEDIATRIC OPHTHALMOLOGY

Growth and Development of the Child's Eye

Children are different from adults in many significant ways. The infant eye, for example, is not simply a small adult eye. Because pathology in the infant eye may be indicated by variations in the size or proportion of its structures, the normal dimensions and proportions must be learned by ophthalmologists responsible for children's eye care.

The palpebral fissure at birth Is almost as long as in childhood, yet a newborn's vertical fissure is only half the size of an adult's. The diameter of the eye at birth is about 66% of that in adulthood. The eye grows rapidly during the first 2 years of life; growth then slows until puberty, when further enlargement occurs. Infants often have astigmatism during their first months of life, and most young children are hyperopic. Absence of hyperopia during early childhood is usually a harbinger of myopia, which increases as growth progresses.

As the axial length of the eye increases (Fig 1), the lens flattens (Fig 2). At birth, the anterior–posterior length of the eye is about 17 mm, increasing to approximately 24 mm in adulthood. The anterior chamber depth at birth is 2.3–2.7 mm, which is shallower than in adults as a result of the steep anterior lens surface in children.

The average corneal horizontal diameter is 9.5–10.5 mm in newborns and 12 mm in adults. The radius of corneal curvature is 6.6–7.4 mm in newborns and 7.4–8.4 mm in adults (Table 1). Keratometry values change markedly in the first year of life, but later remain relatively stable (Fig 3). The infant sclera is about half of its adult thickness and strength.

Developmentally, blue-eyed newborns may deposit additional pigment in their anterior iris stroma, and eye color may gradually darken to green or brown during the first months of life. The dilator pupillae muscle is not well developed at birth, resulting in miotic pupils in infants. The fovea matures during the first months of life, while myelinization of the optic nerve is usually completed shortly after birth. Only 3%–10% of infant eyes have asymmetrical cupping of their optic discs or optic discs whose cup/disc ratio is greater than 0.3.

Excellent visual acuities have been documented in infants. Visually evoked cortical potentials from the occipital cortex, recorded while the infant fixates on patterns of graded size, indicate that 6-month-old infants have already developed 20/20 visual acuity. In the early months of life, behavioral tests such as the forced preferential looking test have documented somewhat lower visual acuities than indicated by electrophysiological recordings. Thus, tests that measure responses from the occipital cortex differ somewhat from tests that may also include responses from the visual association areas of the cortex.

The pediatric eye is a growing eye, which differentiates it in many ways from the adult eye. Further, the developing immune system predisposes children to

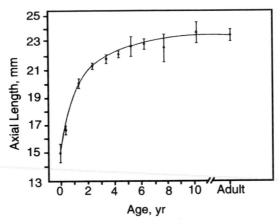

FIG 1—Axial length plotted with respect to age. Dots represent mean values for age group indicated; bars represent standard deviations. (Figures 1–3 reproduced by permission from Gordon RA, Donzis PB. Refractive development of the human eye. *Arch Ophthalmol.* 1985;103: 785–789. Copyright ©1985, American Medical Association.)

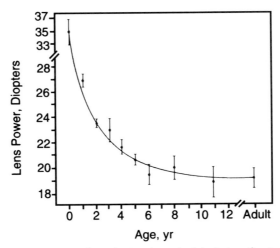

FIG 2—Mean values (dots) and standard deviations (bars) for lens power as determined by modified SRK formula, plotted with respect to age.

reactions to inflammation and diseases that are distinctly different from those of adults. Similarly, because the central nervous system is in its formative period, it is particularly vulnerable to growth abnormalities and developmental interruptions. Thus, many interrelated influences are at work in pediatric ophthalmology. BCSC Section 2, *Fundamentals and Principles of Ophthalmology,* includes an extensive discussion of embryology and development.

TABLE 1

DIMENSIONS OF NEWBORN AND ADULT EYES

	NEWBORN	ADULT
Anterior–posterior length (mm)	17	24
Corneal horizontal diameter (mm)	9.5–10.5	12
Radius of corneal curvature (mm)	6.6–7.4	7.4–8.4

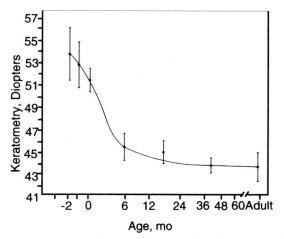

FIG 3—Keratometry values plotted with respect to age on logarithmic scale. Negative number represents months of prematurity; dots, mean value for age group indicated; and bars, standard deviations.

CHAPTER XV

Congenital Anomalies

Many details and definitions pertaining to genetics, chromosomal anomalies, and developmental embryology are discussed and illustrated in BCSC Section 2, *Fundamentals and Principles of Ophthalmology*. See the glossary on the next page for terms frequently associated with dysmorphology and congenital anomalies.

Major congenital anomalies occur in 2%–3% of live births. The etiologies include monogenic causes, chromosomal anomalies, multifactorial disorders, environmental agents, and unidentified causes. Unfortunately, the latter category, unknown etiology, accounts for 50% or more of these malformations. Regardless of etiology, from a developmental point of view congenital anomalies may be organized into the following categories (examples are given in parentheses):

- *Agenesis:* developmental failure (anophthalmos)
- *Hypoplasia:* developmental arrest (eyelid coloboma)
- *Hyperplasia:* developmental excess (distichiasis)
- Abnormal development (cryptophthalmos)
- Failure to divide or canalize (congenital nasolacrimal duct obstruction)
- *Dysraphia:* failure to fuse (choroidal coloboma)
- Persistence of vestigial structures (persistent pupillary membrane, remnant hyaloid artery)

A *malformation* implies a morphological defect present from the onset of development or a very early stage. A disturbance to a group of cells in a single developmental field may cause multiple malformations. Multiple causations may result in similar field defects and patterns of malformation. A single structural defect or factor can lead to a cascade, or domino effect, of secondary anomalies referred to as a *sequence.* However, sequence does not always imply a single causative factor. The Pierre Robin group of anomalies (cleft palate, glossoptosis, micrognathia, respiratory problems) may represent a sequence caused by abnormal descent of the tongue and is noted in many syndromes (such as Stickler or fetal alcohol) and chromosomal anomalies. By contrast, a *syndrome* implies a single cause even if the etiologic agent is not yet identified. An *association* represents defects noted to occur together in a statistically significant number of patients, such as, for example, the CHARGE association (ocular **c**oloboma, **h**eart defects, choanal **a**tresia, mental **r**etardation, and **g**enitourinary and **e**ar anomalies). An association may represent a variety of yet-unidentified causations. Two or more minor anomalies in combination significantly increase the chance of an associated major malformation.

Cohen MM Jr. *The Child with Multiple Birth Defects.* 2nd ed. New York: Oxford University Press; 1997.

Smith DW, Jones KL. *Smith's Recognizable Patterns of Human Malformation*. 5th ed. Philadelphia: Saunders; 1997.

Wyllie AH. The genetic refulatio of apoptosis. *Curr Opin Genet Dev.* 1995;5:97–104.

Glossary

The following additional terms are frequently used in discussions of congenital anomalies and dysmorphology:

Apoptosis   An orderly sequence of events in which cells shut down and self-destruct without causing injury to neighboring cells that need to remain for the development of the embryo. Persistent hyperplastic primary vitreous is a likely example of a defect in apoptosis in the eye's development. Also called *programmed cell death.*

Congenital anomalies   Includes all forms of developmental defects present at birth, whether caused by genetic chromosomal or environmental etiologies.

Deformation   Abnormal form, shape, or position of a part of the body caused by a mechanical process, such as intrauterine compression.

Developmental field   A group of cells that respond as a coordinated unit to embryonic interaction defects in development, resulting in multiple malformations.

Disruption   A morphological defect resulting from the extrinsic breakdown of, or interference with, an originally normal developmental process.

Dysplasia   Abnormal organization of cells into tissue(s) and its morphological result; the process (and consequence) of abnormality of histogenesis, e.g., collagen formation in the joints and zonular fibers of a patient with Marfan syndrome.

Neurocristopathy   A constellation of malformations or a craniofacial syndrome involving structures that are primarily derived from neural crest cells (e.g., Goldenhar syndrome).

Teratogen   Any agent that can produce a permanent morphological or functional abnormality. This category includes not only drugs and environmental agents such as ionizing radiation but also viruses and other pathogenic organisms (e.g., rubella virus, *Toxoplasma gondii*) and metabolic abnormalities (e.g., diabetes).

CHAPTER XVI

Eyelid Disorders

Congenital eyelid disorders can result from abnormal differentiation of the eyelids and adnexa, developmental arrest, intrauterine environmental insults, and other unknown factors. Examples of these groups are discussed below.

Cryptophthalmos This rare condition results from failure of differentiation of eyelid structures. The skin passes uninterrupted from the forehead over the eye to the cheek and blends in with the cornea of the eye, which is usually malformed (Fig XVI-1).

Congenital coloboma of the eyelid The upper eyelid is usually involved in this condition. It varies from a small notch to the absence of the entire length of the eyelid, which may be fused to the globe (Fig XVI-2). The eye of an infant with a congenital coloboma should be observed for drying, but often the defect is well tolerated. Surgical closure of the eyelid defect is usually required eventually.

Ankyloblepharon Fusion of part or all of the eyelid margins is known as *ankyloblepharon.* A variant is *ankyloblepharon filiforme adnatum,* in which the eyelid margins are connected by fine strands. An association with trisomy 18 has been observed. Treatment is surgical.

Congenital ectropion Eversion of the eyelid margin usually involves the lower eyelid secondary to a vertical deficiency of the skin. A lateral tarsorrhaphy may be needed for mild cases. More severe cases may require a skin flap or graft.

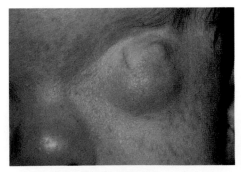

FIG XVI-1—Cryptophthalmos, left eye.

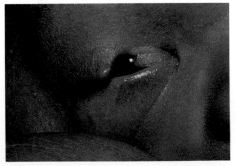

FIG XVI-2—Congenital eyelid coloboma, right eye. The eyelid is fused to the globe.

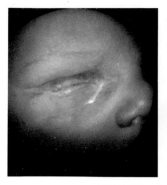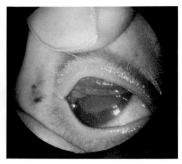

FIG XVI-3—Congenital tarsal kink.

Congenital entropion   The lower eyelid is usually involved in this condition. The distal portion of the lower tarsus is bent or rotated inward, causing the lashes to abrade the cornea. Corneal damage is uncommon; however, if corneal integrity is compromised, surgical repair should be performed as soon as possible.

Epiblepharon   This horizontal fold of skin adjacent to either the upper or lower eyelid may turn the lashes against the cornea, most commonly by the lower eyelid. The cornea often tolerates this condition surprisingly well, and in the first several years of life epiblepharon resolves spontaneously. In severe cases simple excision of the fold of skin/muscle is necessary.

Congenital tarsal kink   The origin of this condition is unknown. The child is born with the upper eyelid bent back and open. The upper tarsal plate often has an actual 180° fold. As with large congenital colobomas, the cornea may be exposed and traumatized by the bent edge, resulting in ulceration. Minor defects can be managed by manually unfolding the tarsus and taping the eyelid shut with a pressure dressing for 1–2 days. More severe cases require surgical incision of the tarsal plate or even excision of a V-shaped wedge from the inner surface to permit unfolding (Fig XVI-3).

Distichiasis   A partial or complete accessory row of eyelashes growing out of or slightly posterior to the meibomian gland orifices is known as distichiasis. The abnormal lashes tend to be thinner, shorter, softer, and less pigmented than normal cilia and are, therefore, often well tolerated. Treatment is indicated if the patient is symptomatic or if evidence of corneal irritation is present (Fig XVI-4).

Euryblepharon   Enlargement of the lateral part of the palpebral aperture with downward displacement of the temporal half of the lower eyelid is known as euryblepharon.

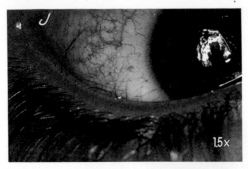

FIG XVI-4—Distichiasis. An accessory row of eyelashes is shown exiting from the meibomian gland orifices. (Reproduced by permission from Byrnes GA, Wilson ME. Congenital distichiasis. *Arch Ophthalmol.* 1991;109:1752–1753. Copyright ©1991, American Medical Association.)

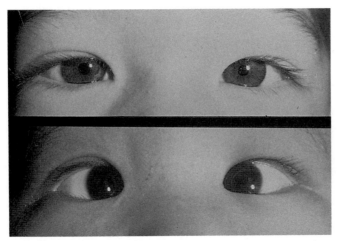

FIG XVI-5—Epicanthus, bilateral. *Top,* Epicanthus tarsalis. *Bottom,* Epicanthus palpebralis. (Reproduced by permission from Crouch E. *The Child's Eye: Strabismus and Amblyopia.* Slide script. San Francisco: American Academy of Ophthalmology; 1982.)

Epicanthus This crescent-shaped fold of skin running vertically between the eyelids and overlying the inner canthus is shown in Figure XVI-5. There are three types of epicanthus:

□ *Epicanthus tarsalis:* the fold is most prominent in the upper eyelid

□ *Epicanthus inversus:* the fold is most prominent in the lower eyelid

□ *Epicanthus palpebralis:* the fold is equally distributed in the upper and lower eyelids

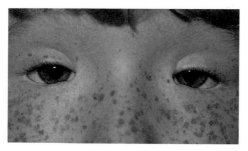

FIG XVI-6—Blepharophimosis, epicanthus inversus, telecanthus, and ptosis.

Epicanthus may be associated with blepharophimosis or ptosis, or it may be an isolated finding. Surgical correction is only occasionally required.

Telecanthus Wide intercanthal distance with a normal interpupillary distance is known as telecanthus. It is frequently associated with craniofacial syndromes such as Waardenburg syndrome. This condition tends to improve with time but can be corrected surgically. Telecanthus should not be confused with *hypertelorism,* which indicates increased separation between the bony orbits.

Palpebral fissure slants Slight upward or downward slanting of palpebral fissures is normally seen on a familial basis or in groups such as individuals of Asian descent. However, certain craniofacial syndromes frequently have a characteristic upward (e.g., Down syndrome) or downward (e.g., Treacher Collins syndrome) slanting (see Figure XXVIII-3).

Blepharophimosis, epicanthus inversus, telecanthus, and ptosis This complex of findings frequently occurs together as an isolated but often autosomal dominant disorder. The palpebral fissures are shortened horizontally and vertically *(blepharophimosis)* with poor levator function and no eyelid fold (Fig XVI-6). Repair of the ptosis, usually with frontalis slings, is often needed early in life. Since the epicanthus and telecanthus may improve with age, repair of these defects should be delayed.

Ptosis (blepharoptosis) This term describes eyelid droop; the condition can be congenital or acquired. Acquired ptosis has been classified according to its various causes (Table XVI-1). Evaluation of ptosis should include a thorough history that includes the date of onset and reviews any ocular disorders in the family. A complete examination, including slit-lamp examination and refraction, should be performed. Astigmatic errors are occasionally associated with ptosis, and they may persist after eyelid surgery. The eyelid is evaluated by describing the upper fold, and the amount of ptosis is documented by measuring the height of the palpebral fissure. Levator function is measured while blocking the effect of the frontalis muscle. Elevation of the ptotic eyelid with jaw movement, or *jaw winking,* may be present. Both tear function and corneal sensitivity should be evaluated, as exposure and drying will be

TABLE XVI-1

CLASSIFICATION OF PTOSIS

Pseudoptosis

Congenital ptosis

Acquired ptosis

   Myogenic

      Myasthenia gravis

      Progressive external ophthalmoplegia

   Neurogenic

      Horner syndrome

      Third nerve palsy

   Mechanical

---

compounded by surgical repair. If Bell's phenomenon is poor, the cornea can decompensate very quickly after ptosis repair. A documentary photograph of the patient is desirable.

Correction of ptosis in a child can often be delayed until the patient is several years old, although consistent chin-up head posturing may justify very early surgery. In rare cases a completely closed eyelid must be elevated to avoid occlusion amblyopia. Surgical techniques include levator resection, tucking of the levator aponeurosis, and eyelid suspension anchored into the frontalis muscle. When levator function is less than 4 mm, frontalis suspension surgery is usually performed. When obtainable, autogenous fascia lata is the preferred material for frontalis suspension surgery. However, some surgeons report good results with silicone rods or human donor fascia lata, although a 50% recurrence rate by 8–10 years postoperatively when human donor fascia lata is used has been documented. The long-term success using autogenous fascia lata has not been adequately studied.

In jaw winking, discussion with the family regarding their concerns about the ptosis versus the eyelid excursion is important. The eyelid excursion is the greater concern in some patients, and they may elect to sacrifice the levator and use a sling to elevate the eyelid.

BCSC Section 7, *Orbit, Eyelids, and Lacrimal System,* discusses the eyelids, their disorders and management, in greater detail.

Crawford JS. Congenital eyelid anomalies in children. *J Pediatr Ophthalmol Strabismus.* 1984;21:140–149.

Kohn R. Additional lacrimal findings in the syndrome of blepharophimosis, epicanthus inversus, and telecanthus. *J Pediatr Ophthalmol Strabismus.* 1983;20:98–100.

Wilson ME, Johnson RW. Congenital ptosis. Long-term results of treatment using lyophilized fascia lata for frontalis suspensions. *Ophthalmology.* 1991;98:1234–1237.

CHAPTER XVII

Infectious and Allergic Ocular Diseases

Intrauterine and Perinatal Infections of the Eye

The maternally transmitted congenital infections discussed in this section can cause ocular damage in several ways:

☐ Through direct action of the infecting agent, which damages tissue

☐ Through a teratogenic effect resulting in malformation

☐ Through a delayed reactivation of the agent after birth, with inflammation that damages developed tissue

These infections can cause continuous tissue damage; therefore, long-term evaluation is required to determine their full impact. Most perinatal disorders have an exceedingly broad spectrum of clinical presentation, ranging from "silent" disease to life-threatening tissue and organ damage. Only the common types of congenital infections are included in this chapter. They can be remembered by the acronym TORCH, standing for toxoplasmosis; other (an expanding list of pathogens including syphilis, varicella, HIV, and parvovirus B19); rubella; cytomegalic inclusion disease; and herpes simplex virus.

Stamos JK, Rowley AH. Timely diagnosis of congenital infections. *Pediatr Clin North Am.* 1994;41:1017–1033.

Toxoplasmosis

Toxoplasma gondii, the etiologic agent of toxoplasmosis, is an obligate intracellular protozoon parasite capable of infecting a wide variety of animal hosts, including humans. The parasite reproduces by endogeny until the cell is full of organisms, at which time it bursts and the protozoa are released into the bloodstream. The release of organisms causes inflammation from associated antigens. If the cell does not burst, then the encysted organisms can remain viable inside the cell for as long as 25 years. The toxoplasma organism exists in three forms: the oocyst; tissue cyst; and tachyzoite, or proliferative form. The Greek word *toxon,* meaning bow, is suggested by the shape of the proliferative form.

Toxoplasmosis is highly prevalent in North America, where the percentage of patients with antibodies increases with age. Fewer than 10% of individuals under 5 years of age are immunologically positive, compared to about 60% in the 80-year-old group. Approximately 70% of the obstetric population has had no toxoplasmosis infection and is, therefore, at risk.

Cats are the definitive host for *T gondii,* and they are thought to be important in the transmission of the disease to humans and other animals by means of oocysts shed in their feces. The oocysts become infective after 1–4 days at room temperature and remain infective for up to 1 year. Humans usually become infected by ingesting the oocysts or tissue cysts of toxoplasma that reside in the brain and muscle tissue of infected animals. Eating raw or rare meat is a common route of transmission and is hazardous for seronegative pregnant women, who should also take sanitary precautions when cleaning up after cats.

A significant proportion of women who seroconvert during pregnancy will transmit the disease to their offspring. Approximately 1 per 1000 newborns is infected. Although only about 10% of congenitally infected neonates will have serious systemic disease, more than 80% of congenitally infected individuals not treated as infants develop chorioretinal lesions by adolescence. The earlier the disease is acquired in pregnancy, the greater the risk to the fetus. Toxoplasmosis in siblings of infected patients is rare.

Most cases of ocular toxoplasmosis seen in adults represent congenital infection. An acquired basis should not be seriously considered unless seroconversion of previously negative undiluted serum is demonstrated.

Toxoplasmosis has a particular affinity for the central nervous system, including the retina. Pathologically, the organism produces a localized necrotizing retinitis overlying a secondary choroiditis that may be necrotizing or granulomatous. Tissue cysts develop at the borders of lesions and may rupture, liberating proliferative organisms any time in life by mechanisms that are poorly understood.

In neonates the disease occurs in a continuous clinical spectrum ranging from no signs or findings to severe disease, including retinochoroiditis, abnormal cerebrospinal fluid, vomiting, diarrhea, anemia, convulsions, intracranial calcifications, jaundice, fever, hepatosplenomegaly, hydrocephalus, microcephalus, and retardation. Retinochoroiditis is found in about 80% of severely affected individuals. It is usually bilateral and frequently involves the macula (Fig XVII-1). Lesions sometimes develop after birth. Most retinal lesions appear inactive when first visualized. The typical inactive toxoplasmic lesion is a pigmented, flat scar. New lesions that develop near the scar are white and elevated, exuding cells and protein into the vitreous when active. Microphthalmos and cataracts are rare. Satellite foci are highly characteristic of toxoplasmosis.

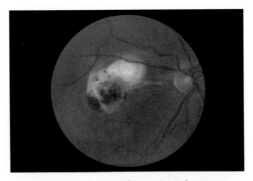

FIG XVII-1—Toxoplasmosis, right eye.

Diagnosis If congenital toxoplasmosis is suspected, a funduscopic examination and CT scan of the brain should be performed because chorioretinitis and cerebral calcifications are frequently present in symptomatic infants. The diagnosis can be confirmed by serologic tests for antibodies. Immunoglobulin G (IgG)–specific antibodies can be measured with the Sabin-Feldman dye test, the indirect immunofluorescent antibody test, or the enzyme-linked immunosorbent assay (ELISA). IgM-specific antibodies are measured with the double-sandwich IgM ELISA or the IgM immunosorbent agglutination assay (ISAGA).

Passively transferred maternal antibodies decrease steadily from the infant's serum and may be virtually absent 4–6 months after birth. IgM antibodies from the mother do not cross the placental barrier. Therefore, the finding of specific IgM antibodies in the newborn is usually diagnostic. Antibody titers in newborns tend to be high; titers in adults with ocular toxoplasmosis tend to be low. The presence of any antibody (even in undiluted serum) in an adult is significant, but it implies only previous contact with antigen. A negative titer is evidence against the diagnosis of ocular toxoplasmosis.

Tuberculosis and syphilis can closely mimic ocular toxoplasmosis. A serological test for syphilis, a chest x-ray, and tuberculin skin test are, therefore, advisable when toxoplasmosis is suspected. Additional conditions that can resemble ocular toxoplasmosis include nocardiosis, sporotrichosis, cryptococcosis, choroidal dystrophies, histoplasmosis, congenital hypertrophy of the retinal pigment epithelium, macular colobomas, traumatic scars, Best disease, and toxocariasis. In newborns the differential diagnosis of toxoplasmosis should rule out cytomegalic inclusion disease, herpetic infection, retinoblastoma, Coats disease, candidiasis, AIDS, and Aicardi syndrome.

Treatment Treatment of the acutely infected pregnant woman may prevent transmission of the infection to the fetus, resulting in a 50% decrease in the incidence of congenital infection. Data regarding the efficacy of postnatal treatment of infants with congenital toxoplasmosis appear promising. Treatment is recommended for infants younger than 10 weeks of age with congenital toxoplasmosis and for older patients with any active-appearing retinal lesion diagnosed as toxoplasmosis.

The mainstays of treatment for active disease are pyrimethamine, sulfadiazine, folinic acid, and steroids. The first two drugs are folic acid antagonists. Steroids have an anti-inflammatory effect but should not be given without antitoxoplasma drugs, because suppression of immune mechanisms may allow unchecked proliferation of tissue cysts. The clinical response to drug therapy is rarely dramatic. Because no drugs yet investigated can sterilize retinal tissue cysts, reactivation of ocular disease after treatment is always possible. Treatment schedules for children vary somewhat and current drug and dosage recommendations should be consulted. See Table XXIII-4 on p 261; see also discussion of toxoplasmosis in BCSC Section 9, *Intraocular Inflammation and Uveitis*. The drugs used to treat ocular toxoplasmosis can have substantial systemic side effects; consultation with a physician fully cognizant of their use and contraindications is therefore desirable.

Mets MB, Holfels E, Boyer KM, et al. Eye manifestations of congenital toxoplasmosis. *Am J Ophthalmol.* 1996;122:309–324.

Wilson CB, Remington JS. Toxoplasmosis. In: Feigin RD, Cherry JD, eds. *Textbook of Pediatric Infectious Diseases.* 4th ed. Philadelphia: Saunders; 1997.

Rubella

The rubella virus is the cause of rubella (German measles). The human is the only known host. The virus was first isolated in 1962, and rubella was made a reportable disease in the United States in 1966. Live virus vaccine introduced in 1969 has markedly reduced the frequency of this disease. The approximate incidence of infection in newborns in the United States is 1 per 100,000 live births. Before widespread immunization began, rubella was typically a childhood disease; antibodies are found in less than 20% of individuals under 4 years of age but more than 90% of individuals over 35 years of age. About 10%–15% of women in the childbearing years are susceptible to rubella. The disease is distributed worldwide, and epidemics have occurred regularly at intervals of 6–9 years.

The portal of entry for the rubella virus is thought to be the upper respiratory system. The earlier in pregnancy the infection is contracted, the greater the risk to the fetus. If the disease is acquired by the mother during the first 8 weeks of gestation, the fetus has a 50% chance of becoming infected, and infected infants have about an 80% chance of developing defects. The fetal infection rate drops to 28% for maternal infections acquired between weeks 21 and 24, and defects are uncommon in these infants. Maternal infections occurring even later rarely cause fetal infections or defects.

Congenitally infected infants may shed virus for months to years after birth. Virus shedding from the pharynx, urine, conjunctiva, feces, and lens aspirate during congenital cataract surgery constitutes a significant health hazard to seronegative pregnant women. Extreme caution must be practiced in situations of unavoidable contact between such women and infants.

Ocular pathology consists of

☐ Nuclear or total cataract

☐ Unilateral or bilateral mild microphthalmos

☐ Chronic nongranulomatous iridocyclitis with focal necrosis of the pigment epithelium of the ciliary body

☐ Irregular degeneration of the retinal pigment epithelium

Other ocular abnormalities may include transient corneal opacification, congenital glaucoma, and iris hypoplasia.

Diagnosis   Clinical and laboratory findings are both useful in diagnosis. The range of nonocular clinical findings in symptomatic, congenitally infected newborns is large, including growth retardation, hearing defects, hepatosplenomegaly, pulmonary artery hypoplasia, encephalitis, patent ductus arteriosus, interstitial pneumonitis, brain radiolucencies, and thrombocytopenia. Hearing defects, usually of the nerve deafness type, are thought to be the most common abnormality of congenital rubella syndrome. Microcephaly and mental retardation occur in the more severely affected patients.

The most common ocular abnormality in congenital rubella is cataract. The typical rubella cataract is most dense centrally without a sharp demarcation between the nuclear and peripheral opacifications. Microphthalmos is common but not severe. When both eyes are microphthalmic, the size reduction may be easily overlooked. Affected irides fail to dilate normally to mydriatics and cycloplegics. Congenital glaucoma and transient corneal opacifications occur, although it is rare for an eye to have both congenital glaucoma and congenital cataracts. Late compli-

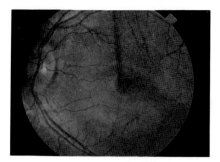

FIG XVII-2—Fundus photograph of 6-year-old with rubella syndrome (ERG normal).

cations include glaucoma and subretinal neovascularization. A diffuse salt-and-pepper retinopathy is often seen (Fig XVII-2). It may be central or peripheral and does not significantly affect vision. The differential diagnosis of salt-and-pepper retinopathy also includes syphilis, measles, varicella, and influenza.

Serological diagnosis is based upon the presence of IgG- or IgM-specific antibodies. The dominant fetal antibody present at birth in rubella-infected infants is maternal IgG. Therefore, positive fetal hemagglutination inhibition, fluorescent, complement fixation, and neutralizing antibody tests in newborns do not necessarily indicate fetal infection. However, IgM does not pass the placenta, and the finding of IgM antibody in cord sera does establish fetal infection. The virus itself is most frequently isolated from pharyngeal swabs and is present in many tissues of the body, including the lens of the eye. Lens aspirates may be sent for virus cultures when the diagnosis has not been established by other means.

Treatment   Rubella infection requires treatment tailored to individual pathology. Cataract surgery is often complicated because of inadequate mydriasis and microphthalmos. The postoperative course is usually characterized by moderate to severe inflammation with a marked tendency for pupillary membrane formation. Associated glaucoma may also require surgical management. Impaired language development secondary to hearing loss and mental retardation may require special education and hearing aids. The eradication of rubella now seems possible as a result of availability of live attenuated virus vaccine.

Griffith BP, Booss J. Neurologic infections of the fetus and newborn. *Neurol Clin.* 1994;12:541–564.

Wolff SM. The ocular manifestations of congenital rubella. *Trans Am Ophthalmol Soc.* 1972;70:577–614.

Zimmerman LE. Histopathologic basis for ocular manifestations of congenital rubella syndrome. *Am J Ophthalmol.* 1968;65:837–862.

Cytomegalic Inclusion Disease

The virus that causes cytomegalic inclusion disease (CID) is cytomegalovirus (CMV), which is thought to be relatively host-specific. It is a virus of the herpes family. Other members of this group include the herpes simplex virus, the varicella-zoster virus, and the Epstein-Barr virus. The human CMV is capable of infecting a wide variety of human tissues, including those of the central nervous system. Like the herpes simplex virus, CMV probably persists in human tissues for years.

The prevalence of antibody increases with age. From 60% to 90% of women of childbearing age have antibody. Neonatal infection may be a result of

□ Viremia in the mother from subclinical primary infection

□ Reinfection

□ Reactivation of latent maternal infection

Maternal viremia is thought to be the most common method of transmission to the fetus. Since at least 10% of the cervices of pregnant women harbor virus, transmission may occur during birth. It may also occur after birth from contact with oropharyngeal and breast fluids, but postnatal transmission routes have not been documented.

Prevention is not yet possible because of incomplete knowledge concerning epidemiology and pathogenesis. About 1% of all newborns are infected with cytomegalovirus, making this the most common congenital infection among humans. Symptoms are seen in approximately 10% of newborns with congenital CMV infection. The remaining 90% of newborns without clinical evidence of infection are asymptomatically infected, but 10%–15% of these children develop sequelae. Congenitally infected infants may excrete virus for several years after birth. Congenitally infected consecutive births have been reported but are uncommon.

Retinochoroiditis is the most frequent ocular abnormality in congenital CMV infection, involving about 15% of infants with symptomatic infection. Because progression of retinitis can occur, periodic ophthalmoscopic assessments, in addition to hearing and neurologic evaluation, are recommended. CMV retinopathy can occur, rarely, in children with AIDS. However, congenital infections of the eye have not been reported at birth as manifestations of in utero infections with human immunodeficiency virus.

Histologically, the infected retinal cells are enlarged (cytomegalic) and contain intranuclear and cytoplasmic inclusion bodies. Retinal necrosis may be a prominent feature. A secondary granulomatous choroiditis is usually present.

Diagnosis and treatment Diagnosis is based on clinical examination and confirmatory laboratory findings. In adults newly acquired generalized disease may mimic the infectious mononucleosis syndrome, but most cases are asymptomatic. Most adult patients with CMV retinitis are immunologically compromised, for example, because of AIDS or immunosuppression for renal transplantation.

In neonates the systemic disease has a broad spectrum of clinical signs. The most severely affected infants have fever, hepatosplenomegaly, jaundice, anemia, thrombocytopenia, petechial hemorrhages, encephalitis, pneumonitis, and sensorineural deafness. Abnormal EEGs, seizures, periventricular calcifications, psychomotor retardation, and microcephaly are common in these patients.

The ophthalmic manifestations of cytomegalovirus are highly variable and nonspecific. Strabismus, nystagmus, cataracts, microphthalmos, uveitis, optic disc

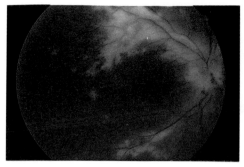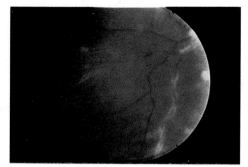

FIG XVII-3—Active CMV retinochoroiditis in a premature infant, right eye.

anomalies, optic nerve atrophy, anophthalmos, and Peters anomaly have all been reported. Retinochoroiditis occurs in about 15% of severely affected neonates (Fig XVII-3). The retinal lesions are usually multiple, located centrally or peripherally, and are commonly bilateral. White opacities are seen in acute infections. Retinal hemorrhages may be prominent; atrophy of the retinal pigment epithelium and retina develop later. Laboratory studies to rule out this disorder should probably be obtained for any newborn with congenital ocular defects not explained by other causes.

Diagnosis is made by recovery of virus from body fluids including urine, maternal cervical secretions, saliva, and aqueous humor. Methods for demonstrating the presence of the antibody include indirect hemagglutination, complement fixation, and immunofluorescent tests. The finding of IgM-specific antibody in the neonate is strong presumptive evidence of infection. Liver biopsies and studies of exfoliated cells in the urine may also be diagnostic. Periventricular calcifications may occasionally be found on CT scans of the brain. The differential diagnosis is similar to that of toxoplasmosis. Ganciclovir is currently the drug most frequently used for CMV retinitis in infants, but foscarnet can also be given.

Holland GN. An update on AIDS-related cytomegalovirus retinitis. In: *Focal Points: Clinical Modules for Ophthalmologists.* San Francisco: American Academy of Ophthalmology; 1991;9:5.

Nicholson DH. Cytomegalovirus infection of the retina. *Int Ophthalmol Clin.* 1975; 15:151–162.

Stagno S. Cytomegalovirus. In: Remington JS, Klein JO, eds. *Infectious Diseases of the Fetus and Newborn Infant.* 4th ed. Philadelphia: Saunders; 1995.

Herpes Simplex Virus

Herpes simplex virus (HSV) can persist for years in the infected host. HSV infections often recur despite the presence of neutralizing antibodies, and the mechanisms for this recurrence are not fully understood. Physical and emotional stress, ultraviolet irradiation, menstruation, and fever may trigger reappearance of eye, skin, or mouth lesions.

All members of the herpesvirus family have similar characteristics and infect a wide range of animals including humans. Intranuclear inclusions are present in infected cells. The two major types of herpesvirus are HSV-1 and HSV-2, which differ from one another antigenically, biologically, and epidemiologically. Most nongenital herpetic infections are associated with HSV-1, which is generally transmitted by close personal contact and frequently affects the eye, skin, and mouth. Most genital and neonatal herpetic infections are associated with HSV-2, which is commonly transmitted venereally.

The source of perinatal herpes simplex infection is usually maternal. In those cases with a known source, infection by way of the maternal cervix is most common. Often herpetic cervicitis has no signs or symptoms. The frequency of virus-positive cervices in late pregnancy is 1–4 per 1000. It is believed that most neonatal HSV infections are acquired at the time of delivery. In the presence of active genital disease, the risk of congenital infection is about 50% following vaginal delivery. Transplacental infection following maternal viremia is uncommon. Occasionally, a nongenital source of infection from the mother is the cause, or infection may be contracted, rarely, from nonmaternal sources.

In severely affected eyes histologic examination reveals a necrotizing retinitis. The choroidal response is secondary to the retinal inflammation. Intranuclear inclusions may be evident on light microscopy, and electron microscopy may reveal virus particles.

Asymptomatic neonatal herpetic infection is rare. Symptomatic disease in the neonate can develop at any time during the first month of life. The most common features of neonatal HSV infection are vesicular skin lesions, ulcerative mouth sores, and keratoconjunctivitis. Infection is localized to the central nervous system (CNS), skin, eyes, or oral cavity in one third of cases. It is disseminated in two thirds of cases, with or without CNS involvement. Disseminated forms of infection involve the liver, adrenal glands, and lungs (thus resembling bacterial sepsis). A 75%–80% mortality is associated with the disseminated form and a 50% mortality with disease that is localized to the CNS. The long-term prognosis for any infant who survives disseminated HSV infection is poor, primarily because of the likelihood of serious, permanent neurologic sequelae.

A small percentage of infants with neonatal herpes have eye involvement, including conjunctivitis, keratitis, retinochoroiditis, and cataracts. The keratitis can be epithelial (punctate, dendritic, or geographic) or stromal in type. Retinal involvement is typically severe and may show massive yellow-white exudates with severe vitreous reaction. Large or small localized lesions may also occur either centrally or peripherally. There is no recognized characteristic picture. Eye involvement may occur alone without other clinical manifestations.

Diagnosis   Diagnosis is best made by virus isolation from vesicular fluid, nose and eye swabs, buffy coat of the blood, and cerebrospinal fluid. The demonstration of intranuclear inclusions and multinucleated giant cells in skin along with conjunctival, oral, or genital lesions may be diagnostic. In most instances serological studies are not helpful during the acute phase of the disease. Rising titers, however, suggest infection.

Treatment   Therapy for disseminated herpes includes administration of acyclovir or vidarabine. Epithelial keratitis may be treated with topical antiviral agents (vidarabine, trifluridine, idoxuridine) or debridement. If the conjunctiva or eyelids are affected, topical antivirals are often used prophylactically, but this practice is controversial. Cesarean section has been advised for delivery in the presence of active genital herpes in the mother. The procedure should be performed no later than 4 hours after rupture of the amniotic membranes to limit retrograde infection of the fetus.

Bale JF Jr, Murph JR. Congenital infections and the nervous system. *Pediatr Clin North Am.* 1992;39:669–690.

Parrish CM. Herpes simplex virus eye disease. In: *Focal Points: Clinical Modules for Ophthalmologists.* San Francisco: American Academy of Ophthalmology; 1997;15:2.

Whitley RJ. Herpes simplex virus infections. In: Remington JS, Klein JO, eds. *Infectious Diseases of the Fetus and Newborn Infant.* 4th ed. Philadelphia: Saunders; 1995.

Syphilis

Syphilis is caused by the spirochete *Treponema pallidum,* and sexual contact is the usual route of transmission. All cases must be reported. Fetal infection occurs following maternal spirochetemia. The longer the mother has had syphilis, the lower the risk of transmitting the disease to her child. If the mother has contracted primary or secondary disease, about one half of her offspring will be infected. In cases of untreated late maternal syphilis (the most common form), about 70% of infants are healthy.

Clinical signs develop during the first few months of life. Congenitally acquired infection can lead to neonatal death or premature delivery. Congenital syphilis should be considered in premature births of unexplained cause, large placenta, persistent rhinitis, intractable rash, unexplained jaundice, hepatosplenomegaly, pneumonia, anemia, generalized lymphadenopathy, and metaphyseal abnormalities or periostitis on x-ray.

Chorioretinitis appearing as a salt-and-pepper granularity of the fundus occurs in some infants (Fig XVII-4). A pseudo–retinitis pigmentosa picture may be seen, and, rarely, anterior uveitis and/or glaucoma may develop. Widely spaced, peg-shaped teeth, eighth nerve deafness, and interstitial keratitis constitute *Hutchinson's triad.* Other manifestations include saddle nose, short maxilla, and linear scars, called *rhagades,* around body orifices.

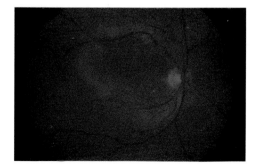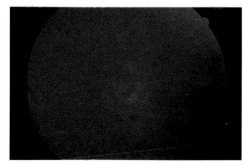

FIG XVII-4—Syphilitic retinitis and vasculitis, bilateral.

Diagnosis Darkfield examination of the exudate from skin lesions may be diagnostic. The VDRL (venereal disease research laboratory) and FTA-ABS (fluorescent treponemal antibody absorption) tests are the most widely performed serological tests. The FTA-ABS is more sensitive and specific. Neither of these tests differentiates between passively transferred maternal and actively produced fetal antibodies. IgM antibody does not cross the placenta. Thus, a positive IgM–FTA-ABS test is strong evidence of congenital infection.

Treatment Treatment of congenital syphilis is usually with parenteral aqueous penicillin G. Dosages, routes of administration, duration of treatment, or alternative antibiotics should be determined in consultation with an expert in pediatric infectious diseases.

Ingall D, Dobson SRM, Musher D. Syphilis. In: Remington JS, Klein JO, eds. *Diseases of the Fetus and Newborn Infant.* 4th ed. Philadelphia: Saunders; 1995.

Starling SP. Syphilis in infants and young children. *Pediatr Ann.* 1994;23:334–340.

Ophthalmia Neonatorum

Ophthalmia neonatorum, or neonatal conjunctivitis, is characterized by redness, swelling, and discharge from the conjunctiva during the newborn period. The prevalence is unknown, but the disease is no longer common in the United States and other industrialized countries.

Causes of ophthalmia neonatorum include chemical irritants; bacteria; chlamydiae; and, rarely, herpes simplex viruses. Almost any of the common bacterial pathogens can cause the condition. *Neisseria gonorrhoeae* is of particular concern because it can rapidly penetrate intact epithelial cells and cause corneal ulceration. Trachoma or inclusion conjunctivitis (TRIC) caused by chlamydiae is the most common conjunctival infection in neonates. Chlamydiae are obligate intracellular parasites susceptible to certain antibiotics (see Treatment and Prevention, below).

Gonococcal and TRIC infections are usually contracted from the maternal genital tract. Approximately 5%–10% of maternal cervices harbor gonococcus or TRIC agents. Routine cervical cultures should be obtained late in pregnancy, and positive cases should be treated to reduce the frequency of gonococcal ophthalmia neonatorum.

Corneal ulcers and endophthalmitis were common complications of gonorrheal ophthalmia neonatorum before the widespread use of silver nitrate prophylaxis and antibiotics. Rarely, TRIC infections can cause conjunctival scarring and micropannus formation, but these conditions do not result in visual loss. Herpetic eye disease in newborns can present as a blepharoconjunctivitis with typical herpetic vesicles on the eyelid margins and may extend, resulting in diffuse chorioretinitis and encephalitis. Each of these diseases can be associated with systemic illness. For example, gonorrheal ophthalmia resulting from premature rupture of the membranes can be associated with neonatal pulmonary infiltrates, meningitis, and sepsis. Septic arthritis may be present 1–4 weeks after birth.

Chlamydial pneumonia presents at 3–13 weeks of age. Not all patients with pneumonia have a clinically evident conjunctivitis, and not all patients with conjunctivitis develop pneumonia. However, a significant proportion of patients with chlamydial conjunctivitis contract pneumonia if untreated. Rhinitis, nasopharyngitis, tracheitis, and otitis media have also been associated with chlamydial infection.

Diagnosis

The incubation periods of the various forms of ophthalmia neonatorum are diverse and unreliable. However, chemical conjunctivitis quickly follows topical silver nitrate instillation. Even though *Neisseria* infection tends to be hyperacute with a purulent discharge and silver nitrate conjunctivitis tends to be mild with a watery discharge, it is not possible to establish etiology on the basis of clinical characteristics alone. The ocular manifestations of various causes of ophthalmia neonatorum overlap considerably, and laboratory studies are essential to establish the specific cause. Inadequate treatment can confuse and delay the correct diagnosis.

Diagnosis is made using stains and cultures. Gram stains of conjunctival exudate may reveal gram-negative intracellular diplococci, characteristic of *Neisseria*. Staphylococci and streptococci can also be identified tentatively from the Gram stain. Giemsa stains of conjunctival scrapings may demonstrate intracytoplasmic inclusions characteristic of TRIC infection. Fluorescent antibody-staining techniques and ELISA are available in some laboratories, and polymerase chain reaction (PCR) assays are being developed to offer rapid diagnosis of chlamydial infections. Cotton-tipped applicators moistened with liquid broth can be used to swab the conjunctival surfaces for culture on blood agar plates, chocolate agar plates, and Thayer-Martin media. The latter preparations should be warmed and then placed in a 37° C incubator with an enriched carbon dioxide environment.

Treatment and Prevention

Infants with probable *Neisseria* infection should be hospitalized. Treatment of nondisseminated infection, including conjunctivitis, is ceftriaxone (25–50 mg/kg IV or IM, not to exceed 125 mg) given once. Disseminated infections require 10–14 days of parenteral antibiotic treatment. Infants with gonococcal conjunctivitis should have their eyes irrigated with normal saline at frequent intervals until the discharge is eliminated. Topical antibiotics provide no added therapeutic benefit. If the cornea is involved, 0.5% atropine drops should be instilled once or twice daily. A serological test for syphilis is advisable, and public health reporting should be completed to assure treatment of the mother and possible contacts.

Chlamydial conjunctivitis in infants is treated with oral erythromycin (50 mg/kg/day in four divided doses) for 14 days. For infants who do not tolerate erythromycin, sulfonamides may be used after the immediate neonatal period. Topical treatment of chlamydial conjunctivitis in infants is unnecessary and will not adequately address possible associated pneumonitis. The parents should also be treated. Other organisms should be treated based on culture results and organism sensitivity to antibiotics.

Karl Sigmund Franz Credé introduced the use of 2% silver nitrate eyedrops in 1881. The 1% solution presently in widespread use has significantly reduced the incidence of gonorrheal ophthalmia neonatorum, but it is not always effective. Additionally, silver nitrate is not effective against TRIC infections. Therefore, tetracycline ointment or erythromycin ointment is more commonly used for prophylaxis after birth.

Povidone-iodine 2.5% ophthalmic solution may prove to be the ideal prophylactic agent because of its low cost and minimal toxicity and the lack of occurrence of bacterial resistance to it. However, widespread use of antibiotic or povidone-iodine prophylaxis may decrease the incidence of chlamydial conjunctivitis but fail

Table XVII-1

Causes of Conjunctival Inflammation in Children

Infectious conjunctivitis
  Bacterial
  Viral
  Chlamydial

Blepharoconjunctivitis

Allergic conjunctivitis

Trauma

Foreign body

Drug, toxin, or chemical reaction

Nasolacrimal duct obstruction

Iritis

Episcleritis or scleritis

to affect the incidence of pneumonitis and may actually increase its severity indirectly. Although conjunctivitis is not present in all infants who have chlamydial pneumonitis, it is often the clinical sign that brings the child to medical attention. There is some suspicion that chlamydial pneumonitis may have long-term effects on pulmonary function. Possibly, then, infections presenting after a prolonged period because the clinical sign of conjunctivitis was lacking could result in further pulmonary compromise.

Holland GN. Infectious diseases. In: Isenberg SJ, ed. *The Eye in Infancy.* 2nd ed. St Louis: Mosby; 1994:493–504.

O'Hara MA. Ophthalmia neonatorum. *Pediatr Clin North Am.* 1993;40:715–725.

Conjunctivitis

A list of common causes of conjunctival inflammation, or red eye, in infants and children is given in Table XVII-1. The majority of cases of acute conjunctivitis in children are bacterial in origin. About 20% of cases are caused by a virus. BCSC Section 8, *External Disease and Cornea,* discusses conjunctivitis in detail.

Bacterial Conjunctivitis

Common clinical findings in children with bacterial or viral conjunctivitis are burning, stinging, foreign body sensation, ocular discharge, and matting of the eyelids. Symptoms and signs may present either unilaterally or bilaterally. The discharge may be serous, mucoid, or mucopurulent.

    Haemophilus influenzae and *Streptococcus pneumoniae (pneumococcus)* are the most frequent causes of acute conjunctivitis in children. Children with conjunctivitis caused by these organisms often have morning crusting and difficulty opening the eyelids. *Staphylococcus aureus* is a less common cause of acute conjunctivitis in

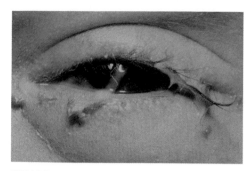

FIG XVII-5—*Neisseria gonorrhoeae* conjunctivitis.

children than in adults. It can produce a chronic conjunctivitis with a phlyctenular keratitis. *Neisseria gonorrhoeae* causes a hyperacute, profusely purulent conjunctivitis (Fig XVII-5). See the section on ophthalmia neonatorum, pp 182–184. The incidence of bacterial conjunctivitis is higher in winter months, and the patient often has an associated upper respiratory tract infection. Other organisms causing conjunctivitis in children include *Streptococcus pyogenes, Moraxella* species, gram-negative rods (e.g., *Pseudomonas* and *Escherichia coli*), *N meningitidis, N catarrhalis,* and *H aegyptius.*

Diagnosis A Gram stain may be useful in differentiating bacterial causes of conjunctivitis from viral and allergic causes. The presence of numerous polymorphonuclear leukocytes along with gram-positive cocci in clusters or gram-negative pleomorphic rods would be highly suggestive of infection with *S pneumoniae* or *H influenzae,* respectively. A Giemsa stain of a conjunctival scraping may be useful in diagnosing cases of chronic conjunctivitis, especially if chlamydial infection or allergy are being considered.

A culture is not required in mild cases of suspected bacterial conjunctivitis in healthy children. Conjunctival cultures should be obtained in patients who do not respond to treatment and in cases with severe inflammation, chronic or recurrent infection, or atypical conjunctival appearance. See p 183 for recommended culture techniques and media.

Treatment Although most cases of bacterial conjunctivitis are self-limited, treatment is nonetheless indicated to shorten the course of the infection, thereby making the patient more comfortable and less likely to infect others. Topical antibiotic treatment should be continued for several days after symptoms have subsided. A drop preparation is generally preferred to an ointment in children because of easier installation.

Because cultures are not routinely performed, broad-spectrum antibiotics are desirable. Trimethoprim/polymyxin B (Polytrim) is probably the most frequently prescribed antibiotic drop for suspected bacterial conjunctivitis. It has a good spectrum of activity for the common pathogens of bacterial conjunctivitis in children and is well tolerated. Sulfacetamide ophthalmic preparations have the advantage of being less expensive but tend to sting more. Topical aminoglycoside preparations should be reserved for more serious ocular infections. Topical fluoroquinolones available for children older than 1 year of age have a good spectrum of activity against both gram-positive and gram-negative organisms, but they should be reserved for more serious infections such as keratoconjunctivitis. Topical steroid or antibiotic-corticosteroid combinations should be avoided for initial therapy because of the risk of potentiating the infection. BCSC Section 2, *Fundamentals and Principles of Ophthalmology,* discusses these medications and others in depth in Part 5, Pharmacology.

Viral Conjunctivitis

Epidemic keratoconjunctivitis This infection is an acute follicular conjunctivitis that is usually unilateral at onset and associated with preauricular lymphadenopathy. The infection is commonly caused by adenovirus type 8, 11, or 19. Initial complaints are foreign body sensation and periorbital pain. A diffuse superficial keratitis is followed by focal epithelial lesions that stain. After 11–15 days subepithelial opacities begin to form under the focal epithelial infiltrates. The epithelial component fades by day 30, but the subepithelial opacities may linger for 3 months to 2 years. In severe infections, particularly in infants, a conjunctival membrane and marked swelling of the eyelids occur that must be differentiated from orbital or preseptal cellulitis (see next section).

The infection is easily transmitted and occurs in epidemic outbreaks. Infected children may need to be kept out of school or child care for up to 2 weeks. Medical personnel who become infected should be excluded from ophthalmic examination areas for at least 2 weeks, and isolation areas should be designated for examination of patients known to have adenoviral infections.

Diagnosis is confirmed by isolation of the agent or increased antibody titer to the specific adenovirus type. The organism can be recovered from the eyes and throat for 2 weeks after onset, demonstrating that patients are infectious during this period. Complications include persistent subepithelial opacities and conjunctival scar formation. Treatment is supportive. Topical steroids administered 3–4 times daily may be useful in reducing symptoms but probably do not alter the course of the disease. Steroid use in adenovirus infections is controversial and seldom considered in children.

Pharyngeal conjunctival fever This common ocular adenovirus infection consists of pharyngitis, fever, and a nonpurulent follicular conjunctivitis. The usual etiology is adenovirus, most commonly type 3. Early signs include foreign body sensation, hyperemia and edema of the conjunctiva with marked tearing, and mild sore throat. Several days later, a bilateral, nontender preauricular lymphadenopathy occurs with eyelid edema and follicular conjunctivitis. Subconjunctival hemorrhages and, rarely, lesions of the cornea may occur. Spontaneous resolution commonly occurs in 2–3 weeks. Treatment is supportive. Antivirals and steroids do not alter the natural course of the disease.

Herpes simplex conjunctivitis This form usually occurs with primary infection by the organism and commonly has an associated herpetic eyelid lesion. Dendritic keratitis may occur as a manifestation of primary or recurrent viral infection. Herpetic blepharoconjunctivitis often occurs on a recurrent basis. Herpetic follicular conjunctivitis usually spares the cornea but may be associated with punctate keratitis or

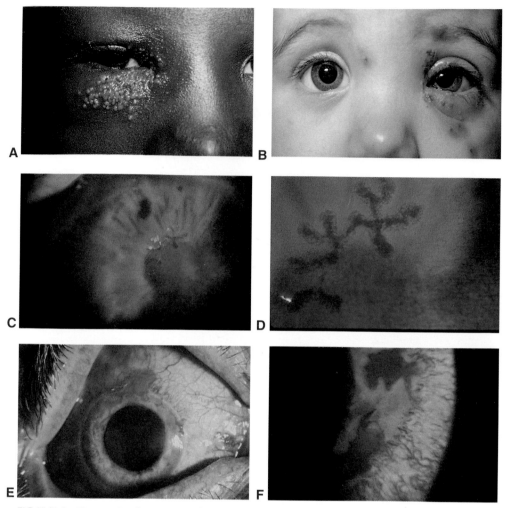

FIG XVII-6—Herpes simplex. *A,* Vesicular lesions, right lower eyelid. *B,* Medial canthal distribution, left eye. *C and D,* Dendritic keratitis demonstrated by stain with rose bengal solution. *E and F,* Dendritic keratoconjunctivitis.

a dendritic ulcer (Fig XVII-6). Most cases are caused by herpes simplex type 1, although type 2 (genital) virus occurs in newborns. Clinically, types 1 and 2 are similar. Treatment includes corneal debridement and/or topical antiviral agents (trifluridine, vidarabine, or idoxuridine).

Herpes zoster   Children are seldom affected by herpes zoster, which rarely produces conjunctivitis. Vesicular lesions may erupt on the periorbital skin with subsequent ocular involvement (Fig XVII-7). Treatment includes steroids for the inflammation and for iritis if present. Systemic acyclovir is currently recommended by

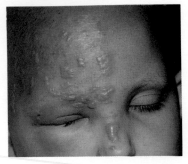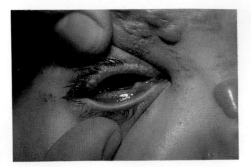

FIG XVII-7—Herpes zoster.

pediatric infectious disease specialists for infants and children with herpes zoster ophthalmicus.

Infectious mononucleosis The etiology of this acute systemic disease is Epstein-Barr virus. The disease usually occurs between ages 15 and 30 years and is benign and self-limited. Findings include fever, widespread lymphadenopathy, pharyngitis, hepatic involvement, and the presence of atypical lymphocytes and heterophil antibodies in the circulating blood. Conjunctivitis occurs in a very high percentage of cases. Treatment is supportive including bed rest, antipyretics, analgesics, and cool compresses to the eyes.

Influenza virus Acute conjunctivitis with superficial punctate or interstitial keratitis, chemosis, and secondary bacterial infection may be caused by influenza virus type A, B, or C. The clinical manifestations include headache, fever, malaise, myalgias, nasal congestion, nausea, cough, and pharyngitis. Treatment is supportive with topical antibiotics to prevent secondary infection.

Mumps virus An acute viremia may lead to ocular involvement. The conjunctival manifestations are chemosis, follicular or papillary conjunctivitis, hyperemia, and subconjunctival hemorrhages. Treatment is supportive with topical antibiotics to prevent secondary bacterial infection.

Rubeola This acute, contagious febrile illness affects primarily young, school-age children. Etiology is a paramyxovirus. Clinical manifestations include maculopapular rash, keratoconjunctivitis, and inflammation of the respiratory tract. Treatment includes antipyretics, analgesics, and cool compresses on the eyelids.

Varicella (chickenpox) This contagious viral exanthem of childhood causes fever and vesicular eruptions of skin and mucous membranes. The etiology is varicella-zoster virus. Clinical manifestations include fever and skin lesions, and ocular involvement during primary childhood varicella is uncommon. Conjunctival vesicles or ulcerations and internal ophthalmoplegia can occur (Fig XVII-8). The cornea may be involved with a dendritic ulcer, opacification, punctate epithelial keratitis, or interstitial keratitis.

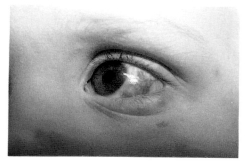

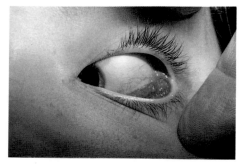

FIG XVII-8—Varicella conjunctivitis, left eye.

FIG XVII-9—Parinaud oculoglandular syndrome, left eye.

Treatment is symptomatic. Topical steroids are contraindicated except for late nonulcerative interstitial keratitis. Topical antibiotics may prevent secondary infection. Intravenous or oral acyclovir may be considered in the treatment of immunocompromised children with chickenpox but should be administered under the direction of an expert in pediatric infectious diseases.

Other Types of Conjunctivitis

Parinaud oculoglandular syndrome   This unilateral granulomatous follicular conjunctivitis is associated with preauricular and submandibular lymphadenopathy (Fig XVII-9). The etiology is usually unknown but has been associated with cat-scratch disease. The cat-scratch bacillus has now been isolated. Other possibilities include *Francisella tularensis, Yersinia pseudotuberculosis* (formerly *Pasteurella pseudotuberculosis), Mycobacterium tuberculosis, M leprae, Treponema pallidum,* and lymphogranuloma venereum.

The pathology includes focal granulomatous lesions in the conjunctiva surrounded by follicles with yellow spots in the center. Clinical manifestations include the granulomas and follicular lesions of the conjunctiva with mucopurulent discharges and swelling. The preauricular lymphadenopathy may be extensive with associated cervical and submandibular lymphadenopathy. The patient usually has fever, malaise, and a history of exposure to animals, especially cats. Diagnosis is confirmed by conjunctival biopsy, which reveals a granuloma with epithelioid cells. Treatment is supportive with antibodies directed at the specific etiologic agent.

Trachoma   Except in areas of the South and on Indian reservations trachoma is uncommon in the United States. Most cases are mild. Clinical manifestations include acute purulent conjunctivitis, follicles, papillary hypertrophy, vascularization of the cornea, and progressive cicatricial changes of the cornea and conjunctiva. Diagnosis is made from corneal scrapings, which reveal cytoplasmic inclusion bodies. Expressed follicle material demonstrates large macrophages and lymphoblasts. Treatment includes topical and/or systemic sulfonamides, erythromycin, and tetracyclines.

Cellulitis

Orbital cellulitis and preseptal cellulitis are both usually more rapidly progressive and more severe in children than in adults. See also BCSC Section 7, *Orbit, Eyelids, and Lacrimal System.*

Impetigo

Impetigo secondary to *S aureus* or group A *Streptococcus pyogenes* is common in children under 6 years of age. The infection may occur in healthy patients but is more common in conditions compromised by poor hygiene. Lesions start as small red maculae that rapidly progress to serous vesicles surrounded by erythema. The ocular adnexa may become markedly erythematous with edema of the preseptal spaces, but no lesions appear on the tarsal or bulbar conjunctiva. Serous material is released from the vesicles, and satellite lesions develop by autoinoculation. Impetigo is highly contagious in infants and must be differentiated from herpes simplex and varicella. Topical antibiotic ointments such as bacitracin may be useful in limiting person-to-person spread of impetigo, but with multiple lesions or involvement of multiple family members, oral antibiotics effective against both *S aureus* and group A streptococci should be given and continued for 10 days to prevent secondary complications.

Preseptal Cellulitis

Preseptal cellulitis, a common infection in children, is an inflammatory process involving the tissues anterior to the orbital septum. Infections may be secondary to trauma or a minor skin abrasion, or they may spread from contiguous structures such as the paranasal sinuses. The cellulitis is frequently associated with upper respiratory tract infections in which inflammatory infiltration of the preseptal area occurs. In severe cases edema and erythema may cause necrosis.

Eyelid edema may extend into the eyebrow and forehead. The periorbital skin becomes taut and inflamed, and edema may appear on the contralateral eyelids. Proptosis is not a typical feature of preseptal cellulitis, and the globe remains normal. Full ocular motility and absence of pain on eye movement distinguish preseptal from orbital cellulitis. *Staphylococcus aureus* is the most common cause for these infections, often following trauma. *Streptococcus pneumoniae* is also a common cause, and its presentation is very similar to *S aureus.*

Haemophilus influenzae cellulitis and conjunctivitis occur most commonly in children between the ages of 6 and 36 months. Since HiB vaccination for *H influenzae* infection began in 1990, the incidence of cellulitis and conjunctivitis caused by this organism has declined dramatically. Fever, irritability, upper respiratory tract infection, and lethargy are the early indications of *H influenzae* infection. A distinct pattern of preseptal cellulitis—a sharply demarcated, reddish purple discoloration of the involved area—distinguishes this entity from other forms of bacterial cellulitis. Profound edema of the upper and lower eyelids may extend into the cheek, and the eyelids may have to be separated by retractors to allow examination of the globe. Chemosis, conjunctival papillary hyperemia, corneal haze, and mucopurulent discharge may also be present. Patients have leukocytosis and paranasal sinusitis; secondary inflammation of the orbit may occur. *H influenzae* is diagnosed by Gram stain and cultures taken from the conjunctiva, nasopharynx, and blood.

Pediatric consultation is important in the management of *H influenzae* cellulitis because a secondary meningitis can occur. Hospitalization is required, and appropriate antibiotics should be given intravenously. Incision and drainage of the preseptal space may be required in severe cases. Complications rarely follow mild preseptal cellulitis.

Orbital Cellulitis

Orbital cellulitis is an infection of the orbit that involves the tissues posterior to the orbital septum. It commonly occurs in association with ethmoid or frontal sinusitis and can also follow penetrating injuries of the orbit. A retained foreign body can trigger orbital cellulitis months after the initial injury. The introduction of CT technology has enabled researchers to recognize *orbital subperiosteal abscess* as a specific entity within the general clinical setting of orbital cellulitis. A subperiosteal abscess occurs as a result of the accumulation of purulent material between the periorbita and the orbital bones, usually as a complication of bacterial sinusitis.

The etiologic agents most commonly responsible for orbital cellulitis vary with age. In general, children younger than 9 years have infections caused by a single, aerobic pathogen. Children older than 9 years may have complex infections with multiple pathogens, both aerobic and anaerobic. *S aureus* and gram-negative bacilli are most common in the neonate. In children between 6 months and 5 years of age *H influenzae* and *Streptococcus pneumoniae* are the most common pathogens, followed by other gram-positive cocci. In older children and adults *S aureus*, *Streptococcus pyogenes, Streptococcus pneumoniae*, and various anaerobic species are common pathogens. Gram-negative organisms are found primarily in immunosuppressed patients.

Diagnosis   Early signs and symptoms of orbital cellulitis include lethargy, fever, eyelid edema, rhinorrhea, headache, orbital pain, and tenderness on palpation. The nasal mucosa becomes hyperemic with a purulent nasal discharge. Increased venous congestion may cause elevated intraocular pressure (IOP). Proptosis, downward and lateral displacement of the globe, and limited ocular rotations suggest subperiosteal abscess formation.

Preseptal cellulitis is distinguished from orbital cellulitis by cutaneous involvement with normal ocular motility and absence of proptosis. Retinoblastoma, metastatic orbital tumor, leukemia, and rhabdomyosarcoma can produce similar pictures (see chapter XXVI). Inflammatory pseudotumor of the orbit rarely produces the marked degree of orbital edema, chemosis, and proptosis characteristic of orbital cellulitis.

Paranasal sinusitis is the most common cause of bacterial orbital cellulitis (Fig XVII-10). In children under 10 years of age the ethmoid sinuses are most frequently involved. In the presence of orbital cellulitis a CT scan is indicated to determine the presence and extent of sinusitis and subperiosteal abscess as well as to rule out a foreign body in a patient with a history of trauma (Fig XVII-11).

Complications of orbital cellulitis include *cavernous sinus thrombosis,* or *intracranial extension* (subdural or brain abscesses, meningitis, periosteal abscess), which may result in death. Cavernous sinus thrombosis can be difficult to distinguish from simple orbital cellulitis. Paralysis of eye movement in cavernous sinus thrombosis is often out of proportion to the degree of proptosis. Pain on motion and tenderness to palpation are absent. Decreased sensation along the maxillary division of cranial nerve V (trigeminal) is helpful for diagnosis. Bilateral involvement is virtually diagnostic of cavernous sinus thrombosis.

Other complications of orbital cellulitis include corneal exposure with secondary ulcerative keratitis, neurotropic keratitis, secondary glaucoma, septic uveitis

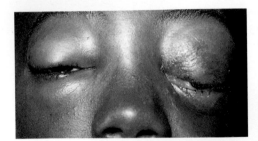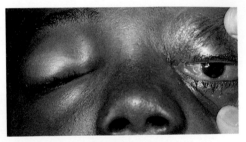

FIG XVII-10—Orbital cellulitis secondary to pansinusitis.

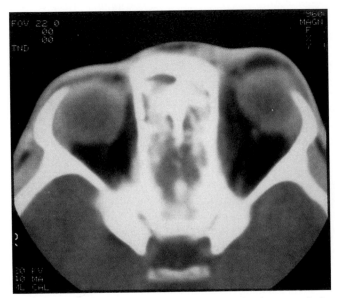

FIG XVII-11—Axial CT image showing a medial subperiosteal abscess of the left orbit associated with ethmoid sinusitis.

or retinitis, exudative retinal detachment, optic nerve edema, inflammatory neuritis, infectious neuritis, central retinal artery occlusion, and panophthalmitis.

Treatment Orbital cellulitis in children is a potentially fatal emergency that requires hospitalization and treatment with intravenous broad-spectrum antibiotics. An orbital CT scan should be performed, and Gram stain and culture of discharge and blood cultures should also be done. If associated sinusitis is present, an otolaryngologist should be consulted. To monitor the patient for disease progression that could require surgical intervention, visual acuity and pupillary function should be assessed every 6 hours.

Currently acceptable anitibiotic regimens, based on the pathogens expected in each age group, would include single-drug therapy with ceftriaxone sodium for children under 9 years of age and ceftriaxone sodium with clindamycin phosphate for children 9 years of age and older because of the increasing prevalence of anaerobes. Other possible combinations include ampicillin sodium/sulbactam sodium or ticarcillin disodium/clavulanate potassium. Because of a changing inventory of available drugs, consultation with a pediatric infectious disease specialist should be considered.

Emergency drainage of a subperiosteal abscess is indicated for a patient of any age with decreased vision or an afferent pupillary defect. Even in the absence of optic nerve dysfunction, surgical drainage may be required for clinical deterioration despite 48 hours of intravenous antibiotics or to relieve significant discomfort.

The patients who tend to do best with medical management alone are those younger than 9 years who have a medial subperiosteal abscess of modest size and no intracranial or frontal sinus involvement.

Harris GJ. Subperiosteal abscess of the orbit. Age as a factor in the bacteriology and response to treatment. *Ophthalmology.* 1994;101:585–595.

Lessner A, Stern GA. Preseptal and orbital cellulitis. *Infect Dis Clin North Am.* 1992; 6:933–952.

Related conditions *Maxillary osteomyelitis* is a rare condition of early infancy. Infection spreads from the nose into the tooth buds with unilateral erythema and edema of the eyelids, cheek, and nose. Infection may spread and cause orbital cellulitis.

Fungal orbital cellulitis (mucormycosis) occurs most frequently in patients with ketoacidosis or severe immunosuppression. The infection causes thrombosing vasculitis with ischemic necrosis of involved tissue (Fig XVII-12). Cranial nerves are often involved, and extension into the central nervous system often occurs. Smears and biopsy of the involved tissues reveal the fungal organisms. Treatment includes debridement of necrotic and infected tissue plus administration of amphotericin. Predisposing factors such as metabolic acidosis should be controlled.

Ocular Allergy

Allergic ocular disease is a common problem in children, often occurring in association with asthma, allergic rhinitis, and atopic dermatitis. Marked itching and bilateral conjunctival inflammation of a chronic, recurrent, and possibly seasonal nature are hallmarks of external ocular disease of allergic origin. Other signs and symptoms may be nonspecific and include tearing, stinging, burning, and photophobia. Three specific types of ocular allergy are discussed below: seasonal allergic conjunctivitis, vernal keratoconjunctivitis, and atopic keratoconjunctivitis.

Seasonal Allergic Conjunctivitis (SAC)

A Type I anaphylactic hypersensitivity reaction, SAC accounts for more than 50% of cases of allergic conjunctivitis. It occurs when a sensitized patient encounters an antigen. Patients tend to be under 30 years old and often have a history of hay fever, eczema, or other atopic disease. The conjunctiva may have a milky, pale appearance, and a watery or mucoid discharge is often present. There may be follicles and

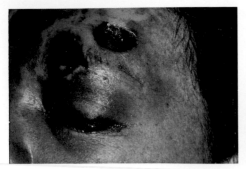

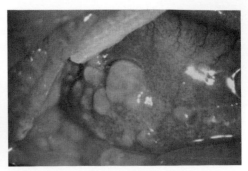

FIG XVII-12—Mucormycosis, left orbit.

FIG XVII-13—Palpebral vernal keratoconjunctivitis, upper eyelid.

mild papillary hypertrophy of the tarsal conjunctiva. Conjunctival scrapings demonstrate eosinophils.

Treatment of SAC may involve nondrug therapy such as environmental measures (air conditioning and electronic air filters to reduce antigen load) and cool compresses to the eyes. Pharmacotherapy includes oral antihistamines such as chlorpheniramine, terfenadine, and loratadine. The latter two are second-generation H_1 receptor antagonists and may cause less drowsiness than other antihistamines because they do not cross blood–brain barriers to any extent. Topical antihistamine-vasoconstrictor combinations are also useful in relieving itching and conjunctival injection. A new antihistamine is levocabastin, a topical H_1 receptor antagonist, which has been shown to be more potent than older preparations. Ketorolac, a topical nonsteroidal anti-inflammatory drug (NSAID), has also demonstrated effectiveness in the treatment of SAC. Finally, mast-cell inhibitors also reduce signs and symptoms of SAC. Cromolyn sodium, the prototype mast-cell stabilizer, is variously effective in the treatment of SAC. Lodoxamide is more potent than cromolyn sodium in the treatment of SAC but is also more expensive.

Vernal Keratoconjunctivitis

The palpebral form of vernal keratoconjunctivitis (VKC) is a recurrent bilateral inflammation of the conjunctiva that occurs on a seasonal basis during spring and summer. This common, self-limiting disease has a wide geographical incidence and occurs most frequently in males between the ages of 6 and 20 years. The exact etiology is unknown but is thought to be an allergic diathesis.

The chief pathologic findings include overgrowth of the subconjunctival tissues in the substantia propria. The tissue is infiltrated with lymphocytes, plasma cells, and eosinophils. With progression large numbers of cells accumulate, forming nodules of tissue that project from the tarsal plate. New blood vessels are formed, producing giant papillae.

Clinically, the palpebral form of VKC preferentially affects the tarsal conjunctiva of the upper eyelid (Fig XVII-13). Changes in the lower eyelid are rare and slight.

In the early stages the eye may be diffusely injected with little discharge, and the conjunctiva appears milky. The most prominent features are photophobia and intense itching. There may be no progression beyond this stage. However, papillae may multiply, covering the tarsal area with a mosaic of flat papules. The conjunctiva is then covered with a milky veil.

The discharge is characteristically thick, ropy, and dirty white. It contains epithelial cells, leukocytes, and large numbers of eosinophils. VKC must be distinguished from trachoma, SAC, and contact lens–induced giant papillary conjunctivitis. VKC differs from trachoma in the following ways:

□ True follicles with germinal centers are rare

□ Eosinophils are numerous

□ Scarring of the tarsus is uncommon; chemosis is common in SAC

Contact lens–induced *giant papillary conjunctivitis (GPC),* which may develop in wearers of either hard or soft contact lenses, can resemble VKC. However, GPC has fewer eosinophils and far less itching and mucus. See also BCSC Section 8, *External Disease and Cornea.*

The *limbal,* or *bulbar,* form of VKC is also bilateral and seasonal, with etiology and pathogenesis similar to the palpebral disease. Intense itching is the most constant clinical feature. The earliest changes are commonly thickening and opacification of the conjunctiva at the limbus, usually most marked at the upper margin of the cornea. The discrete limbal nodules that appear in this thickened conjunctiva are gray, jellylike, elevated lumps with vascular cores. They may increase in number and become confluent. The nodules persist as long as the seasonal exacerbation of the disease lasts. A whitish Trantas dot may occur in the raised lesion, and this pit is filled with eosinophils. In severe cases the limbal lesions spread onto the cornea, forming a pannuslike membrane.

Diagnosis is made clinically. Corneal or conjunctival scrapings reveal numerous eosinophils and eosinophilic granules. A single limbal vernal lesion may simulate a phlyctenule.

Corneal vernal disease is often seen in association with palpebral vernal disease and may be present early in the disorder. Corneal findings are often associated with symptoms such as irritation, itching, increased tearing, foreign body sensation, and marked photophobia. Corneal vernal disease is less common than the palpebral and limbal forms. The superficial punctate keratitis that occurs may stain with fluorescein or rose bengal. The keratitis preferentially affects the upper segment of the cornea, sparing the periphery. In severe cases the entire cornea may appear to be "dusted with flour." Vernal disease of the cornea is distinguished from other forms of keratitis by its association with vernal palpebral conjunctivitis.

Vernal ulcerative keratitis is rare, but it can complicate epithelial involvement. The ulceration is usually transversely oval and located in the upper part of the cornea. At first the ulcer is shallow and nonvascularized, with a whitened rough area of epithelium around the edges and gray opacification of the exposed Bowman's membrane. The ulcer is indolent, with a varying degree of infiltration of adjacent stroma.

Although VKC has no specific treatment, it can be controlled with topical steroids. The lowest concentration for the least amount of time should be used. Cold compresses and oral antihistamines may also be helpful. The prognosis for recovery is excellent, although the course may last several years. Topical cromolyn sodium will sometimes eliminate the need for topical steroids or allow a reduction in the dose, and lodoxamide appears to be very effective in VKC. The NSAID suprofen has also been used successfully in VKC. Immunotherapy with cyclosporine has been successful in patients with VKC uncontrolled with topical steroids and cromolyn sodium. A bandage lens may be required in cases with severe corneal involvement.

Atopic Keratoconjunctivitis

This form of allergic conjunctivitis is a more severe one that occurs most often in the teenage years. This is a more vision-threatening disease than SAC or VKC. Patients have eczematoid eyelid changes, papillary hypertrophy of the tarsal conjunctiva, and corneal vascularization and scarring. Cataracts may occur. Treatment regimens involve the same drugs used for VKC.

el-Defrawy S, Jackson WB. New directions in therapy for ocular allergy. *Int Ophthalmol Clin.* 1996;36:25–44.

Stevens-Johnson Syndrome (Erythema Multiforme)

Erythema multiforme is an acute inflammatory polymorphic disease affecting skin and mucous membranes. All ages may be affected, and the incidence is equal in both sexes. This is a severe disease with a 5%–15% mortality rate. Ocular involvement, which occurs in as many as half of the patients, varies from a mild mucopurulent conjunctivitis to severe perforating corneal ulcers. Unfortunately, in occasional patients with severe late-phase corneal complication, such as ulceration, vascularization, and perforation, blindness may ensue.

This syndrome has been associated with various bacterial, viral, mycotic, and protozoon infections. Vaccines, collagen diseases, and many drugs have also been implicated. The pathogenesis consists of angiitis leading to erythematous lesions that become edematous or bullous and darken, leaving concentric rings in a target shape. When bullae are present, they are subepidermal and without acantholysis.

Clinical manifestations range from mild to severe. A prodrome of chills is followed by pharyngitis, headache, tachypnea, and tachycardia. In several days bullous mucosal lesions develop, especially in the oropharynx. These lesions rupture and ulcerate and become covered by gray-white membranes and a hemorrhagic crust.

Ocular involvement in Stevens-Johnson syndrome begins with edema, erythema, and encrustation of the eyelids. The palpebral conjunctiva becomes hyperemic, and distinct vesicles or bullae may occur. In many instances a concomitant conjunctivitis appears characterized by watery discharge with mucoid strands (Fig XVII-14). Secondary infection, most commonly with *Staphylococcus* species, may develop. In severe cases a membranous or pseudomembranous conjunctivitis may occur as a result of coalescence of fibrin and necrotic cellular debris. Symblepharon formation may occur with severe pseudomembranous conjunctivitis. Primary corneal involvement and iritis are rare ocular manifestations of Stevens-Johnson syndrome.

Late ocular complications occur in about 20% of patients and include structural anomalies of eyelid position (ectropion and entropion), trichiasis, and symblepharon. Dry eye syndrome may also occur as a result of deficiencies in the tear film, either the aqueous layer from scarring of lacrimal duct orifices or, more commonly, the mucin layer from destruction of the conjunctival goblet cells.

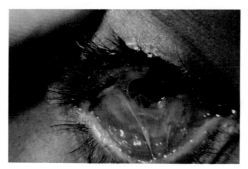

FIG XVII-14—Stevens-Johnson syndrome. Early involvement of conjunctiva, right eye.

Treatment

Early intervention is important in preventing the late ocular complications of Stevens-Johnson syndrome. Systemic therapy with corticosteroids is controversial. Antiviral treatment for cases associated with herpes simplex infection may be required. A discussion of systemic treatment is beyond the scope of this book. A dermatologist and pediatric infectious disease expert should be consulted.

Local measures should be instituted early in the course of the disease. Ocular lubrication with artificial tears and ointments (preferably preservative-free) should be performed regularly. Under topical anesthesia the superior and inferior fornices should be inspected and debrided daily. Lysis of symblepharon with a glass rod can be performed, but this may be ineffective. A symblepharon ring can be useful in severe cases in cooperative patients. Surveillance cultures for microbial infection should be performed as needed. See also BCSC Section 8, *External Disease and Cornea.*

Wilkins J, Morrison L, White CR Jr. Oculocutaneous manifestations of the erythema multiforme/Stevens-Johnson syndrome/toxic epidermal necrolysis spectrum. *Dermatol Clin.* 1992;10:571–582.

Kawasaki Syndrome

Kawasaki syndrome, also known as *mucocutaneous lymph node syndrome,* is a febrile illness primarily affecting children under 5 years of age. The etiology is unknown. The diagnostic criteria are a fever lasting 5 or more days that cannot be explained and at least four of the following:

- Bilateral conjunctival injection
- Mucous membrane changes of injected or fissured lips, injected pharynx, or "strawberry tongue"
- Extremity changes involving erythema of the palms or soles, edema of the hands or feet, or generalized or periungual desquamation
- Rash
- Cervical lymphadenopathy

The most significant complication of Kawasaki syndrome is the formation of coronary artery aneurysm. Coronary artery evaluation by two-dimensional echocardiography is therefore indicated. Anterior uveitis during the acute phase of the illness is common but generally self-limited. Conjunctival scarring can occur, and bilateral retinal ischemia has been observed histopathologically.

Treatment is mainly supportive, and aspirin is considered the drug of choice. Corticosteroid therapy is contraindicated because of its association with an increased rate of coronary artery aneurysm formation.

CHAPTER XVIII

The Lacrimal Drainage System

Tear fluid enters the lacrimal drainage system through the *punctum,* a small (approximately 0.3 mm), round opening located in each eyelid just nasal to and in line with the most medial of the meibomian gland orifices. The lower punctum is more temporal than the upper, and both are tilted slightly inward to contact the surface of the eye. Each punctum opens into a *canaliculus* that runs vertically for 1–2 mm and then turns nasally toward the lacrimal sac, running parallel to the eyelid margin. The canaliculi are lined with stratified squamous epithelium and surrounded by a layer of elastic tissue that permits considerable dilation. The tarsal plate does not extend into the portion of the eyelid containing the canaliculus, which consequently is easily torn. The upper and lower canaliculi join to form a very short *common canaliculus* before entering the lacrimal sac through the *valve of Rosenmüller.*

The *lacrimal sac* occupies the lacrimal fossa, which is formed by the lacrimal bone and the frontal process of the maxillary bone. The medial canthal ligament, which arises from the anterior lacrimal crest, lies in front of the upper portion of the sac. The epithelial lining of the sac is composed of a superficial columnar layer and a deeper layer of flattened cells, as well as numerous mucus-secreting goblet cells. Similar epithelium lines the *nasolacrimal duct (NLD),* which extends downward in a slightly lateral and posterior direction from the sac through a short bony canal to enter the temporal portion of the nose beneath the inferior turbinate at the *valve of Hasner.*

The membranous lacrimal drainage passages arise embryologically from a solid epithelial cord formed by invagination of surface ectoderm, which canalizes toward the end of gestation. Persistence of a thin tissue membrane across the lower end of the duct at birth is very common.

Developmental Anomalies

Atresia of the lacrimal puncta   This anomaly results from failure of the upper end of the developing drainage system to canalize. Symptoms are typically limited to accumulation and overflow of clear tears; mucopurulence is not seen to the degree typical of an obstruction of the lacrimal duct. Often only a thin epithelial membrane obstructs a well-developed canalicular system. The punctal site is easily identified in such cases, and perforating the membrane with a needle, followed by dilation, is usually curative. When the terminal portion of the canaliculus is also atretic, more elaborate surgery is required, ranging from a simple incisional punctoplasty combined with silicone intubation to conjunctivodacryocystorhinostomy in extreme cases. Congenital obstruction elsewhere in the canalicular system may cause symptoms similar to those of punctal atresia.

Cahill KV, Burns JA. Management of epiphora in the presence of congenital punctal and canalicular atresia. *Ophthal Plast Reconstr Surg.* 1991;7:167–172.

Supernumerary puncta   These are occasionally seen nasal to the normal opening; they require no treatment.

Congenital lacrimal fistula   Less common than atresia but more significant, this anomaly is an epithelium-lined tract extending from the common canaliculus or lacrimal sac to the skin surface of the lower eyelid, usually just inferonasal to the medial canthus. Discharge from the fistula is often associated with NLD obstruction and may cease to be a problem after the lower drainage system becomes patent. Persistence of bothersome symptoms necessitates surgical excision of the entire fistulous tract.

Birchansky LD, Nerad JA, Kersten RC, et al. Management of congenital lacrimal sac fistula. *Arch Ophthalmol.* 1990;108:388–390.

Dacryocystocele

Congenital dacryocystocele (sometimes referred to as *mucocele, dacryocele,* or *amniotocele* of the lacrimal sac) is an uncommon condition in which cystic swelling of the lacrimal sac accompanies obstruction of the lacrimal drainage system both above and below the sac. The lower blockage is usually membranous, similar to that responsible for the congenital NLD obstruction described below. Sometimes the upper part of the system is also obstructed anatomically, but often an unusually competent valve of Rosenmüller simply prevents reflux of accumulated fluid from the sac. Most authorities believe the fluid originates as mucus secreted by the epithelium of the lacrimal sac, although lacrimal gland secretions and amniotic fluid have been suggested as alternatives. Bilateral involvement is occasionally seen.

Dacryocystocele presents at birth as a bluish swelling about 1 cm in diameter just below and nasal to the medial canthus. Its appearance is quite distinctive, but the possibility of confusion with hemangioma, dermoid cyst, or encephalocele must be considered. Possible associated bulging of mucosa at the lower end of the NLD into the nasal cavity can significantly compromise the airway. This intranasal finding is sometimes also seen with NLD obstruction in the absence of a clinically apparent dacryocystocele. If the condition does not resolve spontaneously, infection with obvious local inflammatory changes usually develops within the first few weeks of life (Fig XVIII-1).

An uninfected dacryocystocele can sometimes be decompressed by digital massage, which in combination with topical antibiotic administration may lead to resolution without complications. Lacrimal probing should be performed no later than 1 month after birth in persistent cases. Once dacryocystitis develops, systemic antibiotics are indicated, and acute surgical decompression of the sac is usually necessary. This decompression can be accomplished initially by passing a probe or lacrimal needle through a canaliculus into the distended sac, but for permanent and complete relief elimination of associated NLD obstruction may be necessary.

Probing the lower system can be difficult because of the considerable anatomic distortion that frequently accompanies dacryocystocele. Sometimes, intranasal surgery to marsupialize the bulging lower end of the duct is required. Incision and drainage of an infected dacryocystocele through skin should be avoided if possible because of the danger of creating a persistent fistulous tract.

Mansour AM, Cheng KP, Mumma JV, et al. Congenital dacryocele: A collaborative review. *Ophthalmology.* 1991;98:1744–1751.

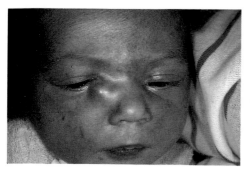

FIG XVIII-1—Congenital dacryocystocele, right eye, in a newborn girl. Note typical location and bluish discoloration of overlying skin.

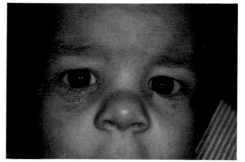

FIG XVIII-2—Congenital nasolacrimal duct obstruction, right eye, in an infant boy. Note wetness and mucus accumulation, without evidence of inflammation.

Nasolacrimal Duct Obstruction

Clinically evident obstruction of drainage below the lacrimal sac occurs in about 5% of full-term newborns. Usually, a thin mucosal membrane at the lower end of the NLD is the cause. Symptoms become manifest by age 1 month in 80%–90% of cases, and they typically consist of epiphora and sticky mucoid or mucopurulent discharge that accumulates on the eyelid margins and lashes (Fig XVIII-2). Bilateral involvement is common. The severity of these manifestations may vary considerably from day to day. Digital pressure applied over the lacrimal sac often, but not invariably, produces reflux of cloudy fluid through the punctum. Culture of the discharge typically indicates the presence of multiple strains of bacteria, but this step is not necessary for clinical management.

The differential diagnosis of congenital NLD obstruction includes the following disorders:

□ Punctal atresia, which is ruled out by inspection

□ Conjunctivitis, which is distinguished by acute history and inflammatory signs

□ Blepharitis, which is characterized by dry crusting on the eyelid margins and is very common in association with Down syndrome

□ Congenital glaucoma, in which epiphora caused by hypersecretion of tears is associated with nasal wetness, a feature absent from the clinical picture of lacrimal obstruction

The clinician can confirm the impatency of the drainage system by instilling 2% fluorescein into the tear film and noting significant retention after 5–10 minutes, with failure of dye to appear in the nose or pharynx after 10–15 minutes.

Nonsurgical Management

Conservative management of congenital NLD obstruction is frequently initiated by the primary care physician and includes administration of topical antibiotics and lacrimal sac massage. The antimicrobial agent should cover a broad spectrum of bacteria. Some clinicians prefer ointment because of its longer retention in the eye; others prefer drops, which are more likely to reach the sac. Application of antibiotic one to four times per day (depending on the degree of purulence observed by the family) can provide temporary relief from symptoms.

Digital massage of the lacrimal sac should be performed several times per day, conveniently done before the time of each diaper change. Massage serves two purposes: it empties the sac, reducing opportunity for bacterial growth; and it applies hydrostatic pressure to the drainage obstruction, which occasionally may open the duct and permanently relieve symptoms. To create sufficient pressure, it is necessary to compress the sac while initially occluding the canaliculi. The parent is instructed to place a finger above the medial canthus and then firmly press and slide downward along this side of the nose. This process should be done several times each at least three or four different times per day.

Congenital NLD obstruction resolves spontaneously with conservative management in a large majority of cases. Published series have shown clearing in 50%–90% of patients during the first 6 months of life. The probability that an affected 6-month-old will become asymptomatic by age 1 year is similarly about 70%. Beyond 1 year the rate of spontaneous resolution is significantly reduced and potential for permanent damage to the lacrimal drainage system from chronic repeated infections increases.

Paul TO. Medical management of congenital nasolacrimal duct obstruction. *J Pediatr Ophthalmol Strabismus.* 1985;22:68–70.

Surgical Management

When symptoms of congenital NLD obstruction persist, surgical probing of the lacrimal system is indicated. This procedure can be attempted in the ophthalmologist's office up to about age 12–15 months or performed in the operating room with mask or endotracheal anesthesia.

The timing of surgery for congenital NLD obstruction is controversial. Early probing (before 12 months of age) reduces the duration of bothersome symptoms, the burden of conservative management, and the potential for secondary infection. The procedure can be done in the office, avoiding the risk of general anesthesia and the expense of using the operating room. However, waiting until age 12 months or later avoids surgery altogether in a majority of cases and allows for the increased control and comfort afforded by the operating-room setting if surgery proves necessary. The decision for a particular patient must be guided by the following factors:

□ The severity of the child's symptoms

□ The ophthalmologist's training, experience, and practice environment

□ The attitude of the primary care physician

□ The wishes and concerns of the family

The success rate of properly performed initial probing for congenital NLD obstruction exceeds 90% in infants up to 12 months old, and no convincing evidence has shown that delaying surgical treatment until 12–15 months of age could be harmful. However, surgery performed after 24 months meets with failure to relieve symptoms with simple probing in as many as one third of cases. Two hypotheses have been proposed to explain this observation:

☐ Persistent obstruction of tear drainage with consequent infection and inflammation leads to scarring that progressively reduces the probability of successful probing over time.

☐ A small proportion of newborns with congenital NLD obstruction have anatomic variants that are both unlikely to resolve spontaneously and unlikely to be relieved by simple probing; as time passes and most other cases improve, this unchanging subgroup comes to represent an increasingly large fraction of the remaining affected population.

Baker JD. Treatment of congenital nasolacrimal system obstruction. *J Pediatr Ophthalmol Strabismus.* 1985;22:34–36.

Katowitz JA, Welsh MG. Timing of initial probing and irrigation in congenital nasolacrimal duct obstruction. *Ophthalmology.* 1987;94:698–705.

Kushner BJ. Congenital nasolacrimal system obstruction. *Arch Ophthalmol.* 1982; 100:597–600.

Robb RM. Treatment of congenital nasolacrimal system obstruction. *J Pediatr Ophthalmol Strabismus.* 1985;22:36–37.

Surgical procedures Before probing begins in an office setting, the unsedated infant is wrapped securely to immobilize the trunk and extremities as well as the head, and a drop of topical anesthetic is instilled. In the operating room administration of inhalation agents by mask can provide adequate anesthesia, although some surgeons and anesthesiologists prefer to protect the airway with endotracheal intubation. Before instruments are introduced, the lacrimal sac is emptied by digital compression, and the eyelid margins are cleansed of accumulated mucus. Observation of reflux from the puncta confirms patency of the canalicular system.

The clinician initiates probing by dilating either the upper or lower punctum. The risk of inadvertently causing significant damage to the canalicular system may be reduced by probing through the upper eyelid but the easier access afforded by the lower eyelid may outweigh this unproved advantage, particularly in the unanesthetized infant. The instrument used for punctal dilation should have a slightly blunted tip and taper gradually up to a diameter of >1 mm. (Some surgeons use the point of a large standard safety pin.) After the instrument is engaged in the punctal opening, it is immediately directed nasalward and advanced parallel to the eyelid margin while digital countertraction is applied to the eyelid. Holding constant pressure in this manner for 10–15 seconds usually suffices to dilate the punctum.

Before passing a probe through the NLD it is possible to "hydrostatically" test the system by introducing a blunt-tipped irrigating needle into the sac, directing it inferiorly as described below for probing, and attempting to force a small amount of saline through the system from a syringe under moderate pressure. Reflux is prevented by compression or plugging of the canaliculi, but the possibility of aspiration and laryngospasm if fluid volume is excessive must be kept in mind. This maneuver can confirm the presence of NLD obstruction and provides an opportunity to relieve it, which may be advantageous if the duct does not follow a straight linear course, a relatively common situation leading to false passage (see below).

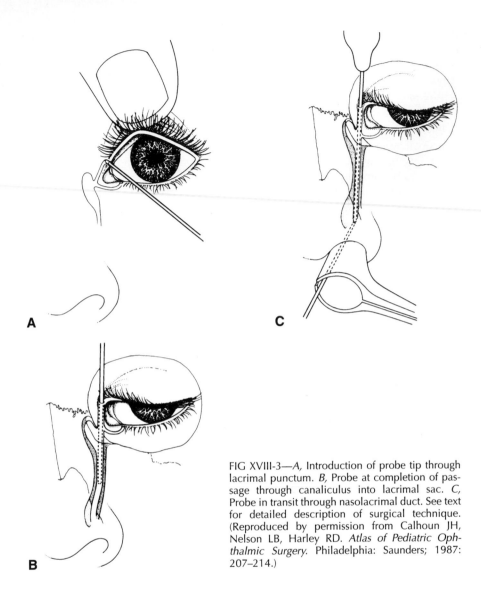

A

C

B

FIG XVIII-3—*A,* Introduction of probe tip through lacrimal punctum. *B,* Probe at completion of passage through canaliculus into lacrimal sac. *C,* Probe in transit through nasolacrimal duct. See text for detailed description of surgical technique. (Reproduced by permission from Calhoun JH, Nelson LB, Harley RD. *Atlas of Pediatric Ophthalmic Surgery.* Philadelphia: Saunders; 1987: 207–214.)

Once the punctum is dilated, a #00, #0, or #1 Bowman probe can be advanced into the sac along the canaliculus parallel to the eyelid margin, while at the same time the eyelid is stretched superotemporally to provide countertraction (Fig XVIII-3). If resistance is encountered (usually the result of kinking rather than anatomic obstruction in the canaliculus), the probe should be pulled back slightly and its direction modified until further advancement becomes possible. The probe should not be forced through the canalicular system. If this maneuver fails, passage in the other eyelid should be tried. Successful passage through the canalicular system is signaled by the feel of the probe tip against the nasal wall of the sac (bone under a thin layer of mucosa), which is quite distinctive. If a soft or spongy resistance is felt at the end of the canaliculus, the probe is probably caught at the valve of Rosenmüller. It should be gently maneuvered with the aid of countertraction on the eyelid and minimal force to get past this area.

When the surgeon is convinced that the nasal wall has been reached, the probe tip is held against the nasal wall of the sac and pivoted roughly 90°, directing it into the NLD and downward toward the floor of the nose, slightly rearward and temporally. Subtle repositioning of the probe, which may be facilitated by bending the probe into a gentle curve, is often required before it can be advanced smoothly. As the probe slides through the NLD, various tactile sensations can be appreciated, the last being a discrete characteristic "pop," which is felt as the lower end of the duct is passed.

Sometimes several minor barriers are overcome along the duct's course, or a sense of constriction is felt throughout its length. In some cases there is no palpable resistance. Occasionally, despite repeated efforts to achieve smooth passage, grating bony resistance is felt, which may indicate that probing will be unsuccessful. (A precise description in the operative report of the feel of probe passage becomes very valuable if later surgery is required.)

The distance traversed in probing from the punctum to the floor of the nasal cavity is approximately equal to the distance from the punctum to the external tip of the nose (less than 3 cm in a 1-year-old). The surgeon who fails to realize that the nasal floor has been reached can inadvertently push the probe through the palate into the oral cavity. To confirm emergence of the probe tip into the nose, a second probe is passed along the nasal floor close against the temporal wall for a distance about equal to the length of the probe segment in the drainage system. The feel of "metal on metal" as the second probe rubs directly against the first should cease as the first probe is slightly withdrawn.

Direct inspection with a nasal speculum and headlamp or a special fiberoptic nasal endoscope can determine the precise position of the probe. After probe withdrawal, irrigation through the drainage system (as described above) should be possible with light pressure on the syringe; recovery of saline colored with fluorescein or methylene blue from the nose with a small suction catheter confirms patency.

Rarely, bony resistance is encountered during probing that cannot be overcome despite all appropriate effort. More often, the probe is misdirected into soft tissue or the maxillary sinus antrum, although proper technique should minimize this problem. If either of these situations occurs, the procedure should be aborted and reattempted on another occasion. The most common undesired outcome of probing is passage into the nose along a route other than the true lacrimal drainage channel. Such *false passage* can result either from faulty manipulation of the probe or from anatomic variations that make it impossible for a straight instrument to follow the channel through its entire length. Detection of false passage can be very difficult or even impossible intraoperatively. Usually, its consequence is simply postoperative persistence or recurrence of symptoms, but occasionally damage to the tissue lining the canaliculus or NLD causes scarring that increases the difficulty of subsequent efforts to relieve drainage obstruction. Significant complications of probing are otherwise rare. Minor bleeding from the nose or into the tears is sometimes noted but requires no treatment.

Postoperative management Optional postoperative medications include antibiotic and corticosteroid drops, alone or in combination, instilled in the eye two to four times per day for a period of several days to a week or longer. Phenylephrine 1/8% nose drops can be used concurrently for 2–3 days to promote tear flow by minimizing edema of the nasal mucosa. Because transient bacteremia can occur after probing, systemic antibiotic prophylaxis should be considered for the patient with congenital heart disease.

Resolution of symptoms is usually immediate and dramatic after probing, but the full effect of the procedure sometimes does not become evident for 1–2 weeks. Recurrence after unsuccessful probing is nearly always obvious within 1 month. A postoperative office visit is not mandatory if the patient's family notifies the surgeon that the problem seems to have resolved.

Relief from symptoms after successful probing is usually complete, but in some cases epiphora still occurs on occasion, particularly outdoors in cold weather or in conjunction with upper respiratory infection. This condition is probably attributable to a patent but narrow lacrimal drainage channel that is overwhelmed by mild hypersecretion or becomes occluded when the nasal mucosa swells. A similar clinical picture is occasionally encountered in an infant or young child without a prior history of complete obstruction. In most cases no treatment is required. Spontaneous improvement is likely as the face grows over time.

If the initial attempt to relieve congenital NLD obstruction with probing is unsuccessful, it is appropriate to repeat the same procedure after an interval of a few weeks. Some surgeons routinely supplement a second probing in the operating room with infracture of the inferior turbinate, which can interfere with tear flow if it is very closely apposed to the lateral wall of the nose. Infracture is accomplished by placing a small periosteal elevator beneath the turbinate or by grasping it with a hemostat, then rotating the instrument to force the turbinate inward until its bony core fractures, without disrupting the overlying soft tissue. The value of this widely practiced maneuver is debatable.

Intubation Silicone intubation of the lacrimal system is usually recommended when simple probing has failed. The silicone tubing is swedged onto a thin probe whose end is modified with a bulbed tip. Once passed into the nose, the tip is engaged with a small specialized hook and withdrawn out the nares. Both the upper and lower eyelids are intubated, leaving a small loop of silicone tubing between the puncta. A variety of measures are employed to secure the ends of the tubing in the nose, such as placing knots in the tubing or passing the tubing through a bolster to prevent retrograde entry into the nasolacrimal duct. Additional modifications, such as placement of suture material in the lumen of the tube to allow the cut ends to be smoothly tied together, have been made. No approach achieves the ideal combination of ease of placement and removal along with high resistance to accidental displacement.

Ideally, the silicone tubing should be left in place for 3–6 months to maximize the probability that the lacrimal drainage system will remain patent after its removal, but shorter periods of intubation can be successful. Occasionally, the tubing becomes dislodged and protrudes excessively out of either the nose or the punctum. In such situations attempts should be made to reposition the tubing if at all possible. Tubing looped out of the punctum can often be repositioned by gentle pressure and threading back through the upper and lower puncta. Ophthalmic ointment on the tubing may facilitate this maneuver. If the tubing is dislocated out of the nose, a cotton-tip applicator or forceps can be used to place it back. Having the child sniff can also be helpful in repositioning tubing. The parents should be cautioned about the possibility of the tube migrating nasally and tearing the punctum. Early removal is necessary in these cases, but having a gentle curve to the tube between the two puncta can usually avoid this problem.

The technique chosen for tube removal depends on the age of the patient, the manner in which the tubing was secured, and its position (in place or partially dislodged). If the ends were secured with a very small knot, the tubing can be removed by cutting and retracting through the punctum. A more cumbersome closure in the nose often requires an anesthesia, since the tube will have to be removed out the nose.

Dacryocystorhinostomy (DCR) may be necessary for those cases in which intubation cannot be accomplished or in which significant symptoms recur when tubing is removed. BCSC Section 7, *Orbit, Eyelids, and Lacrimal System,* discusses DCR and the other procedures covered in this chapter.

Lyon DB, Dortzbach RK, Lemke BN, et al. Canalicular stenosis following probing for congenital nasolacrimal duct obstruction. *Ophthalmic Surg.* 1991;22:228–232.

Migliori ME, Putterman AM. Silicone intubation for the treatment of congenital lacrimal duct obstruction: successful results removing the tubes after six weeks. *Ophthalmology.* 1988;95:792–795.

Sevel D. Insufflation treatment of occluded nasolacrimal apparatus in the child. *Ophthalmology.* 1982;89:329–334.

Welsh MG, Katowitz JA. Timing of Silastic tubing removal after intubation for congenital nasolacrimal duct obstruction. *Ophthal Plast Reconstr Surg.* 1989;5:43–48.

CHAPTER XIX

Diseases of the Cornea and Anterior Segment

This chapter focuses on corneal and anterior segment problems that have their onset during infancy and childhood. To understand how developmental anomalies affect the cornea and anterior segment, it is helpful to review the embryology of these regions of the eye.

Embryology of the Cornea and Anterior Segment

The lens vesicle separates from the surface ectoderm by the sixth week of gestation. The optic cup, which arises from neural ectoderm, has reached the periphery of the lens by this time, and a triangular mass of undifferentiated neural crest cells over-rides the rim of the cup and surrounds the anterior periphery of the lens. Three waves of tissue move forward between the surface ectoderm and the lens. The first of these layers differentiates into the primordial corneal endothelium by the eighth week and subsequently produces Descemet's membrane. The second wave of tissue produces the stroma of the cornea, and the third wave gives rise to the pupillary membrane and the iris stroma. The pigment epithelial layer of the iris develops in later months from neural ectoderm.

By the beginning of the fifth fetal month a complete endothelial lining overlies the primitive anterior chamber, creating a closed cavity. In addition, the iris insertion is now well anterior to the neural crest tissue destined to become the trabecular meshwork. The endothelial lining undergoes fenestration in the final weeks of gestation and the first weeks after birth. The iris insertion also repositions posteriorly to gradually uncover the developing trabecular meshwork. This repositioning, or posterior sliding, probably occurs secondary to differential growth rates and is not merely the result of a cleavage or an atrophy of tissue. At birth the iris insertion has normally reached the level of the scleral spur. Posterior migration of the iris normally continues for about the first year of life.

A spectrum of anterior segment dysgenesis syndromes can result from abnormalities of neural crest cell migration, proliferation, or differentiation. A developmental arrest late in gestation can result in retention of primordial endothelium and incomplete posterior iris migration. BCSC Section 2, *Fundamentals and Principles of Ophthalmology,* discusses these issues in greater detail with illustrations in Part 2, Embryology.

Congenital Corneal Anomalies

Abnormalities of Corneal Size and Shape

The normal horizontal corneal diameter in the newborn is 9.5–10.5 mm. The average 12 mm adult corneal diameter is reached by 2 years of age. Abnormalities of corneal size and shape in childhood include simple megalocornea, keratoglobus, keratoconus, and microcornea. (See also discussion of congenital anomalies in BCSC Section 8, *External Disease and Cornea*.)

Megalocornea   If the horizontal diameter is greater than 13 mm (or 12 mm in the newborn), megalocornea is present. The most common type of megalocornea is *anterior megalophthalmos,* which is X-linked recessive and bilateral. In this condition the normal-sized lens is too small for the enlarged ciliary ring, resulting in subluxation. The iris is hypoplastic with defects visible by transillumination, and the pupil is often ectopic. Elevated IOP and lens dislocation with cataracts often occur in adulthood. *Simple megalocornea* is a rare condition in which both corneas exceed 13 mm in horizontal diameter, but no associated abnormalities are present. This condition must be differentiated from congenital glaucoma.

Keratoglobus   In keratoglobus the cornea is thinner than normal and arcs high over the iris, creating a deeper than normal anterior chamber. Spontaneous breaks in Descemet's membrane may produce acute corneal edema, and the cornea is easily ruptured by minor blunt trauma. Patients with keratoglobus should be advised to wear protective lenses indefinitely. This rare autosomal recessive disorder can be part of the *Ehlers-Danlos type VI syndrome,* which is characterized by generalized thinning and anterior bulging of the cornea accompanied by hyperextensible joints, blue sclera, and gradually progressive neurosensory hearing loss.

Keratoconus   In this condition the central or paracentral cornea undergoes progressive thinning and bulging, so that the cornea takes on the shape of a cone. The disease can present and progress during the adolescent years. There is an association with Down syndrome, other conditions with mental retardation, and atopic disease.

Microcornea   Microcornea is present if the corneal diameter is smaller than 10 mm (or smaller than 9 mm in the newborn) (Fig XIX-1). It may follow a pattern of autosomal dominant inheritance, particularly as part of the oculodentodigital dysplasia syndrome, or it may appear sporadically. Microcornea may be accompanied by many other abnormalities of the eye including cataracts, colobomas, or persistent hyperplastic primary vitreous. It can be seen in nanophthalmos, in which the eye is smaller than normal without other major structural abnormalities.

Anterior Segment Dysgenesis: Peripheral Developmental Abnormalities

The spectrum of developmental anomalies known as *anterior segment dysgenesis* is sometimes referred to as *mesenchymal dysgenesis* and was previously known as *anterior chamber cleavage syndrome* or *mesectodermal dysgenesis.*

Wilson ME. Congenital iris ectropion and a new classification for anterior segment dysgenesis. *J Pediatr Ophthalmol Strabismus.* 1990;27:48–55.

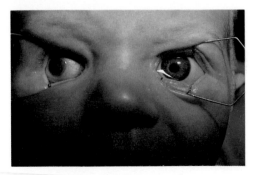
FIG XIX-1—Microcornea, right eye.

Posterior embryotoxon This condition is seen as a central thickening and displacement of Schwalbe's line. It is visible with the slit lamp as an irregular white line just concentric with and anterior to the limbus (Fig XIX-2). Gonioscopically, it appears as a continuous or broken ridge protruding into the anterior chamber. It often has pigmented spots on its inner surface. This anomaly is also referred to as a prominent Schwalbe's ring. It is most often seen in association with Axenfeld-Rieger syndrome but is also found in arteriohepatic dysplasia (Alagille syndrome) and may be an isolated finding in 15% of normal patients.

> Nischal KK, Hingorani M, Bentley CR, et al. Ocular ultrasound in Alagille syndrome: a new sign. *Ophthalmology.* 1997;104:79–85.

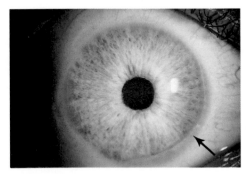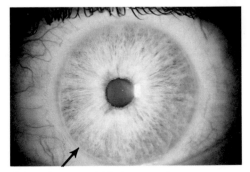
FIG XIX-2—Posterior embryotoxon (arrows), bilateral, in Axenfeld-Rieger syndrome.

Axenfeld-Rieger syndrome This syndrome represents a spectrum of developmental disorders characterized by an anteriorly displaced Schwalbe's line (posterior embryotoxon) with attached iris strands, iris hypoplasia, and anterior chamber dysgenesis leading to glaucoma in late childhood or adulthood in 50% of cases (Figs XIX-3, XIX-4, XIX-5). The conditions previously referred to as *Axenfeld anomaly, Rieger anomaly,* and *Rieger syndrome* often have overlapping findings and have now been grouped into a single entity known as *Axenfeld-Rieger syndrome.*

A glassy, smooth, cryptless iris surface and a high iris insertion are present, sometimes accompanied by iris transillumination. Iris hypoplasia can range from mild stromal thinning to marked atrophy with hole formation, corectopia, and ectropion uveae. Megalocornea or microcornea can occur. Developmental defects of the teeth and facial bones may be associated. Redundant periumbilical skin, hypospadias, and anomalies in the region of the pituitary gland have also been reported. Autosomal dominant inheritance is most common. Mutations in the PAX6 locus of chromosome 11 and on chromosomes 4, 10, and 13 have been identified.

Shields MB, Buckley E, Klintworth GK, et al. Axenfeld-Rieger syndrome. A spectrum of developmental disorders. *Surv Ophthalmol.* 1985;29:387–409.

Walter MA, Mirzayans F, Mears AJ, et al. Autosomal-dominant iridogoniodysgenesis and Axenfeld-Rieger syndrome are genetically distinct. *Ophthalmology.* 1996;103: 1907–1915.

Anterior Segment Dysgenesis: Central Developmental Abnormalities

The basic abnormality in these entities is a localized loss or attenuation of the corneal endothelium or Descemet's membrane, which is usually associated with an overlying stromal and epithelial opacity.

Posterior corneal depression (central posterior keratoconus) This discrete posterior corneal indentation is best detected with a retinoscope or direct ophthalmoscope revealing an abnormal red reflex. It can also be diagnosed with the slit lamp

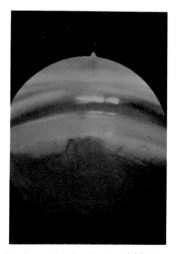

FIG XIX-3—Gonioscopic view in Axenfeld-Rieger syndrome.

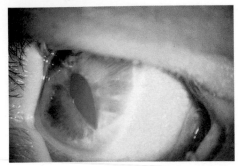
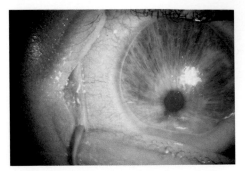

FIG XIX-4—Axenfeld-Rieger syndrome, bilateral.

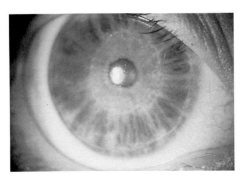
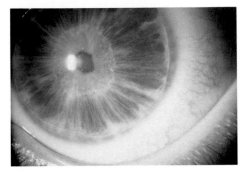

FIG XIX-5—Iridogoniodysgenesis, bilateral.

by moving the beam across the defect to discern increased convexity of the posterior corneal surface. Sometimes pigment deposits appear on the border of the posterior defect. The anterior curvature of the cornea is normal. This defect usually causes irregular astigmatism and can result in amblyopia if the refractive error is not corrected.

Peters anomaly This anomaly consists of a posterior corneal defect with stromal opacity and often adherent iris strands. In many cases the stromal opacity decreases with time. The size and density of the opacity can range from a faint stromal opacity to a dense opaque central leukoma. In extreme cases the central leukoma may be vascularized and protrude above the level of the cornea. The strands from the iris to the borders of this defect vary in number and density. A more severe variety of this condition involves adherence of the lens to the cornea at the site of the central defect (Fig XIX-6). Peters anomaly is the end result of many defects including the genetic Axenfeld-Rieger syndrome and nongenetic conditions such as congenital rubella.

Mulet M, Caldwell D. Corneal abnormalities. In: Wright KW, ed. *Pediatric Ophthalmology and Strabismus*. St Louis: Mosby; 1995:321–348.

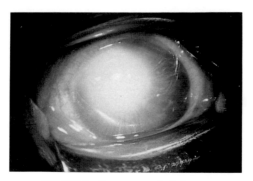

FIG XIX-6—Peters anomaly, left eye.

Combinations of Peripheral and Central Developmental Abnormalities

Central and peripheral abnormalities may be present in the same eye or both eyes of the same patient or in other family members. These lesions may appear sporadically, or they may be inherited in a recognizable pattern. All of these defects, especially those that involve the iris and the anterior chamber angle, predispose a patient to glaucoma. These patients should, therefore, be followed carefully throughout childhood for the development of glaucoma. Many of these defects are also associated with systemic abnormalities. Systemic malformations, especially involving midline body structures such as the pituitary gland and the heart, can occur in association with Peters anomaly.

Hanson IM, Fletcher JM, Jordan T, et al. Mutations at the PAX6 locus are found in heterogeneous anterior segment malformations including Peters' anomaly. *Nat Genet.* 1994;6:168–173.

Traboulsi EI, Maumenee IH. Peters' anomaly and associated congenital malformations. *Arch Ophthalmol.* 1992;110:1739–1742.

Infantile Corneal Opacities

Peters anomaly has already been discussed. Table XIX-1 lists the other possibilities to be considered in a differential diagnosis.

Sclerocornea In this congenital condition the cornea is opaque and resembles the sclera, making the limbus indistinct. The central cornea is clearer than the periphery in nearly all cases. Severe cases show no increased corneal curvature and no apparent scleral sulcus. Sclerocornea often occurs in association with other abnormalities of the eye.

Tears, breaks, or ruptures of Descemet's membrane Such injuries may be caused by forceps trauma to the eye occurring during a difficult delivery. Rupture of Descemet's membrane leads to stromal and sometimes epithelial edema. Other signs of trauma are frequently apparent on the child. In most cases the stromal and epithe-

TABLE XIX-1

DIFFERENTIAL DIAGNOSIS OF INFANTILE CORNEAL OPACITIES

ENTITY	LOCATION AND DESCRIPTION OF OPACITY	OTHER SIGNS	METHOD OF DIAGNOSIS
Sclerocornea	Peripheral opacity, clearest centrally; unilateral or bilateral	Flat cornea	Inspection
Forceps injury	Central opacity; unilateral	Breaks in Descemet's membrane	History
Mucopolysaccharidosis, mucolipidosis	Diffuse opacity; bilateral	Smooth epithelium	Conjunctival biopsy; biochemical testing
Posterior corneal defects	Central opacity; unilateral or bilateral	Iris adherence to cornea; posterior keratoconus	Inspection
Congenital hereditary endothelial dystrophy (CHED)	Diffuse opacity; bilateral	Thickened cornea	Inspection
Dermoid	Temporal opacity; unilateral; raised; hair on surface; keratinized	Associated with Goldenhar syndrome	Inspection
Infantile glaucoma	Diffuse opacity; unilateral or bilateral	Enlarged cornea; breaks in Descemet's membrane	Elevated intraocular pressure
Congenital hereditary stromal dystrophy (CHSD)	Diffuse opacity; bilateral	Stromal opacities, normal thickness, normal epithelium	Autosomal dominant; examine family members

lial edema regresses, but the edges of the broken Descemet's membrane persist indefinitely and can be seen as ridges protruding slightly from the posterior corneal surface. Severe amblyopia may result when the clearing of the corneal opacity is slower than 2 months. The astigmatism induced by the trauma can cause severe amblyopia even if the cornea clears quickly. Improvement with optical correction and patching can often be achieved.

Mucopolysaccharidosis (MPS) and mucolipidosis The varied systemic findings and ultrastructural abnormalities of these lysosomal disorders are beyond the scope of this discussion (see Table XXIX-1 on pp 360–361 and BCSC Section 8, *External Disease and Cornea,* and Section 12, *Retina and Vitreous*). However, corneal clouding and haziness may be present in early life in at least two of these conditions. In MPS IH, or *Hurler syndrome,* corneal clouding occurs by age 6 months, while in MPS IS, or *Scheie syndrome,* it occurs by 12–24 months (Fig XIX-7). In mucolipidosis IV corneal clouding has been reported as early as age 6 weeks. Enzymatic and DNA analyses can identify the metabolic defect in most conditions. Conjunctival biopsies show abnormal cytoplasmic inclusions on electron microscopy.

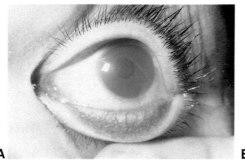 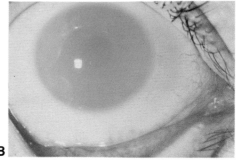

FIG XIX-7—Hurler syndrome. *A,* Early corneal clouding. *B,* Late corneal clouding.

Congenital hereditary endothelial dystrophy (CHED) CHED is an uncommon corneal dystrophy with onset at birth or shortly thereafter. The cornea is diffusely and uniformly edematous secondary to a defect of the corneal endothelium and Descemet's membrane. The edema involves both the stroma and epithelium. The hallmark of CHED is increased corneal thickness. The appearance of the cornea is similar to that seen in congenital glaucoma, but without increased corneal diameter and elevated IOP.

Dermoids A corneal dermoid is a hamartoma composed of fibrofatty tissue covered by keratinized epithelium. Dermoids sometimes contain hair follicles, sebaceous glands, and sweat glands. They can range up to 8–10 mm in diameter and usually straddle the limbus. Dermoids extend into the corneal stroma and adjacent sclera but seldom occupy the full thickness of either cornea or sclera. Most dermoids are on the inferior temporal limbus. Many dermoids produce a lipoid infiltration of the corneal stroma at their leading edge.

Limbal dermoids are often seen with Goldenhar syndrome (see p 353). They are sometimes continuous with subconjunctival lipodermoids that involve the upper outer quadrant of the eye and extend into the orbit under the lateral aspect of the upper eyelid. Large dermoids can cover the visual axis, while small dermoids can produce astigmatism with secondary amblyopia. Surgical excision may result in scarring and astigmatism, which can also lead to amblyopia.

Congenital or infantile glaucoma Glaucoma in an infant can make the cornea hazy, cloudy, opaque, and/or enlarged. Chapter XXI discusses pediatric glaucoma in more detail.

Congenital hereditary stromal dystrophy (CHSD) CHSD is a very rare congenital stationary opacification of the cornea transmitted in an autosomal dominant manner. Flaky or feathery clouding of the stroma, which is of normal thickness, is covered by a smooth, normal epithelium. These features are in contrast to CHED, which has a thickened stroma and epithelial edema.

Treatment

The treatment of congenital corneal opacities is difficult and often visually unrewarding. If bilateral dense opacities are present, keratoplasty should be considered for one eye as soon as possible. If the opacity is unilateral, the decision is more difficult. Keratoplasty should be undertaken only if the family and the physicians involved in the care of the child are prepared for tremendous commitment of time and effort. The team should include ophthalmologists skilled in the management of pediatric corneal surgery, pediatric glaucoma, amblyopia, and strabismus. Contact lens expertise is important for fitting infants with small eyes and large refractive errors. Examinations under anesthesia are required, and infectious keratitis is very common. Social service support is often needed.

Systemic Diseases with Corneal Manifestations in Childhood

The mucopolysaccharidoses have been discussed above. All of the mucopolysaccharidoses except MPS II (Hunter syndrome) may have deposits in the cornea leading to some degree of clinical corneal clouding (see Figure XIX-7).

Cystinosis   This metabolic disease characterized by elevated levels of cystine within the cell is very uncommon. Cystine crystals are deposited in various places throughout the body. In the infantile form of the disease the major presenting symptoms are failure to thrive, rickets, and progressive renal failure called *Fanconi syndrome.* The ocular findings are pathognomonic. Iridescent elongated corneal crystals appear at approximately 1 year of age, first in the peripheral part of the cornea and the anterior part of the stroma. These crystals are also present in the uvea and can be seen with the slit lamp on the surface of the iris (Fig XIX-8). Severe photophobia can make a slit-lamp examination almost impossible without anesthesia. Cystine can be found in conjunctival biopsy specimens. Oral cysteamine has been shown to help the systemic problems but not the corneal crystal deposition. Topical cysteamine drops have had variable results.

> Schneider JA. Cystinosis. In: Buyse ML, ed. *Birth Defects Encyclopedia.* Dover, MA: Center for Birth Defects Information Services; and Cambridge, MA: Blackwell Scientific Publications; 1990:482.

Hepatolenticular degeneration (Wilson disease)   This autosomal recessive inborn error of metabolism results in excess copper deposition in the liver, kidney, and basal ganglia of the brain, leading to cirrhosis, renal tubular damage, and a Parkinson-like defect of motor function. The characteristic copper-colored Kayser-Fleischer ring is limited to Descemet's membrane and is thus separated from the limbus. It may be several millimeters in width. The initial depositions are in the corneal periphery at 12 and 6 o'clock. This arc of depositions spreads, eventually encircling the entire cornea. The ring resolves with treatment. Because it can develop fairly late, the laboratory tests for serum copper and ceruloplasmin are better than an eye examination for early diagnosis.

Congenital syphilis   *Interstitial keratitis* is seen in the first decade of life secondary to untreated congenital syphilis. It presents as rapidly progressive corneal edema followed by abnormal vascularization in the deep stroma adjacent to Descemet's membrane. Intense vascularization may give the cornea a salmon pink color, hence the

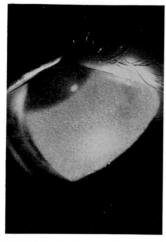

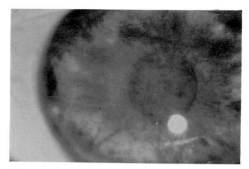

FIG XIX-8—Cystinosis with corneal involvement.

FIG XIX-9—Interstitial keratitis secondary to congenital syphilis.

term *salmon patch*. Blood flow through these vessels gradually ceases over several weeks to several months, leaving empty "ghost" vessels in the corneal stroma (Fig XIX-9). So far, the resurgence of congenital syphilis cases noted in the past 10 years has not led to a resurgence of interstitial keratitis.

Familial dysautonomia (Riley-Day syndrome) This complex autosomal recessive condition occurs largely in children of eastern European Jewish (Ashkenazi) descent. It is characterized by autonomic dysfunction, relative insensitivity to pain, and absence of the fungiform papillae of the tongue. Exposure keratitis and corneal ulcers with secondary opacification are a frequent problem because of the abnormal lacrimation and decreased corneal sensitivity. Preventive measures include supplemental tears and tarsorrhaphies.

Mulet M, Caldwell D. Corneal abnormalities. In: Wright KW, ed. *Pediatric Ophthalmology and Strabismus.* St Louis: Mosby; 1995:321–348.

Robb RM. Ocular abnormalities in childhood metabolic diseases and leukemia. In: Nelson LB, Calhoun JH, Harley RD, eds. *Pediatric Ophthalmology.* 3rd ed. Philadelphia: Saunders; 1991:444–468.

CHAPTER XX

Iris Abnormalities

Aniridia

Aniridia is a panocular, bilateral disorder. The term *aniridia* is a misnomer, since at least a rudimentary iris is always present. Variations range from almost total absence to only mild hypoplasia of the iris. In addition to iris involvement, foveal and optic nerve hypoplasia are present, resulting in a congenital sensory nystagmus and leading to reduced visual acuity, usually 20/100 or worse. Cataracts, glaucoma, and corneal opacification often develop later in childhood, and these may lead to progressive deterioration of visual acuity.

The typical presentation of aniridia is an infant with nystagmus who appears to have absent irides or dilated, unresponsive pupils. Photophobia may also be present. Examination findings commonly include small anterior polar cataracts with attached persistent pupillary membrane strands (Fig XX-1).

A defect in the PAX6 gene on chromosome 11 is the cause of aniridia, which can be sporadic or familial. The familial form is autosomal dominant with complete penetrance but variable expressivity. Two thirds of all aniridic children have affected parents. The PAX6 gene for isolated aniridia, which has been localized to chromosome band 11p13, is probably involved in the complex inductive interactions between the optic cup, surface ectoderm, and neural crest during formation of the iris and other ocular structures. Inadequate gene dosage may thus lead to global impairment of morphogenesis. Both the Embryology and the Genetics chapters of BCSC Section 2, *Fundamentals and Principles of Ophthalmology*, discuss aniridia.

Sporadic aniridia is associated with *Wilms tumor* in as many as one third of cases. The Wilms tumor gene can be detected on DNA analysis. When associated with aniridia, Wilms tumor is diagnosed before age 5 in 80% of cases. All children with sporadic aniridia should undergo chromosomal analysis for the Wilms tumor gene defect. If the results are positive, consultation with an oncologist is needed along with repeated abdominal ultrasonographic and clinical examinations. Familial aniridia patients are rarely at risk for Wilms tumor.

Sporadic aniridia has also been associated with genitourinary abnormalities and mental retardation (ARG triad), a constellation that has been linked with a deletion of the short arm of chromosome 11 (11 p–). Some, but not all, of these patients develop Wilms tumor.

Hanson IM, Fletcher JM, Jordan T, et al. Mutations at the PAX6 locus in aniridia. *Hum Mol Genet.* 1994;2:915–920.

Ivanov I, Shuper A, Shohat M, et al. Aniridia: recent achievements in paediatric practice. *Eur J Pediatr.* 1995;154:795–800.

Mets MB, Erzurum SA. Uveal tract in infants. In: Isenberg SJ, ed. *The Eye in Infancy.* 2nd ed. St Louis: Mosby; 1994:308–317.

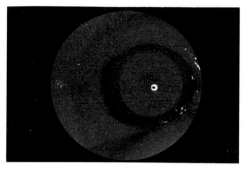

FIG XX-1—Aniridia in an infant. Both the ciliary processes and the edge of the lens are visible. Also present are persistent pupillary membrane fibers and a small central anterior polar cataract.

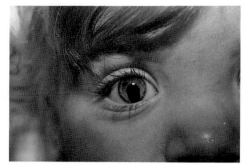

FIG XX-2—Typical iris coloboma, right eye.

Coloboma of the Iris

Iris colobomas are classified as *typical* if they occur in the inferonasal quadrant and can thus be explained by failure of the embryonic fissure to close in the fifth week of gestation. With a typical iris coloboma the pupil is shaped like a light bulb, keyhole, or inverted teardrop (Fig XX-2). Typical colobomas may involve the ciliary body, choroid, retina, and optic nerve. These colobomas are part of a continuum that extends to microphthalmos and anophthalmos. Nystagmus may be present if the optic nerve is involved. Inheritance patterns for isolated microphthalmos and uveal coloboma can be autosomal dominant and recessive.

Atypical iris colobomas occur in areas other than the inferonasal quadrant and are not associated with more posterior uveal colobomas. These colobomas probably result from fibrovascular remnants of the anterior hyaloid system and pupillary membrane.

Although iris colobomas can be associated with almost any chromosomal abnormality, the most common associations are

☐ Trisomy 13

☐ Triploidy

☐ Cat's-eye syndrome

☐ 4p– Wolf-Hirschhorn syndrome

☐ 11q–

☐ 18r (ring)

☐ 13r

☐ Trisomy 18

☐ Klinefelter syndrome

☐ Turner syndrome (rarely)

In addition, many well-characterized syndromes have uveal colobomas associated with them. These include

- CHARGE association (ocular **c**oloboma, **h**eart defects, choanal **a**tresia, mental **r**etardation, and **g**enitourinary and **e**ar anomalies), which accounts for about 15% of cases
- Lenz microphthalmos syndrome
- Goltz focal dermal hypoplasia
- Basal cell nevus syndrome
- Meckel syndrome
- Warburg syndrome
- Aicardi syndrome
- Rubinstein-Taybi syndrome
- Linear sebaceous nevus syndrome
- Goldenhar syndrome

Mets MB, Erzurum SA. Uveal tract in infants. In: Isenberg SJ, ed. *The Eye in Infancy*. 2nd ed. St Louis: Mosby; 1994:308–317.

Wilson ME, O'Neil JW. Pediatric iris abnormalities. In: Wright KW, ed. *Pediatric Ophthalmology and Strabismus*. St Louis: Mosby; 1995:349–365.

Iris Nodules

Lisch Nodules

Lisch nodules are neural crest hamartomas commonly associated with *neurofibromatosis type 1* (NF-1). They are raised and usually tan in color but can be quite variable in appearance (Fig XX-3). The prevalence of Lisch nodules in NF-1 increases with age, being approximately 10 times the patient's age (Fig XX-4). (See also chapter XXVII, Phakomatoses.)

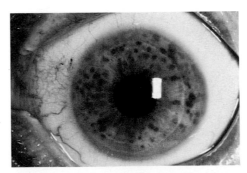

FIG XX-3—Lisch nodules in neurofibromatosis type 1.

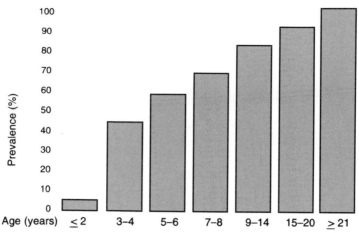

FIG XX-4—Prevalence of Lisch nodules according to age in 167 patients with neurofibromatosis type 1. (Modified from Lubs ML, Bauer MS, Formas ME, et al. Lisch nodules in neurofibromatosis type 1. *N Engl J Med.* 1991;324: 1264–1266.)

Juvenile Xanthogranuloma (JXG)

Juvenile xanthogranuloma is primarily a cutaneous disorder with a predilection for the head and face. Vascular iris lesions may occur as discrete yellowish nodules or as diffuse infiltration causing heterochromia. Spontaneous hyphema can occur. (See also chapter XXVI, Ocular Tumors in Childhood.)

Primary Iris Cysts

Cysts of Iris Pigment Epithelium

Spontaneous cysts of the iris pigment epithelium result from a separation of the two layers of epithelium anywhere between the pupil and ciliary body (Fig XX-5). Clinically, they tend to be stable and rarely cause ocular complications. They appear more frequently in adults.

Central (Pupillary) Cysts

Cysts at the pupillary border are sometimes hereditary. They can be seen at any age and may enlarge slowly but generally remain asymptomatic. Rupture of these cysts can result in *iris flocculi*. Potent cholinesterase-inhibiting eyedrops may produce similar pupillary cysts, especially in young phakic individuals. Discontinuation of the drug or concomitant administration of phenylephrine generally results in improvement.

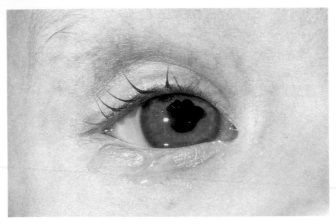

FIG XX-5—Cysts of the pigmented epithelium of the iris.

Cysts of Iris Stroma

Iris stromal cysts occur almost exclusively in infants or young children. They are most likely caused by sequestration of epithelium during embryologic development. The epithelium-lined stromal cysts usually contain goblet cells, and they may enlarge, causing obstruction of the visual axis, glaucoma, corneal decompensation, or iritis from cyst leakage. Numerous treatment modalities have been described, including cyst aspiration and photocoagulation or photodisruption, but the sudden release of cystic contents may result in transient iritis and glaucoma. Because of inherent complications or frequent cyst recurrences with other methods, surgical excision may be the preferred treatment method.

Shields JA. Primary cysts of the iris. *Trans Am Ophthalmol Soc.* 1981;79:771–809.

Sidoti PA, Valencia M, Chen N, et al. Echographic evaluation of primary cysts of the iris pigment epithelium. *Am J Ophthalmol.* 1995;120:161–167.

Brushfield Spots (Wofflin Nodules)

Focal areas of iris stromal hyperplasia surrounded by relative hypoplasia occur in up to 90% of patients with Down syndrome. They are known as *Brushfield spots* in these patients. Essentially identical areas known as *Wofflin nodules* occur in 24% of patients who do not have Down syndrome. Neither condition is pathologic.

Heterochromia Iridis

The differential diagnosis of pediatric heterochromia iridis is extensive. Etiologies can be classified on the basis of whether the condition is congenital or acquired and whether the affected eye is hypopigmented or hyperpigmented (Fig XX-6, Table XX-1).

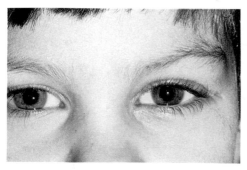

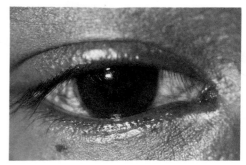

FIG XX-6—Heterochromia iridis. The left iris has become darker after developing a traumatic cataract.

FIG XX-7—Persistent pupillary membrane. Uncorrected visual acuity is 20/40.

TABLE XX-1

PEDIATRIC HETEROCHROMIA IRIDIS

Hypochromic heterochromia

    Horner syndrome (congenital or early in life)
    Incontinentia pigmenti (rare)
    Fuchs heterochromia
    Waardenburg-Klein syndrome
    Nonpigmented tumors
    Hypomelanosis of Ito

Hyperchromic heterochromia

    Oculodermal melanocytosis (associated with glaucoma in nonwhite adults)
    Pigmented tumors
    Siderosis
    Iris ectropion syndrome
    Extensive rubeosis

Modified from Roy FH. *Ocular Differential Diagnosis*. 3rd ed. Philadelphia: Lea & Febiger; 1984.

Persistent Pupillary Membranes

Persistent pupillary membranes (PPM) are the most common developmental abnormality of the iris. They are present in about 95% of newborns, and trace remnants are common in older children and adults. PPM are rarely of any visual significance. However, if especially prominent, they can adhere to the anterior lens capsule, causing a small anterior polar cataract. They may also be associated with various other anterior segment abnormalities (Fig XX-7). See discussion of posterior synechiae at the end of this chapter.

Abnormalities in the Size, Shape, or Location of the Pupil

Congenital Miosis

Congenital miosis, or *microcoria,* may represent an absence or malformation of the dilator pupillae muscle. It can also occur secondary to contracture of fibrous material on the pupil margin from remnants of the tunica vasculosa lentis or neural crest cell anomalies. The condition may be unilateral or bilateral and sporadic or hereditary. A surgical pupilloplasty is needed in severe cases.

The pupil diameter rarely exceeds 2 mm, is often eccentric, and reacts poorly to mydriatic drops. Some patients with eccentric microcoria also have lens subluxation and are therefore part of the spectrum of ectopia lentis et pupillae. Congenital miosis may be associated with microcornea, megalocornea, iris atrophy, iris transillumination, myopia, and glaucoma. It can also be seen with congenital rubella syndrome and hereditary ataxia and in 20% of patients with Lowe oculocerebrorenal syndrome.

> Toulemont PJ, Urvoy M, Coscas G, et al. Association of congenital microcoria with myopia and glaucoma. A study of 23 patients with congenital microcoria. *Ophthalmology.* 1995;102:193–198.

Congenital Mydriasis

Congenitally dilated and fixed pupils with normal-appearing irides have been reported under the names *familial iridoplegia* and *congenital bilateral mydriasis.* Iris sphincter trauma, pharmacologic mydriasis, or acquired neurologic disease affecting the parasympathetic innervation to the pupil must also be considered. Many cases of congenital mydriasis may fall within the aniridia spectrum, especially if the central iris structures from the collarette to the pupillary sphincter are absent.

Dyscoria

The term *dyscoria* refers to an abnormality of the shape of the pupil and is usually reserved for congenital malformations. Acquired inflammatory conditions can lead to posterior synechiae, which can also produce a misshapen pupil. Colobomatous iris defects that produce a dyscoric pupil are discussed above. Iris hypoplasia, especially if sectoral, can produce dyscoria as well as corectopia (see below). Slitlike pupils have been described in the Axenfeld-Rieger syndrome (see Figure XIX-4, p 212), in ectopia lentis et pupillae, and rarely as an isolated condition with normal visual acuity.

Corectopia

Corectopia refers to displacement of the pupil. Normally, the pupil is situated about 0.5 mm inferonasally from the center of the iris. Minor deviations up to 1 mm are usually cosmetically insignificant and should probably not be considered abnormal. Sector iris hypoplasia or other colobomatous lesions can lead to corectopia, and isolated noncolobomatous autosomal dominant corectopia has also been reported. More commonly, however, corectopia is seen in association with lens subluxation, and this combination is referred to as *ectopia lentis et pupillae.* The condition is almost always bilateral, with the pupils and lenses displaced in opposite directions.

The pupils may be oval or slit-shaped, and they often dilate poorly. Iris transillumination may occur, and microspherophakia has been reported. Progressive corectopia can be seen in association with the Axenfeld-Rieger spectrum as well as iridocorneal endothelial (ICE) syndrome.

Polycoria and Pseudopolycoria

True polycoria that must by definition include a sphincter mechanism in each pupil is very rare. The vast majority of accessory iris openings can be classified as *pseudopolycoria*. These iris holes may be congenital or may develop in response to progressive corectopia and iris hypoplasia in Axenfeld-Rieger syndrome or ICE syndrome (Fig XX-8). Pseudopolycoria can also result from trauma or surgery.

Congenital Iris Ectropion

Ectropion of the posterior pigment epithelium onto the anterior surface of the iris is called *ectropion uveae* in much of the literature. This term is a misnomer, because the iris posterior epithelium is derived from neural ectoderm and is not considered part of the uvea. This iris ectropion can occur as an acquired tractional abnormality, often in association with rubeosis iridis, or as a congenital nonprogressive abnormality. The combination of unilateral congenital iris ectropion, a glassy-smooth, cryptless iris surface, a high iris insertion, dysgenesis of the drainage angle, and glaucoma has been referred to as *congenital iris ectropion syndrome* (Fig XX-9). Congenital iris ectropion has been associated in some cases with neurofibromatosis and has been reported more rarely with facial hemihypertrophy and Prader-Willi syndrome.

Wilson ME. Congenital iris ectropion and a new classification for anterior segment dysgenesis. *J Pediatr Ophthalmol Strabismus.* 1990;27:48–55.

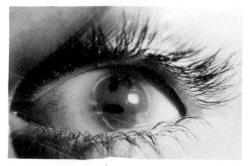 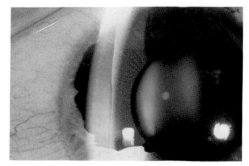

FIG XX-8—Pseudopolycoria that is secondary to Axenfeld-Rieger syndrome.

FIG XX-9—Congenital iris ectropion syndrome. A glassy-smooth, cryptless iris surface is present along with marked ectropion of the posterior pigmented epithelium onto the anterior iris surface.

Iris Transillumination

In albinism iris transillumination results from the absence of pigmentation in the posterior epithelial layers. Iris hypoplasia can also lead to iris transillumination, especially as part of Axenfeld-Rieger or ICE syndrome. Iris transillumination has also been reported in Marfan syndrome, ectopia lentis et pupillae, and microcoria. Patchy areas of transillumination can also be seen after trauma, surgery, or uveitis.

Posterior Synechiae

Congenital adhesions between the iris margin and lens capsule may occur in association with cataracts, aniridia, intrauterine inflammation, or other developmental abnormalities. They can also be isolated, benign remnants of the tunica vasculosa lentis. Acquired posterior synechiae secondary to iridocyclitis occur more frequently. Pediatric sarcoidosis may have inflammatory iris nodules (Koeppe or Busacca) associated with posterior synechiae.

CHAPTER XXI

Pediatric Glaucomas

Pediatric glaucomas constitute a heterogeneous group of diseases, which may result from an intrinsic disease or structural abnormality of the aqueous outflow pathways (*primary glaucoma*) or from abnormalities originating in other regions of the eye (*secondary glaucoma*). A variety of systemic abnormalities are also associated with pediatric glaucoma.

Primary Congenital Glaucoma

Primary congenital open-angle glaucoma is also commonly referred to as *congenital,* or *infantile, glaucoma.* Primary congenital glaucoma occurs in about 1 out of 10,000 births and results in blindness in 2%–15% of cases. Visual acuity is lower than 20/50 in at least 50% of cases. It is bilateral in about two thirds of patients, and occurs more frequently in males (65%) than in females (35%). No specific racial or geographic prevalence has been identified.

While only 25% of affected infants are diagnosed at birth, more than 80% have disease onset within the first year of life. If this disease presents later in childhood (after about age 3–4 years), it is considered *primary juvenile open-angle glaucoma,* a disease that appears to have a different genetic origin (see below) and often responds to therapy classically used for adult open-angle glaucoma (see BCSC Section 10, *Glaucoma*).

> Buckley EG. Primary congenital open angle glaucoma. In: Epstein DL, Allingham RR, Schuman JS, eds. *Chandler and Grant's Glaucoma.* 4th ed. Baltimore: Williams & Wilkins; 1997:598–608.

> deLuise VP, Anderson DR. Primary infantile glaucoma (congenital glaucoma). *Surv Ophthalmol.* 1983;28:1–19.

Genetics

Most cases of primary congenital glaucoma occur sporadically, but an autosomal recessive form with variable penetrance has been identified. A major locus for recessively inherited primary congenital glaucoma (GLC3 gene) has recently been identified on the short arm of chromosome 2 (2p21). The association of congenital glaucoma with abnormalities of other chromosomes has previously been reported in the regions of 6p21, 6p25, 11p, and 11q. Autosomal dominant juvenile-onset primary open-angle glaucoma has been mapped to the long arm of chromosome 1.

When no family history of congenital glaucoma exists, an affected parent has approximately a 5% chance of having an affected child. If the first child is affected, the risk of a second child being affected is approximately 5%, rising to approximately 25% per subsequent offspring if two siblings are affected. Primary congenital glaucoma does not appear to be associated with adult primary open-angle glaucoma; the incidence of steroid-induced intraocular pressure (IOP) elevation is no higher in parents of affected children than in controls.

Broughton WL, Fine BS, Zimmerman LE. Congenital glaucoma associated with a chromosomal defect. A histologic study. *Arch Ophthalmol.* 1981;99:481–486.

Sarfarazi M, Akarsu AN, Hossain A, et al. Assignment of a locus (GLC3A) for primary congenital glaucoma (buphthalmos) to 2p21 and evidence for genetic heterogeneity. *Genomics.* 1995;30:171–177.

Pathophysiology

The basic pathologic defect in primary congenital glaucoma remains obscure. Although Barkan originally proposed a thin imperforate membrane that covered the anterior chamber angle and blocked aqueous outflow, it is now generally believed that the site of obstruction is the trabecular meshwork itself. This disease may represent a developmental arrest of anterior chamber tissue derived from neural crest cells during the late embryologic period.

Anderson DR. The development of the trabecular meshwork and its abnormality in primary infantile glaucoma. *Trans Am Ophthalmol Soc.* 1981;79:458–485.

Walton DS. Primary congenital open angle glaucoma: a study of the anterior segment abnormalities. *Trans Am Ophthalmol Soc.* 1981;77:746–768.

Clinical Manifestations and Diagnosis

Primary congenital glaucoma usually presents in the neonatal or infantile period with a combination of signs and symptoms. Epiphora, photophobia, and blepharospasm constitute the classic "clinical triad" of primary congenital glaucoma. Other symptoms include clouding and/or enlargement of the cornea (Fig XXI-1).

Corneal edema results from elevated IOP and may be gradual or sudden in onset. It is often the presenting sign in infants younger than 3 months of age. Microcystic edema initially involves the corneal epithelium, but later extends also to the stroma, often accompanied by one or more curvilinear breaks in Descemet's membrane *(Haab's striae).* Although edema may resolve with IOP reduction, a scar will remain permanently at the site of Haab's striae. *Photophobia, epiphora,* and *blepharospasm* result from the glare and epithelial abnormalities associated with corneal edema and opacification.

Corneal enlargement occurs with gradual stretching of the cornea as a result of elevated IOP and often appears in slightly older infants up to about 2–3 years of age. The normal newborn has a horizontal corneal diameter of 9.5–10.5 mm; a diameter of >11.5 mm is suggestive of glaucoma. By 1 year of age, normal corneal diameter is 10–11.5 mm; a diameter >12.5 mm suggests abnormality. Any child with a corneal diameter >13 mm should be suspected of having glaucoma.

The signs and symptoms described for primary congenital glaucoma can also occur in infants with other primary developmental and secondary glaucomas, as a nonspecific result of expansion of the infant eye when faced with high IOP. Nonglaucomatous conditions may also cause some of the signs and the symptoms seen in primary congenital glaucoma (Table XXI-1) (see also BCSC Section 10, *Glaucoma*).

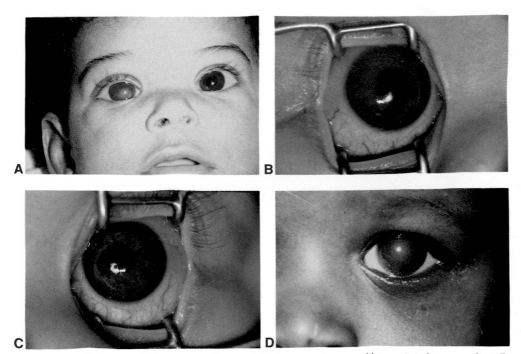

FIG XXI-1—*A,* Congenital glaucoma, right eye. *B,* Right cornea larger and hazy. *C,* Left cornea clear. *D,* Late congenital glaucoma, left eye.

Diagnostic examination A full ophthalmic examination of every child suspected of glaucoma is imperative. Vision will often be poorer in the affected eye in unilateral cases and may be poor in both eyes when bilateral glaucoma is present. The child's ability to fix and follow and the presence of nystagmus should also be noted. *Refraction,* when possible, often reveals myopia and/or astigmatism from eye enlargement and corneal irregularity.

Corneal inspection. The cornea should be examined for size, possible edema, and Haab's striae. A penlight, millimeter ruler, direct ophthalmoscope, and retinoscope are useful. Even a half-millimeter difference in corneal diameter between the eyes can often be noted by inspection. Haab's striae are often seen well against the red reflex after pupil dilation (Fig XXI-2).

Tonometry and intraocular pressure. The best IOP measurements are those taken on a cooperative child using topical anesthesia, since IOP may be falsely elevated in a struggling child and unpredictably altered (usually lowered) when systemic sedatives and anesthetics are administered. A useful technique is to bring the child in slightly hungry and then bottle feed at the time of pressure measurement. The Perkins applanation tonometer and the Tonopen are useful in infants and young children, and Goldmann applanation readings can frequently be achieved in older children.

In primary congenital glaucoma unanesthetized IOP commonly ranges between 30 and 40 mm Hg, and it is usually greater than 20 mm Hg even under anesthesia.

TABLE XXI-1

DIFFERENTIAL DIAGNOSIS OF SIGNS IN PRIMARY CONGENITAL GLAUCOMA

Conditions sharing signs of epiphora and red eye
Conjunctivitis
Congenital nasolacrimal duct obstruction
Corneal epithelial defect/abrasion
Ocular inflammation (uveitis, trauma)

Conditions sharing signs of corneal edema or opacification
Corneal dystrophy
  Congenital hereditary endothelial dystrophy
  Posterior polymorphous dystrophy
Obstetrical birth trauma with Descemet's tears
Storage disease
  Mucopolysaccharidoses
  Cystinosis
Congenital anomalies
  Sclerocornea
  Peters anomaly
Keratitis
  Maternal rubella keratitis
  Herpetic
  Phlyctenular
Idiopathic (diagnosis of exclusion only)

Conditions sharing sign of corneal enlargement
Axial myopia
Megalocornea

Conditions sharing sign of optic nerve cupping (real or apparent)
Physiologic optic nerve cupping
Optic nerve coloboma
Optic atrophy
Optic nerve hypoplasia
Optic nerve malformation

(Reproduced with modification from Buckley EG. Primary congenital open angle glaucoma. In: Epstein DL, Allingham RR, Schuman JS, eds. *Chandler and Grant's Glaucoma.* 4th ed. Baltimore: Williams & Wilkins; 1997:598–608.)

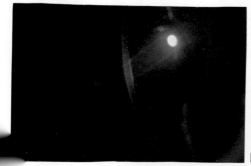

B

FIG XXI-2—*A,* Breaks in Descemet's membrane, right eye. *B,* Retroillumination, same eye.

The normal IOP in infants and young children is lower than that of normal adults; mean IOP is between 10 and 12 mm Hg in newborn infants and reaches approximately 14 mm Hg by age 7–8 years. Asymmetric IOP readings in a quiet or anesthetized child should also raise suspicion of glaucoma in the eye with the higher IOP. Conscious sedation with chloral hydrate (100 mg/kg PO or PR up to 1000 mg maximum dose) allows IOP readings that are minimally altered from those in an awake state. Conscious sedation should be performed with close monitoring of the child's vital signs and oxygenation by pulse oximetry.

Anterior segment examination. After tonometry has been attempted, the portable slit lamp allows detailed inspection of the anterior segments. An abnormally deep anterior chamber and relative peripheral iris stromal hypoplasia are characteristic of primary congenital glaucoma.

Gonioscopy provides important information regarding the mechanism of glaucoma. It is best performed using a Koeppe contact lens and portable slit lamp or loupes. Often a preliminary examination can be performed on a quiet infant in the office, with more detailed assessment possible in the operating room under anesthesia. Figure XXI-3 gives examples of gonioscopic photographs of adult patients. The anterior chamber angle of a *normal* infant differs from that of an adult in the following ways:

☐ The trabecular meshwork is more lightly pigmented

☐ Schwalbe's line is often less distinct

☐ The uveal meshwork is translucent so that the junction between scleral spur and cilary body band is often well seen

In congenital glaucoma the iris often shows an insertion more anterior than that of the normal angle, and the translucency of the uveal meshwork is altered, making cilary body band, trabecular meshwork, and scleral spur indistinct. (The membrane described by Barkan may indeed be these translucent uveal meshwork cells.) The scalloped border of the iris pigmented epithelium is often unusually prominent, especially when peripheral iris stromal hypoplasia is present. Juvenile open-angle glaucoma patients, by contrast, usually demonstrate a normal-appearing open angle.

Optic nerve examination. The optic nerve, when it can be seen, usually shows an increased cup/disc ratio, which can improve with successful treatment and lowering of IOP. The pattern of generalized enlargement of the optic cup seen in very young patients with glaucoma has been attributed to stretching of the optic canal and backward bowing of the lamina cribrosa, which can be reversible (Fig XXI-4). In most cases of primary congenital glaucoma the cup/disc ratio exceeds 0.3; in contrast, 97% of normal newborn eyes show a cup/disc ratio of less than 0.3. Cup/disc asymmetry between two eyes of an infant is also suspicious for glaucoma on the more cupped side.

Buckley EG. Primary congenital open angle glaucoma. In: Epstein DL, Allingham RR, Schuman JS, eds. *Chandler and Grant's Glaucoma.* 4th ed. Baltimore: Williams & Wilkins; 1997:598–608.

Shaffer RN, Weiss DI. *Congenital and Pediatric Glaucomas.* St Louis: Mosby; 1970.

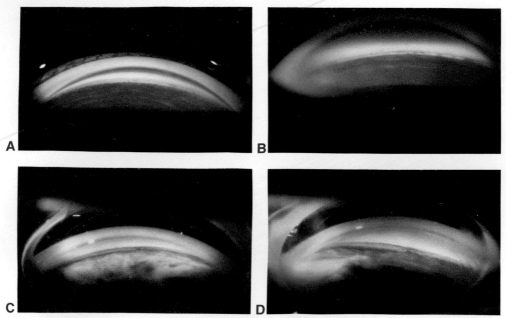

FIG XXI-3—Gonioscopy in adults. *A,* Normal open angle. Gonioscopic photograph shows trace pigmentation of the posterior trabecular meshwork and normal insertion of the iris into a narrow ciliary body band. The Goldmann lens was used. *B,* Normal open angle. This gonioscopic view using the Goldmann lens shows mild pigmentation of the posterior trabecular meshwork. A wide ciliary body band with posterior insertion of the iris can also be seen. *C,* Narrow angle. This gonioscopic view using the Zeiss lens without indentation shows pigment in inferior angle but poor visualization of angle anatomy. *D,* Same angle as shown in *C.* Gonioscopy with a Zeiss lens with indentation shows peripheral anterior synechiae in the posterior trabecular meshwork. Pigment deposits on Schwalbe's line can also be seen. (Photographs courtesy of Elizabeth A. Hodapp, MD.)

Natural History

In almost all cases of untreated primary congenital glaucoma the disease progresses and leads to blindness. The cornea becomes irreversibly opacified and may vascularize. It may continue to enlarge through the first 2–3 years of life, reaching a diameter up to 16–17 mm. As the entire eye enlarges, pseudoproptosis and an "ox eye" appearance, called *buphthalmos,* may result. Scleral thinning and myopic fundus changes may occur, and spontaneous lens dislocation can result. Optic nerve cupping also increases and may finally lead to complete blindness.

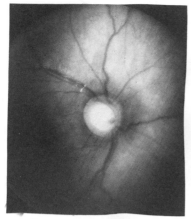 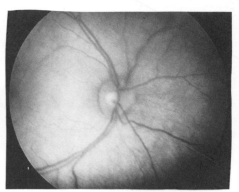

FIG XXI-4.—Optic nerve changes after treatment for congenital glaucoma. *Left,* Preoperative enlarged optic disc cup. *Right,* Resolution of disc cupping after pressure is reduced by goniotomy. (Photographs courtesy of Sharon Freedman, MD.)

Other Primary Developmental and Secondary Pediatric Glaucomas

Primary Developmental Glaucomas

In addition to primary congenital open-angle glaucoma, other primary developmental glaucomas can present at birth or shortly after. The ophthalmologist and pediatrician should carefully examine the newborn or infant with glaucoma to uncover associated ocular and systemic abnormalities, such as

- Congenital rubella
- Oculocerebrorenal (Lowe) syndrome
- Sturge-Weber syndrome (nevus flammeus, or port-wine stain, of the face on the affected side)
- Neurofibromatosis
- Homocystinuria

Infantile glaucoma can present with the following ocular abnormalities:

- Aniridia
- Axenfeld-Rieger syndrome
- Congenital iris ectropion
- Peters anomaly
- Sclerocornea
- Posterior polymorphous dystrophy
- Congenital hereditary endothelial dystrophy

See BCSC Section 10, *Glaucoma,* Table X-2.

Treatment of infants with primary developmental glaucomas should usually follow the same guidelines as those for primary congenital glaucoma (see Treatment below). In some cases (e.g., aniridia and Axenfeld-Rieger syndrome), secondary glaucoma may also occur later in childhood, and treatment again resembles that for other secondary glaucomas in childhood.

Secondary Glaucoma

Secondary glaucomas in children may result from trauma, inflammation, or uveitis (e.g., juvenile rheumatoid arthritis). Aphakic glaucoma after congenital cataract surgery, secondary angle-closure glaucoma in cases of cicatricial retinopathy of prematurity, and glaucoma associated with childhood intraocular neoplasm (e.g., retinoblastoma, juvenile xanthogranuloma, and medulloepithelioma) are secondary glaucomas specific to children. Less commonly, secondary glaucoma can result from some of the same causes as in adults, such as steroid use. In general, secondary glaucoma in children is managed as it is managed in adults. Those eyes with angle closure usually require peripheral iridectomy or lensectomy, while medical therapy is attempted first with other secondary glaucomas.

Aphakic glaucoma deserves special comment. Acute or subacute angle closure with iris bombé is rare; it usually occurs soon after surgery but can have delayed onset (more than 1 year). The treatment is surgical iridectomy, often with goniosynechialysis and anterior vitrectomy. The incidence of the more common open-angle glaucoma after removal of congenital cataracts varies from 15% to 30%, with a mean time to onset of 5 years after surgery. The risk of glaucoma seems higher in infants operated prior to 1 year of age, in those with initial corneal diameter <10 mm, and in those with persistent hyperplastic primary vitreous (PHPV). Children who are aphakic are at lifelong risk for developing glaucoma and need careful examination (including IOP evaluation) on a regular basis.

Egbert JE, Wright MM, Dahlhauser KF, et al. A prospective study of ocular hypertension and glaucoma after pediatric cataract surgery. *Ophthalmology*. 1995;102: 1098–1101.

Hoskins HD Jr, Shaffer RN, Hetherington J. Anatomical classification of the developmental glaucomas. *Arch Ophthalmol.* 1984;102:1331–1336.

Walton DS. Unusual pediatric glaucomas. In: Epstein DL, Allingham RR, Schuman JS, eds. *Chandler and Grant's Glaucoma.* 4th ed. Baltimore: Williams & Wilkins; 1997:623–638.

Treatment

While it is true that juvenile open-angle glaucoma and most secondary glaucomas of childhood are managed in much the same way as similar conditions in adults, differences in approach do exist. Management of adult glaucoma is more likely to delay surgery until medical options have been pursued.

Surgical Therapy

Surgical intervention is the treatment of choice for primary congenital glaucoma and most of the other primary developmental glaucomas presenting in infancy and early childhood. BCSC Section 10, *Glaucoma*, also covers the procedures discussed in this chapter.

Angle surgery is the preferred initial surgical intervention in these cases. *Goniotomy,* in which an incision is made in the trabecular meshwork under direct gonioscopic visualization, is often preferred when the cornea is clear; *trabeculotomy,* which uses an external approach to identify, cannulate, and then connect Schlemm's canal with the anterior chamber by tearing through the poorly functioning trabecular meshwork, is preferable in cases of poor visualization of the angle.

Usually, at least two angle surgeries are performed prior to proceeding with an additional surgical modality. IOP is controlled with one or two angle surgeries in approximately 80% of infants with primary congenital glaucoma presenting from 3 months to 1 year of age. If angle surgery is unsuccessful and medical therapy (see below) is inadequate to control IOP and glaucoma, additional options include trabeculectomy with antifibrotic therapy (e.g., mitomycin) or glaucoma implant procedures.

Trabeculectomy with the use of mitomycin-C is successful in approximately 50%–95% of children. The reported success rate may vary tremendously with characteristics of the patient and the eye. Patients younger than 1 year of age and those who are aphakic may not fare as well. The long-term risk of leaking and endophthalmitis may be particularly high with mitomycin-augmented trabeculectomy in children; both complications have already occurred.

The reported success of glaucoma *implant surgery* with the Molteno, Baerveldt, and Ahmed implants has varied between 54% and approximately 80%–85%. While most of these children must remain on adjunctive topical medical therapy to control IOP after surgery, their blebs are thicker and may be less prone to leaking and infection than those of mitomycin-augmented trabeculectomy.

Cycloablation with the Nd:YAG laser, diode laser, or by cyclocryotherapy is generally reserved for extremely resistant cases or those not amenable to the intraocular surgeries noted above. These techniques decrease ciliary body production of aqueous humor. Cyclocryotherapy (freeze treatment to the ciliary body through the sclera) has a reported success of about 33%. Repeat applications are the rule, and risk of phthisis and blindness is significant (approximately 10%). Transscleral laser cycloablation with the Nd:YAG or the diode laser has also been used in refractory cases. Short-term success is about 50% with a retreatment rate of ~70% with either laser.

Medical Therapy

The menu of glaucoma medications available for use continues to expand. See also BCSC Section 10, *Glaucoma.*

Carbonic anhydrase inhibitors have been used for many years as aqueous suppressants in children, and they may be quite effective. Acetazolamide (Diamox), the most commonly used agent, is effective at oral doses of 10–20 mg/kg per day, divided in three or four doses. Care must be taken to watch for weight loss, lethargy, or metabolic acidosis, although most children tolerate this medication well.

The topical carbonic anhydrase inhibitor dorzolamide (Trusopt) has recently become available as a 2.0% solution. Preliminary studies using dorzolamide (Trusopt) tid indicate that this drug is effective in many cases, although it produces a smaller reduction in IOP (<15%) than does full-dose oral acetazolamide in the same child (~20%).

Topical beta-blocker therapy has been used in children since 1978, and it can also effectively lower IOP about 20%. The major risks of this therapy are respiratory distress caused by apnea or bronchospasm and bradycardia, which is noted to occur mostly in very tiny infants and in children with a history of bronchospasm. Timolol (or its equivalent) or betaxolol (Betoptic S) should be prescribed as 0.25% bid for initial therapy. The parent should be instructed how to perform nasolacrimal occlusion with these drugs.

Miotic therapy is rarely effective in cases of primary congenital glaucoma, perhaps because of the high iris insertion in these cases. Long-acting or slow-release miotics such as pilocarpine (Pilopine gel and Ocusert) or echothiophate (Phospholine Iodide) can be helpful, particularly in cases of juvenile open-angle glaucoma and some secondary childhood glaucomas.

Adrenergic agents such as epinephrine or dipivefrin (Propine) are not usually effective in children, particularly when a nonselective beta blocker is already in use. The alpha$_2$-adrenergic agonist apraclonidine (Iopidine) has been useful when short-term IOP reduction is essential, but it shows a high incidence of tachyphylaxis and allergy in young children.

The *prostaglandin derivative* latanoprost (Xalatan) has recently become available at a strength of 0.005% for use at bedtime. Very preliminary experience shows an excellent systemic safety profile and variable IOP reduction with this medication in pediatric patients with glaucoma.

> Freedman SF. Medical and surgical treatments for childhood glaucomas. In: Epstein DL, Allingham RR, Schuman JS, eds. *Chandler and Grant's Glaucoma.* 4th ed. Baltimore: Williams & Wilkins; 1997:609–622.
>
> Freedman SF, Buckley EG. Goniotomy and trabeculectomy. In: Buckley EG, Freedman SF, Shields MB. *Atlas of Ophthalmic Surgery, Vol III: Strabismus and Glaucoma.* St Louis: Mosby; 1995.
>
> Freedman SF, Walton DS. Approach to infants and children with glaucoma. In: Epstein DL, Allingham RR, Schuman JS, eds. *Chandler and Grant's Glaucoma.* 4th ed. Baltimore: Williams & Wilkins; 1997:586–597.

Prognosis and Follow-up

If primary congenital glaucoma presents at birth, the prognosis for IOP control and visual preservation is quite poor, with at least half of these eyes becoming legally blind. With a corneal diameter >14 mm at diagnosis the visual prognosis is similarly poor. Up to 80%–90% of cases in the "favorable prognostic group" (onset 3–12 months) can be controlled with angle surgery. The remaining >10% of these, and many of the remaining cases of primary and secondary glaucomas, often present a lifelong challenge.

Visual loss in childhood glaucoma is multifactorial. It may result not only from corneal scarring and opacification or optic nerve damage but also from significant myopic astigmatism and associated anisometropic and strabismic amblyopia, especially in unilateral cases. Myopia results from axial enlargement of the eye in the setting of high IOP, while astigmatism often results from unequal expansion of the anterior segment, corneal scarring and opacification, or dislocation of the lens. Careful assessment of vision, refraction, and amblyopia therapy are needed to optimize visual function in these children.

Diligent follow-up is needed in all cases of childhood glaucoma, and it should also be performed in cases where glaucoma may be suspected but cannot yet be confirmed. After any given surgical intervention or change in medical therapy, the control of IOP should be assessed within 1–2 weeks. The status of the cornea in terms of its size and clarity, the appearance of the optic nerve, and the refractive error can all often provide clues regarding improved IOP control. If IOP cannot be determined in the office, a sedated examination with chloral hydrate, or occasionally an examination under anesthesia, may be needed. The IOP should be considered not as an isolated finding but rather in conjunction with other features of the examination. If the IOP is <20 mm Hg under anesthesia, but clinical evidence shows persistent corneal edema or enlargement, progressive optic nerve cupping, or myopic progression, then further intervention should be pursued despite the IOP reading. By contrast, an IOP in the 20 mm Hg range in a young child who shows evidence of clinical improvement may be followed carefully in the short term without any other intervention.

Careful repeated follow-up of all parameters associated with glaucoma in children is the only way to ensure disease control and optimal preservation of visual function. Even those children apparently "cured" after angle surgery can relapse years later with elevated IOP and subsequent visual loss. Visual fields can be helpful in following disease progression in older children, but they are rarely useful in children younger than 6–8 years of age. Optic nerve photographs should be taken whenever possible, and these can be helpful for comparison during later examinations. As discussed above, refractive error and corneal size and clarity are also helpful to follow as evidence for ocular stability over time. Serial axial length measurement may be followed as well, but it is no more reliable than corneal diameter measurement.

CHAPTER XXII

Childhood Cataracts and Other Pediatric Lens Disorders

The normal lens includes a central embryonal nucleus surrounded by secondary fibers forming the fetal nucleus, which has anterior and posterior Y-sutures. Occasionally, development of the lens is abnormal, resulting in structural variations described below. Cataracts or other abnormalities of the lens often cause retinal images to be blurred, and amblyopia is a common consequence. BCSC Section 11, *Lens and Cataract,* also covers the conditions and procedures discussed in this chapter.

Structural or Positional Lens Abnormalities

Congenital aphakia Absence of the lens at birth is rare. This condition is usually associated with a markedly abnormal eye.

Spherophakia A lens that is spherical and smaller than a normal lens is called spherophakic. This condition is usually bilateral. The lens may dislocate, causing secondary glaucoma (Fig XXII-1).

Coloboma A lens coloboma involves flattening or notching of the lens periphery (Fig XXII-2). This abnormality is usually located inferonasally. Zonular fibers are commonly absent in the colobomatous area, and an associated ciliary body coloboma may be present.

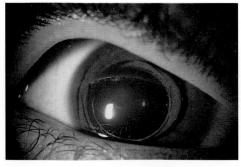

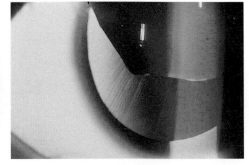

FIG XXII-1—Spherophakia with lens dislocation into anterior chamber, left eye.

FIG XXII-2—Lens equator flattening (with dislocation), which may be referred to as lens coloboma.

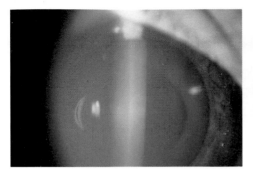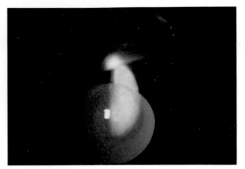

FIG XXII-3—Posterior lenticonus.

Lenticonus   *Anterior* or *posterior lenticonus* describes a central ectasia of the lens surface that is often associated with lens opacities. Anterior lenticonus may be associated with nerve deafness and nephritis (Alport syndrome). Decreased vision is common with posterior lenticonus. The underlying lens defect may be congenital, but the cataract is frequently developmental and comes to the ophthalmologist's attention at a later age than a truly congenital cataract (Fig XXII-3).

Dislocation   When the lens is not in its normal anatomic position, it is said to be *dislocated.* The degree of dislocation can vary from partial to complete. Other terms for this condition include *ectopia lentis, luxation,* and *subluxation,* but the term dislocated will be used in this discussion to avoid confusion. A dislocated lens often results in decreased vision from large errors of refraction. Diplopia and/or photophobia may be present. The condition is usually bilateral when inherited, but it can be unilateral when caused by trauma or glaucoma. The family history may mention decreased vision or visual disturbances. On clinical examination the anterior chamber is deep, and tremulous movement of the iris (iridodonesis) is common. Transillumination of the peripheral iris may be possible. The lens equator may be apparent in the pupillary space, and zonular fibers may be visible.

Refraction through the phakic and aphakic space should be completed together with a careful slit-lamp examination. Gonioscopy is undertaken to reveal associated anomalies of the iridocorneal angle, and ophthalmoscopy is important to rule out retinal lesions. Corneal astigmatism is common in Marfan syndrome (see below), and it can be documented by keratometry. Axial A-scan measurements are useful prognostically because the incidence of retinal detachment increases with abnormally large eyes. Patients with lens abnormalities may benefit from evaluation by a pediatrician or a geneticist.

Lens dislocation can occur as an isolated disorder or in association with other ocular or systemic abnormalities. Trauma accounts for a higher percentage of lens dislocation than any other cause. Spontaneous lens dislocation has been reported in

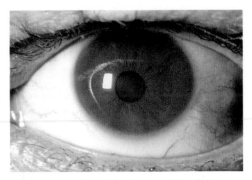

FIG XXII-4—Ectopia lentis et pupillae, left eye.

aniridia and, rarely, with exfoliation syndrome and buphthalmos. Associated systemic disorders include

□ Marfan syndrome

□ Homocystinuria

□ Weill-Marchesani syndrome

□ Hyperlysinemia

□ Sulfite oxidase deficiency

□ Syphilis

□ Ehlers-Danlos syndrome

Simple ectopia lentis is usually bilateral and symmetric with upward temporal lens displacement. Autosomal dominant inheritance is most common. The onset may be congenital or may occur between 20 and 65 years of age. Glaucoma is most common in the late-onset type. The best optical correction, phakic or aphakic, should be prescribed. If the lens edge crosses the pupillary space, a trial of mydriasis may be useful. Lensectomy with vitrectomy instrumentation may be considered if the vision cannot be satisfactorily corrected with spectacles or a contact lens.

Ectopia lentis et pupillae, or lens and pupillary displacement, is a congenital anomaly distinguished by slit- or oval-shaped pupils (Fig XXII-4). The condition is usually bilateral but not symmetric. Glaucoma and cataracts may be present. Inheritance is autosomal recessive, and the family history is essential. Errors of refraction should be treated.

Marfan syndrome   This disorder has a prevalence of 1 in 10,000. Inheritance is autosomal dominant, but 15% of cases have no family history. Marfan syndrome is caused by mutations in the fibrillin gene on chromosome 15. These patients are characteristically tall with long limbs and fingers (arachnodactyly). Loose, flexible joints, scoliosis, and chest deformities are common. Cardiovascular complications include aortic dilation, dissecting aneurysm, and floppy mitral valve. Enophthalmos with flat malar areas is apparent. Visual acuity is often reduced from associated lens dislocation, which is present in 50%–80% of patients and usually bilateral and upward (Fig XXII-5). Myopia and corneal astigmatism are common. Peripheral trans-

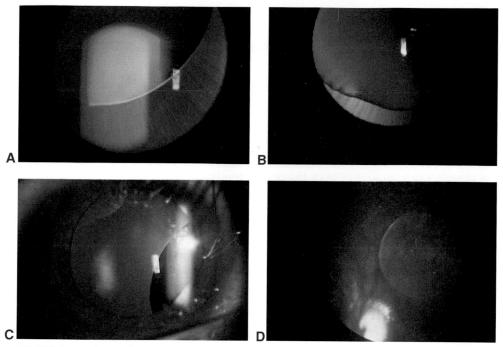

FIG XXII-5—Marfan syndrome. *A and B,* Superotemporal displacement of lenses, bilateral. *C,* Inferonasal displacement, right eye. *D,* Lens dislocation into vitreous, left eye.

illumination of the iris is seen in 10% of cases, and pectinate ligaments are occasionally seen in the anterior chamber angle.

Patients with Marfan syndrome require a thorough history and physical and ocular examinations together with annual echocardiograms. Propranolol may be prescribed to reduce myocardial contractility if the aorta is dilated. Refractive errors should be corrected and lensectomy may improve vision in some cases. Antibiotic prophylaxis is indicated to prevent endocarditis associated with surgery. A-scan axial length measurement is helpful to document patients with a high risk of retinal detachment as a consequence of increased axial length.

Homocystinuria This rare autosomal recessive condition results in mental retardation in 50% of cases. Thrombotic vascular occlusions are common and associated with increased anesthetic risk. These patients are unusually tall with osteoporosis, scoliosis, and chest deformities. They often have blue irides. Partial or complete vascular obstruction is present in various organs, and hypertension, cardiac murmurs, and cardiomegaly are seen. Lens dislocation is present in 90% of these patients, usually inferior and bilateral (Fig XXII-6). Progressive myopia may be the first sign of lens dislocation. Glaucoma may result if the lens dislocates into the anterior chamber. The zonular fibers have been shown to be histopathologically deficient.

Diagnosis is confirmed by an analysis of the serum homocysteine level. Management includes both a general and an ocular history and examination. Surgery should be avoided if possible because of the increased anesthetic risks of

TABLE XXII-1

ETIOLOGY OF PEDIATRIC CATARACTS

Bilateral cataracts

Idiopathic
Hereditary cataracts (autosomal dominant most common,
    also autosomal recessive or X-linked)
Genetic and metabolic diseases
    Down syndrome
    Hallermann-Streiff syndrome
    Lowe syndrome
    Galactosemia
    Marfan syndrome
    Trisomy 13–15
    Hypoglycemia
    Alport syndrome
    Myotonic dystrophy
    Fabry disease
    Hypoparathyroidism
    Conradi syndrome
Maternal infection
    Rubella
    Cytomegalovirus
    Varicella
    Syphilis
    Toxoplasmosis
Ocular anomalies
    Aniridia
    Anterior segment dysgenesis syndrome
Toxic
    Corticosteroids
    Radiation (may also be unilateral)

Unilateral cataracts

Idiopathic
Ocular anomalies
    Persistent hyperplastic primary vitreous (PHPV)
    Anterior segment dysgenesis
    Posterior lenticonus
    Posterior pole tumors
Traumatic (rule out child abuse)
Rubella
Masked bilateral cataract

Visual function can be assessed by history, observation of the fixation and following reflexes, behavioral testing, and electrophysiologic exams. Detailed evaluation of the normally symmetric red reflexes is easily accomplished in a darkened room by shining a bright direct ophthalmoscope into both eyes simultaneously. This test, which is called the *illumination test, red reflex test,* or *Bruckner test,* can easily be used for routine ocular screening by nurses, pediatricians, and family practitioners.

Slit-lamp examination clarifies the morphology of the cataract and may help determine, along with associated findings, the etiology and prognosis. For example,

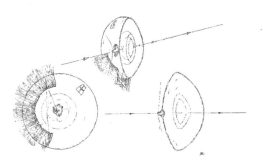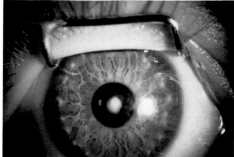

FIG XXII-8—Anterior polar cataract. (Illustration courtesy of Alan Y. Chow, MD.)

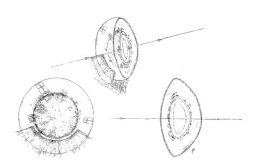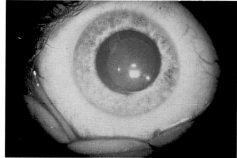

FIG XXII-9—Lamellar cataract. (Illustration courtesy of Alan Y. Chow, MD.) Note that in photograph on the right the opacity surrounds the nucleus and is outside the Y-sutures.

most *anterior polar cataracts* are small, measuring less than 1–2 mm, and are usually not progressive (Fig XXII-8). Surgery is seldom required, and the visual prognosis is excellent.

Lamellar cataracts are characterized by layers of opacification peripheral to the Y-sutures with a clear nucleus (Fig XXII-9). They are generally bilateral, 5 mm or more in diameter, of variable density, and found in normal-sized eyes. These cataracts are often inherited, and they are considered acquired and progressive rather than truly congenital. Some of these children have visually insignificant cataracts and do not require surgery or require it late. Visual prognosis is very good.

Nuclear cataracts are typically congenital, dense axial opacities of 3 mm or more (Fig XXII-10). They are frequently associated with mild to moderate microphthalmos and inherited as autosomal dominant traits. Visual results are generally only fair even if surgery is done early and poor if done late.

Posterior lenticonus/lentiglobus presents as a posterior lens opacity associated with bulging of the posterior lens capsule (Fig XXII-11). Although frequently mistaken for a congenital cataract, this opacity is usually acquired in infancy and is slow-

TABLE XXII-2

EVALUATION OF PEDIATRIC CATARACTS

Family history (autosomal dominant or X-linked)

Pediatric physical examination

Ocular examination including
    Corneal diameter
    Iris configuration
    Anterior chamber depth
    Lens position
    Cataract morphology
    Posterior segment
      Rule out posterior mass
      Rule out retinal detachment
      Rule out optic nerve stalk to lens
    Intraocular pressure

Laboratory studies
    Bilateral cataracts
      Urine for reducing substance after milk feeding
      TORCH titer and VDRL
      Optional: Urine for amino acids, blood for calcium and
        phosphorus, red-cell galactokinase level
    Unilateral cataract
      TORCH titer

unilateral opacities that might have been visually insignificant in infancy and progressed later in childhood can be removed at almost any age with good results. Detailed history concerning age of onset of visual signs and symptoms or ocular status on previous eye examinations can be helpful in assessing prognosis. Occasionally, vision can be improved and surgery postponed by chronic dilation of the pupil and patching of the better eye.

Surgery The surgical approach to pediatric cataracts is different from that in adults and depends on whether a posterior chamber intraocular lens (PC IOL) is being considered. In children up to the age of 2 years in whom contact lenses or spectacles are the preferred means of aphakic optical correction, lensectomy is performed through a small limbal incision using a vitreous-cutting instrument or a manual aspirating device. Some surgeons prefer to use a vitreous-cutting instrument through a pars plana or pars plicata approach. Irrigation can be provided by an integrated infusion sleeve or by a separate cannula for bimanual surgery. Lens cortex and nucleus are generally soft, and ultrasonic phacoemulsification is not required. Tough, fibrotic plaques are best handled by increasing vitrectomy port size, increasing suction, and reducing cutting speed or by manually removing them with intraocular scissors and forceps. A large, round anterior capsulectomy is easily performed either before or, preferably, after complete cortical removal.

Since posterior capsule opacification occurs rapidly—sometimes even within weeks—in nearly all infantile cataract extractions, and since even a slight opacification can be amblyogenic, a controlled moderate posterior capsulectomy and anterior vitrectomy should be performed at the time of surgery. Most investigators have found no adverse effect from primary posterior capsulectomy. This technique allows for rapid, permanent establishment of a clear visual access for retinoscopy and prompt fitting and monitoring of aphakic optical correction, which is important in the age group subject to amblyopia. Sufficient peripheral posterior capsular remnants should be left, if possible, to facilitate secondary PC IOL implantation at a later date.

For children older than 2 years of age PC IOL implantation is preferred by some surgeons for both unilateral and bilateral cataracts. Although long-term risks of PC IOLs are unknown, accumulating evidence of PC IOLs in children to date has been favorable.

When an implant is to be used, the main adjustment in childhood cataract surgery involves the management of the anterior and posterior capsules. A controlled opening in the anterior capsule (by capsulorrhexis, or by "vitrectorrhexis," with a vitreous-cutting instrument) is important to help ensure "in-the-bag" placement of the PC IOL. Capsular fixation of the implant is believed to be far superior to sulcus fixation in terms of safety and stability of the lens. The posterior capsule can be left intact if it is clear at the end of the procedure and if the child is considered cooperative for an Nd:YAG laser capsulotomy (generally 4 years and older). Alternatively, the posterior capsule can be opened primarily in conjunction with a limited anterior vitrectomy prior to IOL placement. Some surgeons prefer to close the anterior wound after IOL placement and perform a posterior capsulotomy through a pars plana approach.

Recently, a procedure known as *posterior capsulorrhexis with optic capture* has been described. This procedure entails capturing the PC IOL optic through the opening created by posterior curvilinear capsulorrhexis. The lens haptics remain in the capsular bag, but the optic is positioned posterior to the capsular bag. Published experience with this technically challenging procedure is limited.

Medical therapy Intensive therapy with topical corticosteroids is advisable after childhood cataract surgery because of significant postoperative inflammation. A short course of oral corticosteroids is advocated by some clinicians, particularly if a PC IOL has been implanted. Mydriasis is obtained for at least 1 month with atropine or cyclopentolate therapy.

Amblyopia management Amblyopia therapy, if necessary, should begin as soon as possible after surgery. For patients left aphakic, corrective lenses—contact lenses for unilateral or bilateral aphakia or spectacles for bilateral aphakia—can be dispensed as early as 1 week after surgery. Patching of the better eye is frequently indicated in cases of unilateral cataracts or asymmetric bilateral cataracts. The amount of patching should be titrated to the degree of amblyopia and the age of the child. Part-time occlusion in the neonatal period may allow stimulation of binocular vision and may help to prevent the occurrence of associated strabismus.

Prognosis for Children with Cataracts

The prognosis for children with unilateral and bilateral congenital and infantile cataracts has improved markedly in the last 15 years. Prior to 1980 most studies demonstrated posttreatment visual acuities of no better than 20/200–20/800 for unilateral congenital cataracts and no better than 20/80–20/100 in bilateral. Improvements in cataract extraction technique and contact lens technology have resulted in many recent reports of 20/20–20/40 visual acuities in patients with bilateral and even unilateral congenital and juvenile cataracts if diagnosed and treated early.

Birch EE, Stager DR. The critical period for surgical treatment of dense congenital unilateral cataract. *Invest Ophthalmol Vis Sci.* 1996;37:1532–1538.

Brady KM, Atkinson CS, Kilty LA, et al. Cataract surgery and intraocular lens implantation in children. *Am J Ophthalmol.* 1995;120:1–9.

Ruttum MS. Childhood cataracts. In: *Focal Points: Clinical Modules for Ophthalmologists.* San Francisco: American Academy of Ophthalmology; 1996;14:1.

CHAPTER XXIII

Uveitis in the Pediatric Age Group

The causes of uveitis can be divided into two general classes: infectious and non-infectious. *Noninfectious* causes can be exogenous (e.g., blunt trauma, allergy) or endogenous (e.g., sympathetic ophthalmia, phacoantigenic uveitis). *Infectious* agents that can cause uveitis include bacteria, viruses, rickettsiae, fungi, protozoa, and parasites.

Uveitis is uncommon in children younger than 16 years of age, and only 5%–8% of the total number of cases are pediatric. Classifying the uveitis as anterior, intermediate, or posterior is useful in assessing possible etiologies. An etiologic agent can be found in about 50% of children with *anterior uveitis. Intermediate uveitis* usually defies precise etiologic definition. *Posterior uveitis* in children represents approximately 50% of the cases of childhood uveitis. Many of these cases are attributed to ocular toxoplasmosis, but etiologies are not determined in as many as a third of them. Half involve primarily the posterior pole.

The agents that cause uveitis all induce similar mechanisms of ocular inflammation, including vascular dilation with accompanying ciliary injection, and increased vascular permeability with fluid leakage into extravascular spaces, causing aqueous flare. Leukocytes and other cells migrate into these spaces, giving rise to inflammatory cells in the aqueous and causing keratic precipitates, hypopyon, cells behind the lens, and cells in the vitreous as well as red blood cells in the anterior chamber.

Clinically, inflammation of the anterior segment results in pain, redness, increased lacrimation, and decreased visual acuity. Ciliary injection will produce a violescent hue in the circumlimbal area. Increased protein content in the anterior chamber is seen as flare. Cells may be detected in the anterior chamber by slit-lamp examination.

Deposition of cellular debris on the endothelial surface of the cornea may produce a keratic precipitate. Posterior and peripheral anterior synechiae may form. In addition, pigment may be seen on either the anterior or posterior surfaces of the lens as well as in the anterior third of the vitreous. Intraocular pressure may be either subnormal or elevated, depending on the severity of the disease.

Inflammation in the posterior segment is often accompanied by reduced visual acuity. Metamorphopsia, micropsia, and macropsia may be noted, and the patient may have floaters. Slit-lamp examination of the vitreous and retina reveals multiple cells and often a distinct retinitis or choroiditis as well as cellular cuffing of the vessels. Cystoid macular edema, optic nerve inflammation, neovascularization, and retinal pigment epithelial changes may all be associated with posterior uveitis along

TABLE XXIII-1

DIFFERENTIAL DIAGNOSIS OF UVEITIS

Anterior uveitis

Juvenile rheumatoid arthritis
Trauma
Sarcoidosis
Herpes zoster
Sympathetic ophthalmia
Herpes simplex
Syphilis
Lyme disease
Unknown etiology (one half of cases)

Intermediate uveitis (pars planitis)

Sarcoidosis
Tuberculosis
Toxocariasis
Lyme disease
Unknown etiology (majority of cases)

Posterior uveitis

Toxoplasmosis
Presumed ocular histoplasmosis
Toxocariasis
Herpes simplex
Syphilis
Sympathetic ophthalmia
Lyme disease
Unknown etiology (one third of cases)

with those signs and symptoms already described for anterior uveitis. For the differential diagnosis of uveitis, see Table XXIII-1. See also BCSC Section 9, *Intraocular Inflammation and Uveitis,* for more information on the conditions covered in this chapter.

Dunn JP. Uveitis in children. In: *Focal Points: Clinical Modules for Ophthalmologists.* San Francisco: American Academy of Ophthalmology; 1995;13:4.

Anterior Uveitis

In approximately 50% of children presenting with anterior uveitis it is not possible to determine the cause. Many ophthalmologists prefer to postpone work-up of anterior uveitis unless it is chronic, recurrent, or unresponsive to initial therapy.

Juvenile Rheumatoid Arthritis

Juvenile rheumatoid arthritis (JRA) is the most common cause of anterior uveitis in children. JRA comprises a group of diseases characterized by chronic synovitis asso-

TABLE XXIII-2

SUBGROUPS OF JUVENILE RHEUMATOID ARTHRITIS

TYPE OF ONSET	% OF JRA PATIENTS	NUMBER OF JOINTS AFFECTED	% WITH UVEITIS
Pauciarticular	50	≤4	20–30
Polyarticular	30	>4	2–5
Systemic	20	variable	1–2

ciated with a number of extra-articular manifestations. Three broad clinical groups are recognized today:

□ Systemic disease (Still disease)

□ Pauciarticular disease

□ Polyarticular disease

These three classes of JRA differ in many features, including the likelihood of iridocyclitis. Characteristics of these groups are listed in Table XXIII-2.

The prevalence of JRA in North America and Europe is 64–113 per 100,000 children. An estimated 240,000 children in the United States have JRA, and 190,000 are at risk for the development of JRA-associated iridocyclitis. Onset may be at any age but is rare before the second year of life. JRA is a major cause of long-term illness and disability in children.

JRA is characterized by a chronic, nonsuppurative synovial inflammation. Increased secretion of joint fluid causes joint effusions. With continued synovitis the articular cartilage and other joint structures are destroyed. Bone deformity then occurs.

Iridocyclitis is most frequently associated with the pauciarticular form of JRA. At particular risk for the development of anterior uveitis are girls with early onset of pauciarticular JRA (i.e., 2–3 years of age), a positive antinuclear antibody (ANA) test, and a negative rheumatoid factor. Approximately 25% of patients in this group will develop anterior uveitis. Patients with polyarticular disease are at lower risk of developing iridocyclitis. In children with the systemic form of JRA, iridocyclitis is rare.

Diagnosis The etiology of rheumatoid arthritis and the mechanism of anterior uveitis remain unknown. Correlation between the course of arthritis and uveitis may be weak, although 90% of JRA patients who develop uveitis will do so within 7 years of the onset of arthritis. In occasional instances uveitis is diagnosed before the onset of joint symptoms. No strong correlation between JRA, iridocyclitis, and human leukocyte antigen (HLA) haplotypes, including HLA-B27, has been found.

The uveitis associated with JRA is usually asymptomatic and chronic. It is characterized by anterior chamber cell and flare. Prolonged inflammation may lead to posterior synechiae, band keratopathy, cataract, hypotony, and glaucoma (Fig XXIII-1). Vitritis and macular edema occur infrequently. Visual loss in JRA may be associated with multiple factors, including amblyopia in susceptible patients.

The differential diagnosis of arthritis and uveitis in children includes sarcoidosis, Lyme disease, psoriatic arthritis, juvenile Reiter syndrome, and inflammatory

mydriatic agent is also required, and surgical intervention may be necessary to remove the inflammation-inciting agent if one is identified.

Sarcoidosis

A chronic, multisystem disease of obscure origin, sarcoidosis is characterized by weight loss, fever, abdominal pain, and anorexia. The disorder occurs 10–15 times more frequently in blacks than in whites, and females outnumber males two to one. Most pediatric cases have been reported from rural communities in the southeastern United States. The etiology is unknown.

The hallmark lesion in sarcoidosis is the noncaseating epithelioid cell tubercle. This tubercle comprises epithelioid cells, multinucleated giant cells of the Langhans type, and a thin rim of lymphocytes. The lung is the most frequently involved organ, and pulmonary signs such as parenchymal infiltrates, miliary nodules, and hilar lymphadenopathy may vary. Liver involvement, cutaneous lesions, and uveitis also occur.

The anterior segment can demonstrate pronounced flare, cells, iris nodules, broad posterior synechiae, large mutton-fat keratic precipitates, and secondary glaucoma. Posterior segment involvement may reveal multiple round, gray-yellow lesions close to the vessels with perivascular cuffs known as *candle wax drippings*, or *taches de bougie*. Snowball opacities may appear in the inferior vitreous. Other ocular lesions include keratoconjunctivitis sicca, band keratopathy, conjunctival nodules, phlyctenular conjunctivitis, and papilledema. When retinal involvement occurs, incidence of central nervous system disease increases.

No specific diagnostic tests are available. Abnormal chest x-rays are noted in 80% of patients with ocular sarcoidosis. The angiotensin-converting enzyme (ACE) may be elevated in systemic sarcoidosis, but some authors report spurious results in children. Hypercalcemia is noted in about 10% of the patients. Serum lysozyme elevation and serum protein electrophoresis with an increased alpha$_2$ globulin fraction are also highly suggestive of sarcoidosis. Biopsy of conjunctival or skin nodules may help to confirm the diagnosis. The differential diagnosis includes tuberculosis and pulmonary mycoses.

Systemic treatment of sarcoidosis is mainly symptomatic and supportive. Corticosteroids may help suppress the acute manifestations. Ophthalmic care includes administration of topical corticosteroids and cycloplegic-mydriatic agents. It may be necessary to use artificial tears, and systemic corticosteroids are often required as well. The natural history of sarcoidosis in children is not well established. The disease is usually chronic, although spontaneous recovery may occur.

Herpes Zoster

Herpes zoster uveitis is caused by the varicella-zoster virus and associated with typical vesicular skin lesions. The uveitis is an example of a latent virus reactivation, which usually develops during convalescence from a varicella infection such as chickenpox, a common infection in children. The exact incidence of concurrent uveitis is unknown. Lymphocytic infiltration of the endoneurium and perineurium of the ciliary nerves occurs as well as a periarteritis.

Clinically, the cornea may develop a superficial geographic or dendritic keratitis resembling herpes simplex. In addition, a deep stromal or disciform keratitis may occur along with ulceration, corneal thinning, and perforation. Synechiae formation and secondary glaucoma may occur. Other problems include extraocular muscle palsy, chorioretinitis, optic neuritis, and scleritis. Phthisis bulbi may occur in long-standing cases.

Topical corticosteroids and cycloplegics are essential in the treatment of the disease. If herpes zoster infection develops while the patient is immunosuppressed, sufficient antibody formation may be undermined. Consequences can be dissemination of the herpesvirus, systemic illness, encephalitis, and death. Therefore, topical rather than systemic steroid therapy is recommended for children who are immunosuppressed. Oral acyclovir given early in the course of zoster infection has been shown to reduce the duration of viral shedding. Vision-threatening disease such as chorioretinitis or optic neuritis should be managed with intravenous acyclovir and prednisone.

Herpes Simplex

Herpes simplex iritis or iridocyclitis presents either with or without involvement of the cornea; however, it is more commonly associated with herpetic keratitis (see also chapter XVII). When deep corneal involvement occurs, severe herpetic uveitis may be accompanied by hyphema. In addition, hypopyon with synechiae formation and poor pupillary dilation can complicate herpes simplex uveitis. Eye involvement occurs in approximately 13% of herpetic infections in newborns, and those affected may harbor posterior lesions. Newborns with systemic herpes simplex virus infection may have late-onset, severe, necrotizing retinitis. The pathogenesis of the intraocular inflammation may be caused by replication of the virus, hypersensitivity, or toxic reaction to the virus or its product.

Herpetic keratitis may be present without pain if there is no intraocular involvement. However, with the onset of iridocyclitis, pain becomes severe. Choroidal hemorrhage, choroidal and intraretinal exudates, and vitreous opacifications may be present.

The diagnosis of herpetic uveitis is based on the presence or history of a dendritic corneal lesion. It is possible for herpetic uveitis to occur without preceding corneal involvement, although this is rare. It is quite difficult to culture virus from the aqueous or the vitreous.

The use of corticosteroids for treatment of uveitis should be accompanied by an antiviral agent. See also BCSC Section 8, *External Disease and Cornea.*

Sympathetic Ophthalmia

Sympathetic ophthalmia is a bilateral granulomatous panuveitis that occurs after injury or surgery to one eye followed by a latent period with development of uveitis in the uninjured or unoperated eye (called the *sympathizing eye*). The incidence of sympathetic ophthalmia has diminished significantly since the advent of improved wound closure techniques and perhaps because of the practice of removing severely damaged eyes early.

Sympathetic ophthalmia is seen more frequently after perforating trauma than following planned ophthalmic procedures. The etiology is unknown but may involve an autoimmune response to one of the proteins associated with the retina, uveal tract, or both. See also BCSC Section 9, *Intraocular Inflammation and Uveitis.*

Syphilis

Syphilis is a systemic communicable infection characterized by periods of clinical activity followed by prolonged latency (see also chapter XVII). Acquired syphilis requires contact between an infective lesion and a break in the skin or mucosa. *Treponema pallidum,* the spirochete responsible for syphilis, can cross the placenta, and congenital syphilis is contracted from the mother, whose infection is usually latent. Many factors determine whether or not significant clinical abnormalities will appear in the newborn. These factors include fetal delayed sensitivity, immune responses, and the time in gestation when the fetus is infected.

Syphilis may involve any organ, including bone, bone marrow, lungs, liver, spleen, teeth, central nervous system, and eyes. Congenital infection characteristically presents with a salt-and-pepper chorioretinitis affecting both eyes. Optic nerve pallor and iritis may be present. Systemic manifestations of congenital syphilis include failure to thrive; moist lesions appearing on the mouth, anus, and genitalia; hepatosplenomegaly; and severe rhinitis. Clinical manifestations of late congenital syphilis include interstitial keratitis, meningitis, deafness, notched teeth, and saber shins.

The diagnosis of syphilis is based not only on the clinical appearance but also on positive serologic tests including a positive VDRL and a positive FTA-ABS. Dark-field examination of scrapings from lesions may reveal the spirochete itself. Treatment includes systemic administration of penicillin.

Intermediate Uveitis (Pars Planitis)

The term *intermediate uveitis,* which is a diagnosis based on the anatomic location of inflammation, is preferred by the International Committee on Uveitis Nomenclature. It replaces the terms *peripheral uveitis* and *chronic cyclitis. Pars planitis* is now considered a type of intermediate uveitis in which a white opacity (snowbank) occurs over the peripheral retina and pars plana. It is the most common type of intermediate uveitis, making up approximately 85%–90% of cases. The distinction between pars planitis and intermediate uveitis is not always clear in common usage, and the two terms are often used interchangeably. Intermediate uveitis represents 5%–15% of all cases of uveitis and about 25% of uveitis in the pediatric age group. The etiology is most often unknown.

Snowbank formation in the region of the pars plana is made up of mononuclear cells, hyperplastic nonpigmented ciliary epithelial cells, and an occasional fibroblast-like cell (Fig XXIII-2). Fibroglial proliferation is present at the vitreous base, drawing the peripheral retina into the snowbank. The retinal veins are sheathed with lymphocytes.

Intermediate uveitis has a gradual onset, and the course may be mild in as many as 50% of these patients. About 75% of patients have bilateral involvement. Retrolental cells appear in the anterior vitreous. Initially, a peripheral perivasculitis usually occurs along with small exudates adjacent to the inflamed peripheral retinal vessels. These exudates enter the vitreous, giving rise to floaters in the field of vision. Besides floaters, the patient may note blurring of distance vision and difficulties with accommodation. The anterior chamber has a minimal response, but the retrolenticular space and anterior vitreous are filled with freely moving cells. Exudate is seen in the region of the pars plana inferiorly. With time the vitreous exudate extends nasally, temporally, and posteriorly. Cystoid macular edema, optic nerve inflammation, posterior subcapsular cataract, glaucoma, exudative retinal detachment, and even phthisis bulbi may develop.

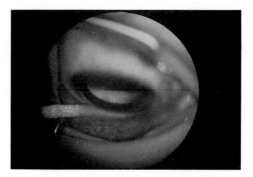

FIG XXIII-2—Intermediate uveitis with inferior snowbank formation, right eye.

Diagnosis The diagnosis is made clinically. Because of the high incidence of bilaterality in intermediate uveitis, unilateral inflammation should cause the clinician to consider sarcoidosis, toxocariasis, peripheral toxoplasmosis, or a retained intraocular foreign body.

Treatment Topical administration or periocular injection of corticosteroids may improve intermediate uveitis considerably. Because the disorder is chronic with recurrences and remissions, treatment should be reserved for those individuals having a moderate decrease in visual acuity, macular edema, or increased vitreous debris. About 10% of these patients will have a self-limited course; 60% will have a prolonged course without exacerbations; and 30% will have a chronic, smoldering course with exacerbations. If treatment with topical and sub-Tenon's injection of corticosteroids every 2–6 weeks does not result in improvement, systemic corticosteroids may be used.

Immunosuppressive agents are considered if systemic steroids are inadequate or if posterior subcapsular cataracts begin to form. Transscleral diathermy and cryotherapy have also been applied. Vitrectomy may be indicated in severe cases.

Hooper PL. Pars planitis. In: *Focal Points: Clinical Modules for Ophthalmologists.* San Francisco: American Academy of Ophthalmology; 1993;11:11.

Posterior Uveitis

More than 50% of pediatric cases of uveitis have posterior inflammation. No etiological agent or disease is documented in about one third of these cases.

Toxoplasmosis

Toxoplasmosis is a parasitic disease with several recognized clinical forms (see also chapter XVII). These include congenital systemic toxoplasmosis, acquired systemic toxoplasmosis, and ocular toxoplasmosis. Congenital systemic toxoplasmosis occurs as three types:

- One form is inactive at birth and goes unrecognized until later inflammation occurs.
- A second type is active at birth, and the clinical picture depends on the timing of the mother's infection during fetal growth. If the mother's infection occurs in the first trimester, death of the fetus usually results. When the infection begins in the second trimester, disease in the fetus is widespread and results in abortion or severe fetal damage. Infection starting in the third trimester is associated with chorioretinitis, encephalomyelitis, and visceral disease in the newborn.
- The third type is known as the recurrent form, and it may be indistinguishable from acquired disease.

Congenital systemic toxoplasmosis occurs in about 1 in every 10,000 births in the United States. Toxoplasmosis is transmitted to the fetus by a mother infected during her pregnancy; however, only about 40% of mothers infected during pregnancy will transmit the disease to the fetus. It is rare for a mother who was infected prior to the pregnancy to transmit toxoplasmosis to the fetus. If one child has been born with toxoplasmosis, the chance of subsequent siblings contracting congenital toxoplasmosis is essentially zero because of maternal immunity.

There are five types of acquired systemic toxoplasmosis:

- Exanthematous
- Meningoencephalitic
- Lymphadenopathic
- Ocular
- Influenzal

The incidence of acquired systemic toxoplasmosis is extremely high throughout the world, and the percentage of affected persons is roughly equal to an individual's age (i.e., 30% of 30-year-olds, 50% of 50-year-olds). Acquired systemic toxoplasmosis may present as an acute exanthem, meningoencephalitis, lymphadenopathy, influenza, or, rarely, simply as retinitis.

Ocular toxoplasmosis also has several forms depending on the structures involved, including papillitis, retinitis, and iridocyclitis. The toxoplasma organisms described in chapter XVII have been identified only in the retina, where they have a predilection for the nerve fiber layer. It is known that the organisms survive best in the tissues of the central nervous system, particularly the brain and retina. Ocular toxoplasmosis may be asymptomatic and can go unrecognized in many individuals. However, toxoplasmosis may cause 30%–50% of all posterior uveitis in the pediatric age group.

Clinically, systemic toxoplasmosis is hallmarked by the *three C's:* convulsions, intracranial calcifications (seen in 5% of infected patients), and chorioretinitis or retinochoroiditis (seen in 80% of these patients). The retinitis is bilateral in 85% of infected individuals.

The presence of ocular toxoplasmosis is usually signaled initially by floaters or by blurred or reduced vision. The anterior segment may show no inflammation in some cases when the disease is confined to the posterior pole. Vitreous opacities may be present with a whitish yellow, slightly raised, indistinct lesion seen in the retina. An exudative focal retinitis involves the anterior layers of the retina in particular. With time these affected areas usually heal, leaving atrophied areas with pronounced pigmentation around their edges.

TABLE XXIII-4

DRUG TREATMENT SCHEDULE FOR TOXOPLASMOSIS

Pyrimethamine (Daraprim)*	4 mg/kg loading dose; then 1 mg/kg/day, given in 2 equal doses per day, for 2–4 days; then 0.5 mg/kg/day for 6 weeks
Folinic acid (leucovorin)	3–9 mg IM daily for 3 days or as required for thrombo- cytopenia or leukopenia (also available for oral use in 5 mg tablet taken daily)
Sulfadiazine (or triple sulfa)	100 mg/kg/day in 4 doses not to exceed 4000 mg/day for 6 weeks
Prednisone	1–2 mg/kg/day for 6 weeks (optional; may be used if macula or optic nerve is threatened)

*Bone marrow depression occurs with pyrimethamine. Peripheral white blood determinations and platelet counts twice a week are recommended to follow the induced leukopenia and thrombocytopenia. Pyrimethamine has teratogenic effects and should not be prescribed for pregnant women.

The disease may run a course of 6 months before healing occurs. Recurrence may first be noted in *satellite lesions.* Recurrence often brings about a very severe anterior uveitis with mutton-fat keratic precipitates, marked cell and flare formation, iris nodules, and posterior synechial development. Papilledema, vitreous precipitates, and glaucoma can all result from toxoplasmosis infection of the eye.

Diagnosis   The diagnosis of toxoplasmosis is based on clinical manifestations and laboratory tests. Other necrotizing lesions of the fundus should be excluded. Laboratory tests include the Sabin-Feldman dye test for specific IgG antibodies, the indirect immunofluorescent antibody test, and the ELISA. Specific IgM antibodies are measured with the double-sandwich IgM ELISA or the IgM immunosorbent agglutination assay (ISAGA).

Treatment   The standard treatment for ocular toxoplasmosis is combination therapy with pyrimethamine and sulfadiazine. Corticosteroid therapy may also be considered in conjunction with antibiotics. Drug treatment schedules for children vary, but the schedule outlined in Table XXIII-4 is typical. Because of significant systemic side effects from these medications, a specialist in pediatric infectious diseases should be consulted. Cryotherapy, photocoagulation, and vitrectomy have also been attempted. The prognosis depends on the patient's immune status, age, and sex; the location of the lesion; and the virulence of the organisms themselves.

Tabbara KF. Ocular toxoplasmosis: toxoplasmic retinochoroiditis. *Int Ophthalmol Clin.* 1995;35:15–29.

Ocular Histoplasmosis

Ocular histoplasmosis is a fungal infection that is benign and asymptomatic 95% of the time. It can be so mild that it goes unnoticed or so serious that it is fatal. Typical symptoms include fever, fatigue, and malaise lasting up to 2 weeks. Histoplasmosis is found worldwide, but it is endemic in the central and eastern United States,

TABLE XXIII-5

MASQUERADE SYNDROMES

SEGMENT	AGE (YEARS)	SIGNS OF INFLAMMATION	DIAGNOSTIC STUDIES*
Anterior segment			
Retinoblastoma	<15	Flare, cells, pseudohypopyon	Aqueous tap for LDH levels and cytology
Leukemia	<15	Flare, cells, heterochromia	Bone marrow, peripheral blood smear, aqueous cytology
Intraocular foreign body	Any age	Flare, cells	X-ray, ultrasound
Malignant melanoma	Any age	Flare, cells	Fluorescein, ultrasound
Juvenile xanthogranuloma	<15	Flare, cells, hyphema	Examination of skin, iris biopsy
Peripheral retinal detachment	Any age	Flare, cells	Ophthalmoscopy
Posterior segment			
Retinitis pigmentosa	Any age	Cells in vitreous	ERG, EOG, visual fields
Reticulum cell sarcoma	15+	Vitreous exudate, retinal hemorrhage or exudates, retinal pigment epithelium infiltrates	Cytology study of aqueous and vitreous
Lymphoma	15+	Retinal hemorrhage or exudates, vitreous cells	Node biopsy, bone marrow, physical examination
Retinoblastoma	<15	Vitreous cells, retinal exudates	Ultrasound, aqueous tap
Malignant melanoma	15+	Vitreous cells	Fluorescein, ultrasound
Multiple sclerosis	15+	Periphlebitis	Neurologic examination

*LDH, lactic dehydrogenase; ERG, electroretinogram; EOG, electro-oculogram.

Other Etiologies

Posterior uveitis can also be caused by herpes simplex, syphilis, sympathetic oph-thalmia, and *Candida albicans* (see BCSC Section 9, *Intraocular Inflammation and Uveitis*).

Masquerade Syndromes

Other conditions can simulate uveitis in the pediatric age group. These *masquerade syndromes* are listed together with their diagnostic features in Table XXIII-5. The eval-uation of uveitis in the pediatric age group should include review of the patient by a pediatrician with particular attention to rheumatic and gastrointestinal disorders, tuberculin skin testing, FTA-ABS, serum protein electrophoresis, chest x-ray, sacro-iliac x-rays (when indicated), and general health. The clinician should also obtain

TABLE XXIII-6

LABORATORY TESTS FOR VARIOUS TYPES OF UVEITIS

Anterior

Complete blood count (to rule out leukemia)
Antinuclear antibody (to subtype JRA)
Serum lysozyme (to rule out sarcoidosis)
Serum protein electrophoresis (to look for alpha$_2$ globulin fraction in sarcoidosis)
FTA-ABS (to rule out syphilis)
HLA-B27 (to rule out ankylosing spondylitis and Reiter syndrome)
ELISA, IFA, for Lyme disease
Tuberculin skin test, chest x-ray (to rule out sarcoidosis and tuberculosis)
GI series (if ulcerative colitis or regional enteritis [Crohn disease] is suspected)
Angiotensin-converting enzyme (ACE)

Intermediate

Serum lysozyme (to rule out sarcoidosis)
Serum protein electrophoresis (to rule out sarcoidosis)
FTA-ABS (to rule out syphilis)
Chest x-ray (to rule out sarcoidosis or tuberculosis)
Tuberculin skin test
ELISA for toxocariasis
Angiotensin-converting enzyme (ACE)

Posterior

ELISA for toxoplasmosis
ELISA for toxocariasis
Serum lysozyme (to rule out sarcoidosis)
Serum protein electrophoresis (to rule out sarcoidosis)
FTA-ABS (to rule out syphilis)
Blood cultures, viral cultures, or antibody levels if cytomegalovirus, herpes simplex
    (especially in a newborn), or rubella is suspected
ELISA, IFA, for Lyme disease
Angiotensin-converting enzyme (ACE)

ocular ultrasound, x-rays to rule out foreign body, and antinuclear antibody determinations when juvenile rheumatoid arthritis is suspected. Laboratory tests for various types of uveitis are listed in Table XXIII-6.

Giles CL. Uveitis in children. In: Nelson LB, Calhoun JH, Harley RD, eds. *Pediatric Ophthalmology.* 3rd ed. Philadelphia: Saunders; 1991:271–291.

CHAPTER XXIV

Vitreous and Retinal Diseases and Disorders

Leukocoria

The term *leukocoria* means "white pupil." The differential diagnosis of leukocoria includes

- Retinoblastoma
- Persistent hyperplastic primary vitreous (PHPV), also known as persistent fetal vasculature (PFV)
- Retinopathy of prematurity (ROP)—stage 5 with total retinal detachment and fibrous membrane
- Posterior cataract
- Choroidal colobomas
- Uveitis
- Toxocariasis
- Congenital retinal folds
- Coats disease
- Vitreous hemorrhage
- Retinal dysplasia
- Other tumors (hamartomas, choroidal hemangiomas, diktyomas, etc.)

The major retinal etiologies will be discussed in this chapter with the exception of retinoblastoma, which is covered in chapter XXVI, Ocular Tumors in Childhood. See also BCSC Section 12, *Retina and Vitreous,* for more information about these conditions.

Persistent Hyperplastic Primary Vitreous (PHPV)

PHPV is a congenital, nonhereditary malformation of the eye that is usually unilateral and not associated with systemic defects. The term *persistent fetal vasculature (PFV)* is more accurate but has not yet supplanted the widespread *PHPV*. The spectrum of severity is broad. Mild cases feature eyes with prominent hyaloid vessel remnants, large Mittendorf's dots, and Bergmeister's papillae. At the other end of the spectrum are microphthalmic eyes with progressive shallowing of the anterior chamber and angle-closure glaucoma from fibrovascular invasion of the lens through a defect in the posterior lens capsule. Peripheral and posterior central retinal detachments may also occur in these more severely involved eyes. The ciliary processes may be elongated and visible through the dilated pupil, and prominent radial ves-

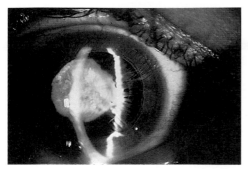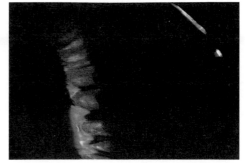

FIG XXIV-1—Persistent hyperplastic primary vitreous. Elongated ciliary processes are adherent to lens.

sels are often noted on the iris surface (Fig XXIV-1). The retrolental plaque is most dense centrally, and it may contain cartilage as well as fibrovascular tissue.

The natural history of the more severely affected untreated eyes is usually one of relentless, progressive cataract formation with concomitant shallowing of the anterior chamber, eventually resulting in angle-closure glaucoma. Retinal detachment, intraocular hemorrhage, and angle-closure glaucoma are the most severe complications in PHPV. The hemorrhages presumably originate in the fibrovascular membrane in the retrolental space. Affected eyes are almost always smaller than the normal fellow eye, although this finding may be apparent only by ultrasound or careful caliper measurement of the corneal diameters. It is important to document microphthalmos, because retinoblastoma is rarely found in microphthalmic eyes. The presence of a cataract is also evidence against the diagnosis of retinoblastoma, although lens opacities may develop in advanced cases.

Many eyes with PHPV can be saved by early cataract surgery combined with membrane excision. In cases with minimal posterior involvement it is even possible to obtain some degree of central vision if early surgical intervention is followed by aggressive contact lens wear combined with patching of the uninvolved eye. The visual prognosis depends on the degree of retinal involvement.

Various surgical approaches to the management of PHPV have been proposed. In most cases, the retrolenticular tissues can be removed by vitreous-cutting instruments. Intraocular hemorrhage is not as common as would be expected. Both limbal and pars plicata/pars plana approaches have been successfully employed. If the macula appears normal, a vigorous effort should be made postoperatively to optically correct aphakia and to patch in the same manner as in the case of a unilateral cataract.

Goldberg MF. Persistent fetal vasculature (PFV): an integrated interpretation of signs and symptoms associated with persistent hyperplastic primary vitreous (PHPV). *Am J Ophthalmol.* 1997;124:587–626.

Haddad R, Font RL, Reeser F. Persistent hyperplastic primary vitreous. A clinicopathologic study of 62 cases and review of the literature. *Surv Ophthalmol.* 1978;23: 123–134.

Karr DJ, Scott WE. Visual acuity results following treatment of persistent hyperplastic primary vitreous. *Arch Ophthalmol.* 1986;104:662–667.

Wright KW, Christensen LE, Noguchi BA. Results of late surgery for presumed congenital cataracts. *Am J Ophthalmol.* 1992;114:409–415.

Retinopathy of Prematurity

Retinopathy of prematurity (ROP) is the current designation for what was previously called *retrolental fibroplasia (RLF)*. ROP includes the acute disease seen in the nursery and the cicatricial disease seen later.

Normally, retinal vascular development begins during week 16 of gestation. Mesenchymal tissue containing spindle cells is the source of retinal vessels. The mesenchyme grows centrifugally from the optic disc, reaching the nasal ora serrata in the eighth month of gestation and the temporal ora serrata up to 1–2 months later. Premature birth may trigger the onset of ROP, in which normal retinal vascular development is altered and abnormal neovascularization occurs. The pathologic process may stop or reverse itself at any point, or the disease may eventually progress to fibroglial proliferation and lead to vitreoretinal traction and retinal detachment.

ROP is rare in infants with a birth weight greater than 2000 g. Premature infants weighing less than 1500 g at birth are at risk of developing serious visual sequelae from ROP, and the risk increases as gestational age and birth weight decrease. In the multicenter trial of cryotherapy for ROP (CRYO-ROP Study) 37% of infants weighing less than 750 g developed severe (stage 3, see below) ROP, while only 21.9% of those weighing 750–999 g and 8.5% of those weighing 1000–1250 g did so.

Administration of supplemental oxygen to the newborn has been implicated as the cause of ROP; however, the variability in severity of and susceptibility to ROP in the extremely premature infant suggests that factors other than hyperoxia play a role in the etiology of this disease. ROP, or a disease process similar to it, has also been reported in infants who did *not* receive supplemental oxygen. Oxygen monitoring is considered standard of care in the intensive care nursery. The loss of life or neurologic function that can occur with oxygen deprivation limits how severely oxygen administration can be cut back in these very ill infants.

Factors other than oxygen have been studied as well. Vitamin E (α-tocopherol) has been proposed as a preventive treatment with conflicting results from several studies. Intraventricular hemorrhage, necrotizing enterocolitis, and death have been associated with high-dose IV vitamin E use. Administration of vitamin E to allow physiologic levels is most often followed. The possibility of premature exposure to light as a factor has also been raised, but not confirmed, in small but controlled studies. Reduction of light in the nursery to allow for better rest is a national trend in the United States.

The ultimate prevention of ROP would be prevention of premature birth itself. Good, early prenatal care can have a great impact on the incidence of premature birth. The cost of prenatal efforts pales in comparison to the measures that may be necessitated by the lack of this care.

Gestational age and birth weight are inversely correlated with the development of ROP. The amount of time in oxygen therapy is a strong correlate, but the level of oxygenation is a weaker correlate. Other characteristics that correlate with the development of ROP are multiple births and transfer after birth to a hospital with a neonatal intensive care unit. ROP is also more prevalent in white newborns.

TABLE XXIV-1

INTERNATIONAL CLASSIFICATION OF ACUTE STAGES
OF RETINOPATHY OF PREMATURITY

Location — Zones II and III are based on convention rather than strict anatomy (see Figure XXIV-7)

Zone I (posterior pole) — Circle with radius of 30°, twice disc-macula distance

Zone II — From edge of zone I to point tangential to nasal ora serrata and around to area near the temporal equator

Zone III — Residual crescent anterior to zone II

Extent — Specified as hours of the clock as observer looks at each eye

Staging the disease

Stage 1 — Demarcation line (Fig XXIV-2)

Stage 2 — Ridge, ± small tufts of fibrovascular proliferation (popcorns) (Fig XXIV-3)

Stage 3 — Ridge with extraretinal fibrovascular proliferation (Fig XXIV-4)

- Mild fibrovascular proliferation
- Moderate fibrovascular proliferation
- Severe fibrovascular proliferation

Stage 4 — Subtotal retinal detachment (Fig XXIV-5)

A. Extrafoveal

B. Retinal detachment including fovea

Stage 5 — Total retinal detachment

Funnel:	Anterior	Posterior
	Open	Open
	Narrow	Narrow

Plus disease — Plus (+) is added when vascular shunting is so marked that the veins are enlarged and the arteries tortuous in the posterior pole (Fig XXIV-6).

Modified from the Committee for Classification of Retinopathy of Prematurity: An international classification of retinopathy of prematurity. *Arch Ophthalmol.* 1984;102:1130–1134.

Among infants who develop ROP, certain diseases are commonly seen, particularly various forms of respiratory distress syndrome including hyaline membrane disease, pulmonary interstitial emphysema, pneumothorax, and bronchopulmonary dysplasia. Other disease entities observed include patent ductus arteriosus, apnea and bradycardia, intracranial hemorrhage, suspected sepsis, anemia, and jaundice.

Classification The 1984 international classification of retinopathy of prematurity describes the disease by stage, zone, and extent. It has functioned very well in the CRYO-ROP Study and will probably be the standard classification for many years (Table XXIV-1, Figs XXIV-2 through XXIV-6). BCSC Section 12, *Retina and Vitreous,* discusses this classification in detail. *Plus disease* refers to arteriolar tortuosity and venous engorgement of the posterior pole.

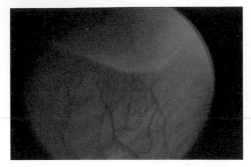 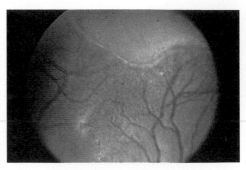

FIG XXIV-2—Late stage 1 ROP. No height to demarcation line. (Reprinted courtesy of Oregon Health Sciences University Ophthalmic Photography Department.)

FIG XXIV-3—Early stage 2 ROP. Demarcation has height and width, creating a ridge. (Reprinted courtesy of Oregon Health Sciences University Ophthalmic Photography Department and CRYO-ROP Cooperative Group.)

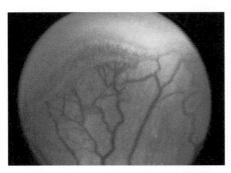 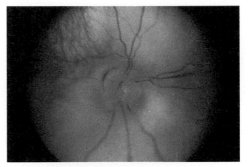

FIG XXIV-4—Stage 3 ROP. Ridge with extraretinal fibrovascular proliferation (top right shows stage 2). (Reprinted by permission from *Arch Ophthalmol*. 1984;102:1134. ©1988 American Medical Association.)

FIG XXIV-5—Stage 4 ROP. Subtotal retinal detachment. (Reprinted by permission from *Arch Ophthalmol*. 1984;102:1132. ©1988 American Medical Association.)

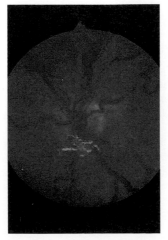

FIG XXIV-6—Classic plus disease.

Management   Fundus examination of the premature infant must be performed with extreme care; these infants are fragile and the examination is stressful. The recommended solution to be used in the examination is Cyclomydril (0.2% cyclopentolate and 1.0% phenylephrine). Phenylephrine 10% (Neo-Synephrine) should *never* be used because of its potential to cause hypertension. Concentrations of cyclopentolate greater than 0.5% should be avoided as well because of induced feeding intolerance. If an examination must be postponed, the postponement and medical reason should be documented in the patient's chart.

It has been recommended that the initial fundus examination for infants weighing less than 1500 g should take place 5–6 weeks after birth, and if no ROP is apparent, the examination should be repeated 2 weeks later (Table XXIV-2). Screening fundus examinations are no longer needed when the retina is fully vascularized (vessels are 1 disc diameter from the ora serrata on the temporal aspect of the retina).

The screening clinician is initially looking for ROP and retinal vessel development. Regardless of the presence or absence of ROP, if the normal retinal vessels do not extend past zone I on early examinations, the chance that treatment will be needed becomes much higher. On follow-up examinations the patient is observed for development of ROP, spontaneous resolution of ROP, or progression to threshold disease. *Threshold disease* is stage 3+ ROP in zone I or II, involving at least 5 contiguous clock-hour sectors or at least 8 interrupted clock-hour sectors (see Table XXIV-2 and Figure XXIV-7). The iris vessels can become visibly congested just prior to the development of threshold disease (Fig XXIV-8).

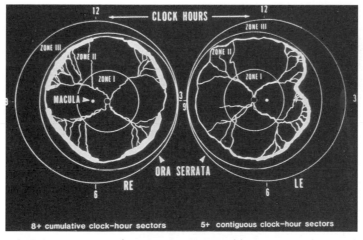

FIG XXIV-7—Diagram of ROP zones. (Reprinted by permission from *Arch Ophthalmol.* 1988;106:472. ©1988 American Medical Association.)

TABLE XXIV-2

EXAMINATION SCHEDULE FOR PREMATURE INFANTS
(BIRTH WEIGHT <1500 G)

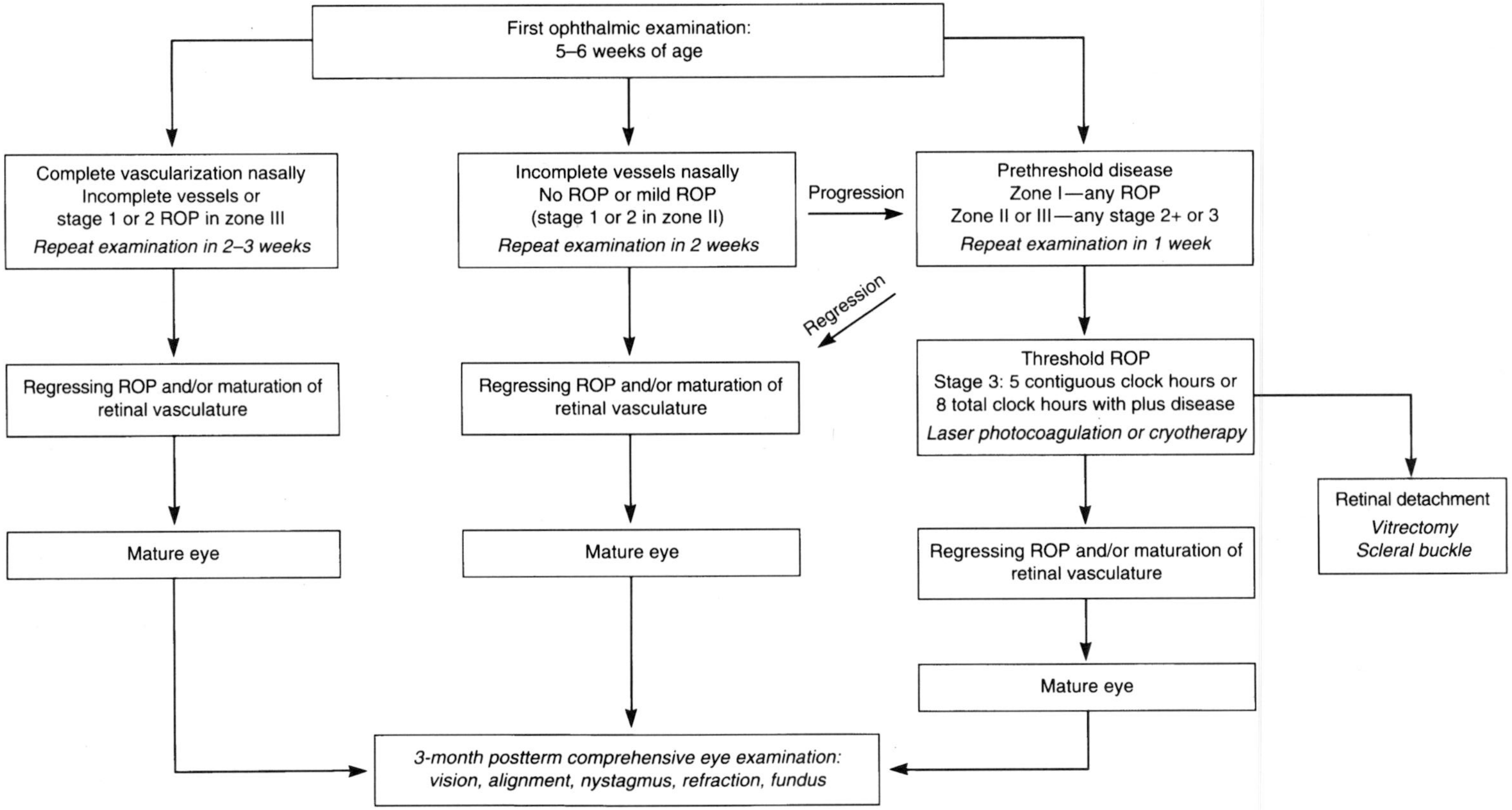

First ophthalmic examination:
5–6 weeks of age

Complete vascularization nasally
Incomplete vessels or
stage 1 or 2 ROP in zone III
Repeat examination in 2–3 weeks

Incomplete vessels nasally
No ROP or mild ROP
(stage 1 or 2 ROP in zone II)
Repeat examination in 2 weeks

Progression

Regression

Prethreshold disease
Zone I—any ROP
Zone II or III—any stage 2+ or 3
Repeat examination in 1 week

Threshold ROP
Stage 3: 5 contiguous clock hours or
8 total clock hours with plus disease
Laser photocoagulation or cryotherapy

Retinal detachment
Vitrectomy
Scleral buckle

Regressing ROP and/or maturation of
retinal vasculature

Regressing ROP and/or maturation of
retinal vasculature

Regressing ROP and/or maturation of
retinal vasculature

Mature eye

Mature eye

Mature eye

3-month postterm comprehensive eye examination:
vision, alignment, nystagmus, refraction, fundus

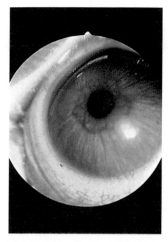

FIG XXIV-8—Congested iris vessels associated with stage 3+ ROP.

The CRYO-ROP Study has shown that 6% of infants with a birth weight less than 1251 g will develop threshold disease and that 45% of these will have vision of 20/200 or worse at 3½ years of age if not treated. If cryotherapy is applied to the avascular areas of retina in these eyes, only 26% of these patients will have vision of 20/200 or worse at 3½ years of age (Fig XXIV-9). Therefore, cryotherapy reduces severe vision loss by about half. At 5½ years of age treated eyes were still much less likely to have very poor vision. However, more of the untreated eyes with quantifiable vision had vision of 20/40 or better than did the treated eyes. Longer-term follow-up studies are necessary to see if this trend persists, particularly after the patients go through teenage years, a common time for secondary retinal detachments in severe ROP. Mild constriction of visual field has been measured in treated eyes; the benefit of preserved acuity outweighs this disadvantage.

The median age at which eyes reached threshold disease in the CRYO-ROP Study was 36.9 weeks postconception; 90% of cases reached threshold between 33.6 and 42 weeks postconception. This age can coincide with the age at which the patient is transferred to another facility or discharged to home. If a child has worsening ROP at this age, considerations of follow-up and treatment possibilities should be included in the discharge plans. Follow-up examinations should be performed according to the schedule presented in Table XXIV-2.

Laser photocoagulation is a newer treatment modality, which has been as effective as cryotherapy in halting threshold disease in the small series published so far. The major advantages of laser over cryotherapy are

□ Greater facility in reaching more posterior locations

□ Less trauma to ocular tissues

□ Less discomfort to the patient

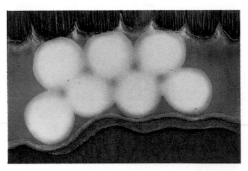

FIG XXIV-9—Cryotherapy as a row at ora serrata extending posteriorly to anterior edge of ridge. (Reprinted by permission from *Arch Ophthalmol.* 1988;106:474. ©1988 American Medical Association.)

Several disturbing reports of cataract formation have arisen, however, particularly with the argon laser.

Although ROP regresses in most cases, sequelae of advanced disease (stage 3) can include both peripheral and posterior retinal changes. Therefore, a child who has had ROP requires periodic ophthalmic examinations beyond the newborn period to reach maximum visual function. Vitreoretinal traction may cause retinal detachment in the first or second decade of life. Retinal folds and dragging of the macula can also occur, causing visual impairment (Fig XXIV-10). Amblyopia may be present as a result of high myopia, macular dragging, or strabismus. Pseudostrabismus caused by dragging of the macula can occur, often giving the appearance of an exotropia as a result of a large angle kappa (Fig XXIV-11). These children need particular attention to their development and education, as they are often multiply handicapped beyond their visual problems.

When the progression of ROP to stage 4 or retinal detachment has not been prevented by laser or cryotherapy, scleral buckling and vitrectomy are also used. The outcome continues to be poor. Anatomical reattachment is achieved in only about 60% of eyes, and a much smaller number recover some vision. Even with laser and cryotherapy treatment, several hundred babies are blinded by this disease in the United States yearly.

Other late changes associated with stage 5 ROP include microphthalmos, cataract, glaucoma, and phthisis bulbi. Glaucoma is caused by peripheral anterior synechiae and angle closure resulting from forward movement of the lens–iris diaphragm. Such eyes are usually blind but may be preserved by cycloplegic agents, steroids, lensectomy, and iridectomy. Enucleation is sometimes necessary for pain relief.

See the end of this chapter, pp 293–294, for the joint statement on ROP screening approved by the American Academy of Pediatrics, the American Association for Pediatric Ophthalmology and Strabismus, and the American Academy of Ophthalmology.

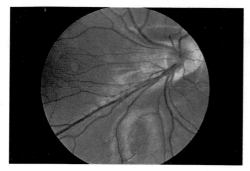

FIG XXIV-10—Cicatricial ROP, right eye.

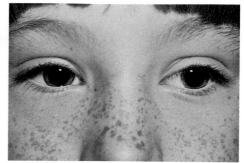

FIG XXIV-11—Pseudoexotropia in a fixating left eye in ROP.

Christiansen SP, Bradford JD. Cataract in infants treated with argon laser photocoagulation for threshold retinopathy of prematurity. *Am J Ophthalmol.* 1995;119:175–180.

The Committee for the Classification of Retinopathy of Prematurity. An international classification of retinopathy of prematurity. *Arch Ophthalmol.* 1984;102:1130–1134.

Cryotherapy for Retinopathy of Prematurity Cooperative Group. Multicenter trial of cryotherapy for retinopathy of prematurity: Snellen visual acuity and structural outcome at 5½ years after randomization. *Arch Ophthalmol.* 1996;114:417–424.

The International Committee for the Classification of the Late Stages of Retinopathy of Prematurity. An international classification of retinopathy of prematurity. *Arch Ophthalmol.* 1987;105:906–912.

Palmer EA. Retinopathy of prematurity. In: *Focal Points: Clinical Modules for Ophthalmologists.* San Francisco: American Academy of Ophthalmology; 1993;11:3.

Silverman WA. The oxygen hypothesis: fruitful predictor or narrow dogma? In: Flynn JT, Phelps DL, eds. *Birth Defects: Original Article Series.* vol 24, no 1. New York: Liss; 1988:203–207.

Coats Disease

Coats disease is an important mimicker of retinoblastoma. The definition of this condition has been narrowed, and Coats disease is now understood to mean the presence of abnormal retinal vessels with a fundus picture showing yellow subretinal exudates. The term *telangiectasia* is frequently used to indicate these anomalous, grapelike clusters of vessels. The macular area is a favored site for exudation. Once the fovea is detached and the subretinal exudate becomes organized, the prognosis for restoration of central vision is poor. See also BCSC Section 12, *Retina and Vitreous.*

In the juvenile form of Coats disease males are affected more frequently than females. This condition is usually, but not always, unilateral. The typical age at diagnosis is 8–10 years, but the disease has also been observed in infants (Fig XXIV-12). The most widely held theory is that the subretinal exudation originates from the leaking anomalous vessels. Hence, the diagnosis of Coats disease requires the presence

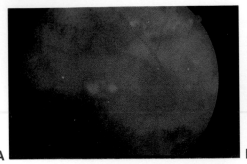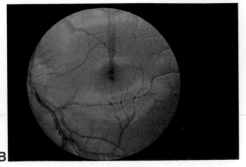

FIG XXIV-12—Coats disease. *A,* Right eye. *B,* Normal left eye.

of the abnormal retinal vessels, which may, on occasion, be small and difficult to find. Fluorescein angioscopy and angiography may be helpful in demonstrating leakage from the telangiectatic vessels and in assessing the effectiveness of therapy.

The differential diagnosis includes angiomatosis retinae, retinoblastoma, PHPV, ROP, toxocariasis, metastatic retinitis, familial exudative vitreoretinopathy, massive retinal fibrosis, Eales disease, sickle cell retinopathy, leukemia, anemia, and cavernous retinal hemangioma.

Treatment is directed at obliterating the abnormal vessels and includes cryotherapy or laser photocoagulation. The disease is stopped when the leaking vessels are destroyed. Eyes with progressive disease develop exudative retinal detachments and subretinal fibrosis. Scleral buckling may be used on eyes with retinal detachments. Some eyes develop intractable glaucoma.

In one study, 22 untreated patients were followed for an average of 5 years. The ocular disease progressed in about half of the patients, while the other half remained stable. Ridley et al (1982) reported on 43 eyes, of which 29 were treated. Of the latter group, 8 (27.5%) deteriorated, 15 (52%) stabilized, and 6 (20.5%) improved. Aggressive treatment of the abnormal vessels and prolonged follow-up were recommended.

Morales AG. Coats' disease: natural history and results of treatment. *Am J Ophthalmol.* 1965;60:855–865.

Ridley ME, Shields JA, Brown GC, et al. Coats' disease. Evaluation of management. *Ophthalmology.* 1982;89:1331–1387.

Tarkkanen A, Laatikainen L. Coats' disease: clinical, angiographic, histopathological findings and clinical management. *Br J Ophthalmol.* 1983;67:766–776.

Hereditary Retinal Disease

Nystagmus is the most definitive presenting sign of a hereditary retinal disorder in the preverbal child. The onset of nystagmus typically occurs between 8 and 12 weeks of age. Poor visual function can also be the presenting abnormality in a young child, and school-age children with retinal disease often fail a vision screening. Work-up requires a complete ophthalmologic examination and an electroretino-

TABLE XXIV-3

ETIOLOGIES OF NYSTAGMUS IN FIRST 3 MONTHS OF LIFE

Primary sensory retinal abnormality

Leber congenital amaurosis
Achromatopsia
Blue-cone monochromatism
Congenital stationary night blindness
  (X-linked and autosomal recessive)

Vitreoretinal abnormality

Norrie disease
Familial exudative vitreoretinopathy

Foveal hypoplasia

Associated with albinism
Associated with aniridia
Isolated

Optic nerve hypoplasia

Optic nerve hypoplasia
Optic nerve coloboma
Optic atrophy

Infectious disease

Congenital toxoplasmosis
Cytomegalovirus
Rubella
Syphilis

Congenital motor nystagmus

Generalized central nervous system disorder

Aicardi syndrome
Others

gram (ERG). Older children can be examined further with electro-oculogram (EOG), color vision, visual fields, and dark adaptation testing.

Table XXIV-3 outlines the etiologies of nystagmus in the first 3 months of life. Optic nerve disorders, infectious diseases, and congenital motor nystagmus are discussed elsewhere in this book (see chapters XII, XVII, and XXV). Hereditary retinal diseases with onset late in childhood are much like adult hereditary retinal diseases and are thoroughly covered in BCSC Section 12, *Retina and Vitreous.*

Leber Congenital Amaurosis

Leber congenital amaurosis is an autosomal recessive disorder that affects both rods and cones. It presents with decreased vision during the first year of life, usually manifesting as nystagmus beginning in the second or third month. Vision ranges from 20/200 to bare light perception in most patients. Hyperopic refraction and sluggish pupillary responses are characteristic findings on examination. Ophthalmoscopic

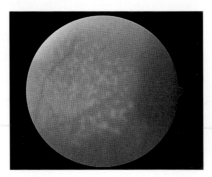

FIG XXIV-13—Leber congenital amaurosis, marbleized fundus type.

appearance is highly variable, ranging from a normal appearance, particularly in infancy, to one resembling classic retinitis pigmentosa with bone spicules, attenuation of arterioles, and disc pallor. Other reported fundus findings include irregularity of the retinal pigment epithelium, extensive chorioretinal atrophy, macular "coloboma," white dots (similar to retinitis punctata albescens), marbleized retinal appearance, and disc edema (Fig XXIV-13). Additional ocular abnormalities include oculodigital reflex (eye poking), cataracts, keratoconus, and keratoglobus. There is a significant incidence of neurologic and renal disorders in these patients. See "Familial Oculorenal Syndromes" later in this chapter.

Given such variability, the diagnosis of Leber congenital amaurosis cannot be based on fundus appearance alone and requires an ERG. However, electroretinography can be technically difficult to perform in infants, and there is a maturation of the response. Thus, an ERG can appear very abnormal in a child who is later normal.

The characteristic clinical picture in this disorder is of an infant in the first 6 months of life presenting with nystagmus and an ERG that is nearly or essentially flat. Histologic examination shows diffuse absence of photoreceptors. No treatment is available. Recently a defect in the guanylate cyclase 2D membrane enzyme, which helps control the level of the intracellular second messenger cGMP, has been identified in some but not all families with this disorder. It has long been suspected that more than one biochemical defect leads to a similar phenotype.

Both *Refsum disease* (infantile phytanic acid storage disease) and *Bassen-Kornzweig syndrome* (abetalipoproteinemia) have been reported to present as Leber congenital amaurosis. Because these are potentially treatable metabolic disorders (reduction of phytanic acid intake and vitamin A and E therapy, respectively), it is recommended that the evaluation of a new patient with findings of Leber congenital amaurosis include a complete blood lipid profile, inspection of peripheral smear for acanthocytes (Bassen-Kornzweig syndrome), and measurement of serum phytanic acid levels.

Lambert SR, Taylor D, Kriss A. The infant with nystagmus, normal appearing fundi, but an abnormal ERG. *Surv Ophthalmol.* 1989;34:173–186.

Achromatopsia

Infants with achromatopsia can be difficult to distinguish initially from those with Leber congenital amaurosis, but they develop better visual functioning and photophobia over time. Complete achromatopsia, or rod monochromatism, is a stationary autosomal recessive disorder in which patients have no color vision, poor central vision, nystagmus, and photophobia. The photophobia is actually a desire to avoid bright light rather than true pain or discomfort, and it may be manifested by squinting or rapid fluttering of the eyelids in normal indoor illumination. It may not appear until several months of age.

Retinal examination is usually normal, with the exception of a decreased or absent foveal reflex. Color vision testing is markedly abnormal, as is the ERG, which shows extinguished photopic responses. Dark glasses or red glasses that exclude short wavelengths may be helpful. Incomplete autosomal recessive forms of achromatopsia occur less often.

> Pokorny J, Smith VC, Pinckers AJ, et al. Classification of complete and incomplete autosomal recessive achromatopsia. *Graefes Arch Clin Exp Ophthalmol.* 1982;219: 121–130.

Blue-Cone Monochromatism

Blue-cone monochromatism is an X-linked stationary cone disorder that may present with nystagmus in the first few months of life. These patients are less severely affected clinically than those with complete achromatopsia. They have a characteristic color vision abnormality and visual acuities that range from 20/60 to 20/200. The fundus examination is essentially normal. Although the short-wavelength cones (blue) are functioning, the photopic ERG is essentially extinguished.

Congenital Stationary Night Blindness (CSNB)

The following classification scheme for congenital stationary night blindness was proposed by Carr (1974). Forms with normal fundi:

- Autosomal dominant
- Autosomal recessive
- X-linked

Forms with abnormal fundi:

- Oguchi disease: yellow sheen after light exposure that disappears following dark adaptation
- Fundus albipunctatus: yellow-white dots, normal vessels

Both autosomal recessive and X-linked forms of CSNB can present in early infancy with nystagmus and normal fundi. These forms are often also associated with myopia and decreased acuity in the range of 20/200. The retina appears normal, although some temporal pallor of the optic nerve may be present. The ERG shows two characteristic patterns; in both, the scotopic b-wave amplitude is greatly reduced. Dark adaptation is abnormal in all patients. Other forms of CSNB are discussed in BCSC Section 12, *Retina and Vitreous.*

> Carr RE. Congenital stationary night blindness. *Trans Am Ophthalmol Soc.* 1974; 72:448–487.

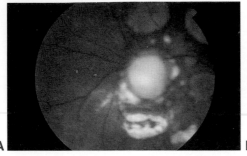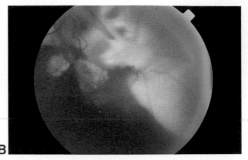

FIG XXIV-14—Aicardi syndrome. *A,* Fundus photograph showing disc and adjacent chorioretinal lacunae. *B,* Peripheral view of same patient showing large chorioretinal lacuna.

Foveal Hypoplasia

Incomplete development of the fovea, or foveal hypoplasia, is another cause of nystagmus in early infancy. It is most often associated with albinism or aniridia but may also be an isolated finding. The ophthalmoscopic appearance shows a decreased or absent foveal reflex with varying degrees of hypoplasia of the macula itself (patients with complete achromatopsia also show decreased foveal reflex). The ERG is normal in these cases. Foveal hypoplasia can be familial and may be related to a defect in the PAX6 gene.

Aicardi Syndrome

Aicardi syndrome is a disorder characterized by round, widespread, depigmented chorioretinal lesions (Fig XXIV-14). Optic nerve head colobomas and microphthalmos also occur. Agenesis of the corpus callosum is seen on CT scan. Affected patients have infantile spasms and severe mental retardation. Aicardi syndrome is an X-linked dominant disorder, lethal in males.

> Carney SH, Brodsky MC, Good WV, et al. Aicardi syndrome: more than meets the eye. *Surv Ophthalmol.* 1993;37:419–424.

> Menezes AV, MacGregor DL, Buncic JR. Aicardi syndrome: natural history and possible predictors of severity. *Pediatr Neurol.* 1994;11:313–318.

Hereditary Macular Dystrophies

The macula can be involved in a hereditary disorder in three possible ways:

- ☐ It may have an abnormal appearance secondary to a hereditary systemic disease (e.g., the cherry-red spot seen in generalized gangliosidosis).

- ☐ It may be involved in a generalized primary retinal disorder, as in some cases of Leber congenital amaurosis. Tests of overall retinal function such as the ERG are abnormal in this situation.

- ☐ The macula alone may be affected by a hereditary disorder including Stargardt disease, Best vitelliform dystrophy, and familial drusen.

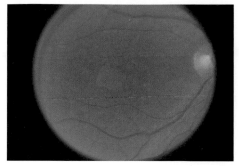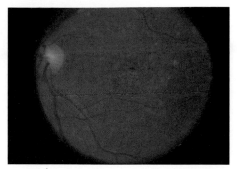

FIG XXIV-15—Stargardt disease, bilateral.

Stargardt Disease (Fundus Flavimaculatus)

Stargardt disease (juvenile macular degeneration) is the most common hereditary macular dystrophy. It is a bilateral, symmetric, progressive condition in which acuity levels off at approximately 20/200. Vision typically begins to deteriorate between ages 8 and 15 years. The fundus appears normal early in the course of the disease, even when some loss of vision has already occurred. The first ophthalmoscopic changes observed are loss of foveal reflex, followed by development of a characteristic bull's-eye lesion. Yellow flecks in the posterior pole are characteristic, but they are not required for the diagnosis (Fig XXIV-15). Eventually, the macula may acquire an atrophic appearance with a peculiar light-reflecting quality that has been described as "beaten bronze." The lesion then enlarges and deepens and may finally show choroidal atrophy with prominent choroidal vessels at its base. The dark choroid sign on fluorescein angiography is very distinctive.

Fundus flavimaculatus   If more retinal flecks develop in the periphery and evidence suggests generalized retinal involvement, the condition is known as *fundus flavimaculatus* (Fig XXIV-16). Early fundus flavimaculatus may be indistinguishable from Stargardt disease, and there are families in which both forms are reported. Final disease classification will depend on genetic studies. ERG abnormalities are seen in fundus flavimaculatus but are not typically seen in Stargardt disease. Most cases show autosomal recessive inheritance, but some dominant families have been reported. In recessive families a defect in a photoreceptor cell–specific transporter gene that is expressed in rods has been found. How this rod defect causes the clinical picture is still under investigation.

Best Vitelliform Dystrophy

The retina may at first appear normal in Best vitelliform dystrophy even though the EOG is abnormal (Fig XXIV-17). The vitelliform stage begins between 4 and 10 years of age and is seen as a yellow-orange cystlike structure, usually in the macula, although the lesion may occur elsewhere and can occasionally be multiple. It is usually 1.5–5.0 disc diameters in size. The "sunny-side up" appearance is associated

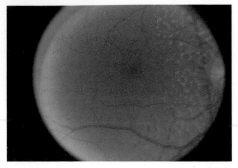
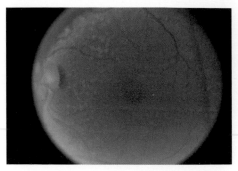

FIG XXIV-16—Fundus flavimaculatus.

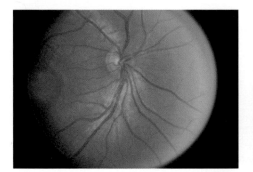
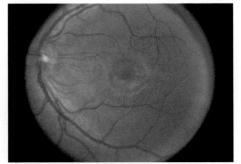

FIG XXIV-17—Best vitelliform dystrophy, bilateral.

with good central vision. With time, the cystic material may become granular, giving rise to the "scrambled egg" stage. Central vision usually remains good.

The contents of the retinal pigment epithelial cyst may rupture and partially resorb, and pseudohypopyon may form with liquefaction of the cystic contents. Eventually, atrophy of the macula ensues. There may be subretinal neovascularization and serous detachment of the retinal pigment epithelium, and subretinal hemorrhage may occur. Most patients see surprisingly well for many years; eventually, however, central vision deteriorates to the level of 20/100 or worse.

The EOG is abnormal in all affected patients and also in carriers. This disorder is one of the few that has an abnormal EOG and a normal ERG. Carriers can be identified by the presence of an abnormal EOG in the absence of morphologic abnormalities. The condition is autosomal dominant and has been mapped to the long arm of chromosome 11.

Familial Drusen

In this dominantly transmitted disorder drusen appear on Bruch's membrane. Decreased central acuity is rare before age 40, but macular drusen are occasionally seen in children. The drusen are small, yellow white, and round or oval. They are similar to the lesions of fundus albipunctatus except that they tend to form grapelike clusters. Complications in adult life include macular edema, hemorrhage, and macular degenerations of various types following subretinal neovascularization.

Hereditary Vitreoretinopathies

The vitreoretinopathies include a broad range of disease entities. Those that are discussed here characteristically present in childhood.

Juvenile Retinoschisis

Foveal retinoschisis is present in almost all cases of juvenile retinoschisis. About 50% of patients have peripheral retinoschisis in addition to foveal involvement. The retinoschisis occurs in the nerve fiber layer. The fovea has a star-shaped or spokelike configuration; vitreous veils or strands are common (Fig XXIV-18); and vitreal syneresis is prominent. Visual acuity is extremely variable but may gradually deteriorate to the finger-counting range. Complications include vitreous hemorrhages and retinal detachments. The ERG shows a reduction of the scotopic b-wave with preservation of the a-wave, while the EOG is normal. The condition is usually transmitted as an X-linked trait.

Stickler Syndrome

Stickler syndrome is an autosomal dominant disease characterized by progressive arthropathy, high myopia, retinal detachment, degenerative joint changes, epiphyseal dysplasia, flat midface, and heart defects. A single family can show great variability in expression of the syndrome, and individuals may manifest only a few of the characteristic findings. In many families a defect in the type II procollagen has been found. Type II collagen is the major structural component of secondary vitreous.

A significant percentage of patients with Stickler syndrome also have the Pierre Robin sequence of cleft palate, small mandible, and backward displacement of the tongue. These patients can be detected in infancy because of their vulnerability to

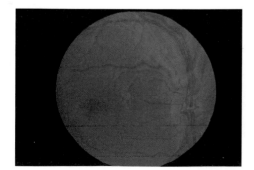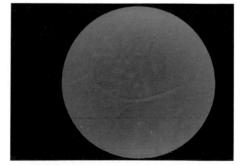

FIG XXIV-18—Juvenile retinoschisis.

serious respiratory and feeding problems, but others with only ophthalmic defects may go unrecognized until later in childhood. The ophthalmic manifestations are not only frequent but also extremely severe and vision threatening. Myopia, usually of a high degree, is the most common finding, and it is often associated with a radial type of retinal degeneration with pigment clumping around the retinal vessels. There is a high incidence of retinal detachment with large retinal breaks and proliferative vitreoretinopathy. Angle anomalies, ectopia lentis, cataracts, ptosis, and strabismus are less frequently associated. The incidence of vitreous loss during cataract surgery is high, as is the rate of subsequent retinal detachments. When possible, retinal folds and breaks should be treated before cataract extraction. Extracapsular techniques may be employed.

Early diagnosis may aid in preventing some of the severe complications of the ocular pathology and allow treatment of mild joint involvement. Although the arthropathy may not be symptomatic initially, these children often show radiographic abnormalities of long bones and joints.

Snead MP, Payne SJ, Barton DE, et al. Stickler syndrome: correlation between vitreoretinal phenotypes and linkage to COL 2A1. *Eye.* 1994;8:609–614.

Vandenberg P. Molecular basis of heritable connective tissue disease. *Biochem Med Metab Biol.* 1993;49:1–12.

Familial Exudative Vitreoretinopathy (FEVR)

Both vitreous traction and posterior vitreous detachment are present in FEVR. The peripheral retina shows lack of vascularization and white areas with and without pressure. Thick peripheral exudates develop both in and under the retina. The combined effect of exudates and vitreous membranes results in retinal traction and subsequent retinal break. Early signs include decreased vision from retinal detachment and cataract. Family members can show marked variation of severity from minimal straightening of vessels and peripheral nonperfusion to total retinal detachment. Differential diagnosis includes ROP and Coats disease.

The disease is usually autosomal dominant as a result of a defect on chromosome 11. X-linked families with a defect in the same gene as Norrie disease and primary retinal dysplasia have also been reported. Cryopexy, photocoagulation, retinal detachment surgery, vitrectomy, and cataract surgery have all been used to manage this disorder.

Norrie Disease

Norrie disease is an X-linked disorder that is characterized by progressive, bilateral, congenital blindness associated with varying degrees of hearing impairment and mental retardation. Affected boys are typically born blind, although the external ocular appearance may initially be normal. During the first few days or weeks of life a yellowish retinal detachment appears bilaterally, followed by a whiter mass behind the clear lens. Over time the lenses, and later the cornea, opacify; and phthisis bulbi ensues by the age of 10 years or earlier. Before endstage is reached the retina shows dysplasia histopathologically. DNA testing is possible for genetic counseling.

Mintz-Hittner HA, Ferrell RE, Sims KB, et al. Peripheral retinopathy in offspring of carriers of Norrie disease gene mutations. Possible transplacental effect of abnormal Norrin. *Ophthalmology.* 1996;103:2128–2134.

Goldmann-Favre Vitreoretinal Dystrophy

Goldmann-Favre vitreoretinal dystrophy consists of vitreous strands and veils as well as foveal and peripheral retinoschisis. The peripheral retina shows changes similar to those seen in retinitis pigmentosa, including optic nerve pallor and attenuation of the retinal vessels. The pigmentary disturbance tends to be in a nummular, rather than a bone spicule, configuration; and in some cases little pigment is seen. Decreased central acuity and night blindness are prominent early findings in the second decade of life, and complicated cataracts subsequently develop. Inheritance is autosomal recessive.

Bloome MA, Garcia CA. *Manual of Retinal and Choroidal Dystrophies.* New York: Appleton-Century-Crofts; 1982.

Brown DM, Weingeist TA. Disorders of the vitreous and the vitreoretinal interface. In: Wright KW, ed. *Pediatric Ophthalmology and Strabismus.* St Louis: Mosby; 1995:467–476.

Systemic Diseases and Disorders with Retinal Manifestations

Diabetes Mellitus

Type I, or *insulin-dependent, diabetes mellitus (IDDM)* was formerly called *juvenile-onset diabetes mellitus.* The prevalence of retinopathy in this condition is directly proportional to the duration of diabetes after puberty. Retinopathy is rarely seen less than 3 years after the onset of diabetes mellitus. Fundus photography or angiography reveals that about 50% of patients have *nonproliferative* (background) retinopathy after 7 years, although only half of these cases can be recognized when examined by direct ophthalmoscopy. The prevalence of retinopathy increases to approximately 90% in patients who have had type I diabetes for 15 years or more. *Proliferative* diabetic retinopathy is rare in pediatric cases and will not be covered in this section. For further discussion see BCSC Section 12, *Retina and Vitreous.*

A variety of nonproliferative changes may be seen in the pediatric age group. These changes are thought to result from obstruction of retinal capillaries and abnormal capillary permeability. Microaneurysms are the first ophthalmoscopic sign; they may be followed by retinal hemorrhages, areas of retinal nonperfusion, cotton-wool spots, hard exudates, intraretinal microvascular abnormalities, and venous dilation. A rapid rise of blood glucose may produce myopia, and sudden reduction of blood glucose can induce hyperopia. Several weeks may be required before a normal refraction is regained.

True diabetic cataracts are rare and probably more common in patients with poorly controlled disease. They resemble a "snowstorm" affecting the anterior and posterior cortices of young patients. Diabetic cataracts are caused by collection of sorbitol within the lens. Sorbitol concentration increases the lens osmolarity, leading to lens swelling and leakage of intralenticular contents. Such cataracts may require surgical treatment.

Management Specific treatment is not indicated for nonproliferative retinopathy in children. A schedule of ophthalmic examinations proposed by the American Academy of Pediatrics includes an initial discussion between the parents and the endocrinologist within the first year after diagnosis of type I diabetes mellitus regarding ocular complications and the need for surveillance. An initial eye examination should be done at 9 years of age if the glucose is poorly controlled or 3 years after puberty if well controlled, with annual follow-up examinations.

Palmberg P, Smith M, Waltman S, et al. The natural history of retinopathy in insulin-dependent juvenile-onset diabetes. *Ophthalmology.* 1981;88:613–618.

Leukemia

Ocular abnormalities are seen in patients with acute lymphoblastic, acute myelogenous, and acute monocytic leukemia. Retinopathy appears less often in children than in adults. A poorer prognosis for children with ocular manifestations has been described in two series. Histopathologically, the choroid is the most frequently affected ocular tissue, but choroidal involvement is usually not apparent clinically. Indirect ophthalmoscopy may sometimes reveal mildly pale fundus areas, but choroidal involvement is more accurately detected by ultrasound.

The most common eye findings are retinal hemorrhages, especially flame-shaped lesions in the nerve fiber layer (Fig XXIV-19). They involve the posterior fundus and can have some correlation with other aspects of the disease such as anemia, thrombocytopenia, or coagulation abnormalities. At times these retinal hemorrhages have white centers similar to the hemorrhages described in pernicious anemia, subacute bacterial endocarditis, scurvy, and septicemia. They can also resemble those associated with intracranial hemorrhages and trauma in infants in that the white centers are fibrin thrombi. However, collections of leukocytes have also been found on histopathology. Other forms of retinal involvement include localized perivascular infiltrations, microinfarction, and discrete tumor infiltrations.

Optic nerve involvement is visible if the disc is infiltrated by leukemic cells (Fig XXIV-20). Translucent swelling of the disc obscures the normal landmarks; with florid involvement, only a white mass is seen in the region of the disc. If the nerve is involved centrally, a papilledema-like fundus picture ensues; such retrolaminar optic nerve involvement results in the loss of central vision. Therefore, a leukemic child with papilledema and a loss of central vision should be considered to have this complication. Early optic nerve involvement in leukemia is a medical emergency

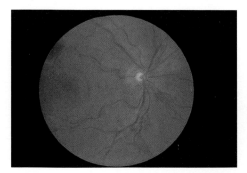 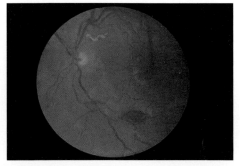

FIG XXIV-19—Retinal hemorrhages in bilateral leukemia.

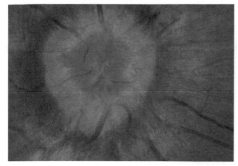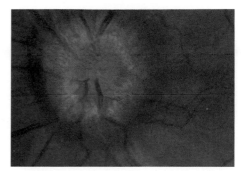

FIG XXIV-20—Leukemic infiltration of optic nerves, bilateral.

because permanent loss of central vision is imminent. Such patients should receive radiation therapy as soon as possible. However, patients receiving cancer chemotherapy may be abnormally sensitive to radiation therapy; blinding optic nerve atrophy has been reported in these patients.

Leukemic infiltrates in the anterior segment may lead to heterochromia iridis, a change in the architecture of the iris; frank iris infiltrates; spontaneous hyphemas; leukemic cells in the anterior chamber; and hypopyon. Keratic precipitates may be seen, and some affected eyes develop glaucoma from tumor cells clogging the trabecular meshwork. Other possible glaucoma mechanisms include posterior synechiae formation, seclusion of the pupil, and pupillary block. Anterior chamber paracentesis for cytologic studies may be diagnostic in cases with anterior segment involvement. Topical steroids and local irradiation are effective for anterior segment complications.

Leukemic involvement of the iris may be confused with juvenile xanthogranuloma (JXG). Methods for distinguishing between these two eye disorders of children include the following:

□ Biopsy of skin lesions of JXG

□ Peripheral blood analysis

□ Bone marrow biopsy

□ Anterior chamber taps for cytologic studies

Leukemic infiltration of the orbit is relatively uncommon and is more characteristic of acute myelogenous leukemia. Orbital involvement may be difficult to distinguish from bacterial or fungal orbital cellulitis. Leukemic orbital infiltration may be best managed by radiation therapy. There is a high correlation between ocular and central nervous system involvement with abnormal cells in the cerebrospinal fluid.

Kincaid MC, Green WR. Ocular and orbital involvement in leukemia. *Surv Ophthalmol.* 1983;27:211–232.

Ohkoshi K, Tsiaras WG. Prognostic importance of ophthalmic manifestations in childhood leukaemia. *Br J Ophthalmol.* 1992;76:651–655.

Rosenthal AR. Ocular manifestations of leukemia. A review. *Ophthalmology.* 1983; 90:899–905.

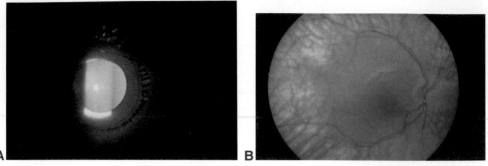

FIG XXIV-21—*A,* Transillumination of iris in albinism, right eye. *B,* Fundus in albinism, right eye.

Albinism

Albinism is a group of various conditions that involve the melanin system of the skin and/or eye (see Table XXIV-4, pp 290–291, and BCSC Section 12, *Retina and Vitreous*). The most common forms are *oculocutaneous albinism* (both tyrosinase positive and negative) and *X-linked ocular albinism.* The primary morbidity for most forms of albinism is ocular, so the ophthalmologist may be the physician who raises the issues of heredity and skin protection from the sun to the family.

The major ophthalmologic findings in albinism are iris transillumination from decreased pigmentation, foveal aplasia or hypoplasia, and a characteristic deficit of pigment in the retina, especially peripheral to the posterior pole (Fig XXIV-21). Nystagmus, light sensitivity, high refractive errors, and reduced central acuity are often present, and visual acuity ranges from 20/40 to 20/200. If a child has significant foveal hypoplasia, nystagmus will begin at 2–3 months of life. The severity of the visual defect tends to be proportionate to the degree of hypopigmentation. An abnormally large number of crossed fibers appear in the optic chiasm of patients and animals with albinism, precluding stereopsis and normal representation of space in the central nervous system. Asymmetric visually evoked cortical potentials (VECP) reflect this abnormality.

All forms of albinism are inherited, and genetic counseling is important. Unlike other recessive disorders, the defective genes responsible for albinism are fairly common, so parents of the patients are usually not related. Some forms of albinism are allelic and others are not. Most children with albinism can attend regular schools with some assistance, but few see well enough to drive. Treatment is nonspecific and includes refraction, tinted glasses, and visual aids for older patients. When either Chédiak-Higashi syndrome or Hermansky-Pudlak syndrome is suspected, hematologic consultation is advised because of the lethal nature of these forms of albinism.

Creel D, Witkop CJ Jr, King RA. Asymmetric visually evoked potential in human albinos: evidence for visual system anomalies. *Invest Ophthalmol.* 1974;13:430–440.

Oetting WS, Summers CG, King RA. Albinism and the associated ocular defects. *Metab Pediatr Syst Ophthalmol.* 1994;17:5–9.

Familial Oculorenal Syndromes

Oculorenal syndromes include *Lowe (oculocerebral) syndrome*. This X-linked recessive disorder with renal defects presents in the first year of life, producing aminoaciduria, metabolic acidosis, proteinuria, hematuria, granular casts in the urine, and rickets. Affected children are mentally retarded, hypotonic, and areflexic. The biochemical defect is in a phosphatase important in Golgi complex vesicular transport. No specific treatment exists.

The most common eye defect is cataract. The lenses are small, thick, and opaque and may demonstrate posterior lenticonus. Congenital glaucoma is often present. Surgery is often difficult, with recurrent cyclitic membranes and recalcitrant glaucoma. Mothers of affected children have punctate snowflake opacities within the lens cortex.

> Lavin CW, McKeown CA. The oculocerebrorenal syndrome of Lowe. *Int Ophthalmol Clin.* 1993;33:179–191.

Alport syndrome is transmitted as an autosomal dominant trait with variable penetrance or as an X-linked disorder. Hematuria begins in childhood. Proteinuria and renal casts develop with hypertension and kidney failure occurring late in the course of the disease. Sensorineural deafness is a prominent feature of this disorder. Anterior lenticonus and anterior polar cataracts are the most common eye abnormalities. The retinal appearance may resemble that of fundus albipunctatus.

> Govan JA. Ocular manifestations of Alport's syndrome: a hereditary disorder of basement membranes? *Br J Ophthalmol.* 1983;67:493–503.

Familial renal-retinal dystrophy is an autosomal recessive inherited condition characterized by interstitial nephritis and pigmentary retinal degeneration. Polyuria, polydipsia, and progressive azotemia is the rule. The eye signs and symptoms are characteristic of retinitis pigmentosa. Some patients who present early in life appear similar to those with Leber congenital amaurosis.

> Clarke MP, Sullivan TJ, Francis C, et al. Senior-Loken syndrome. Case reports of two siblings and association with sensorineural deafness. *Br J Ophthalmol.* 1992;76: 171–172.

> Warady BA, Cibis G, Alon V, et al. Senior-Loken syndrome: revisited. *Pediatrics.* 1994; 94:111–112.

Ocular findings in chronic renal disease are often those of hypertensive retinopathy. Diffuse retinal and disc edema are frequently present. Nonrhegmatogenous bullous retinal detachments, usually involving the inferior retina, may occur. Calcium salts may be deposited in the cornea and conjunctiva. Punctate stippling of the lens capsule is seen in many patients with chronic renal disease, and dense lens opacities develop in some patients. Cataracts frequently form following renal transplantation. Steroid-induced glaucoma is another problem in these patients, either pre- or postoperatively. Cytomegalic inclusion retinitis and *Candida* retinitis may develop following renal transplantation.

TABLE XXIV-4

ALBINISM

DISEASE	OCULAR MANIFESTATIONS	SYSTEMIC MANIFESTATIONS	INHERITANCE
Tyrosinase-negative (OCA1A)	Iris is thin, pale blue; characteristic orange reflex from the iris occurs because of marked transillumination defect; prominent choroidal vessels with poorly defined fovea; nystagmus; head-nodding; frequently myopic astigmatism and strabismus; vision 20/100–20/200; marked photophobia	White hair throughout life; tyrosinase absent, serum tyrosine levels normal; stage I and II melanosomes only; increased susceptibility to skin neoplasia	Autosomal recessive, chromosome 11q14–21
Tyrosinase-positive (OCA2)	Eye color blue, yellow, or brown (age and race dependent); pigment cartwheel effect at pupil and limbus; red reflex minimal to absent in dark race adults; moderate to severe nystagmus; photophobia; moderately severe visual defect; 20/80–20/100	Hair and skin color white at birth, darkening slightly by 2 years; melanosomes to early stage III polyphagosomes; hair bulbs develop pigmentation upon incubation in tyrosine; increased susceptibility to skin neoplasia; hyperkeratoses and freckling in exposed areas of skin	Autosomal recessive, chromosome 15q11.2–q12; P gene
Yellow mutant (Amish) (OCA1B)	At birth complete albinism with blue, translucent irides and albinotic fundal reflex; nystagmus and photophobia; increasing pigmentation with age	White hair and skin at birth; increasing pigmentation with yellow–red hair and light normal skin that tans; biochemically, intermediate reaction between tyrosinase positive and negative; stage III pheomelanosomes: allelic to tyrosinase-negative albinism	Autosomal recessive; allelic with OCA1A
Hermansky-Pudlak syndrome	Eye color blue-gray to brown (age and race dependent); iris normal to cartwheel effect; red reflex present in light-skinned individuals; mild to severe nystagmus and photophobia; slight to moderate decrease in visual acuity; high frequency in Puerto Rico	Platelet bleeding disorder, pulmonary fibrosis; hair color variable, white to dark red-brown; cream-colored skin; melanosis on exposed skin; pigmented nevi and freckles; susceptibility to skin neoplasia; serum tyrosine levels normal to decreased; platelet defect; ceroid storage, cytoplasmic bodies	Autosomal recessive, chromosome 10q2
Brown (OCA3)	Blue to brown irides; transillumination of irides; retinal hypopigmentation; nystagmus; alternating strabismus	Skin and hair light brown; freckles present; areas of hypopigmentation	Autosomal recessive, ? same as autosomal recessive ocular albinism in darker races
Cross syndrome	Gray-blue eye color; cataracts; microphthalmos; severe nystagmus; blindness	White to light blond hair; white to pink skin; pigmented nevi; freckles; scanty melanosomes, stage III, some stage IV; oligophrenia; gingival fibromatosis; athetosis	Autosomal recessive

Type	Ocular findings	Systemic findings	Inheritance
Ocular	*X-linked form:* Marked deficiency of pigment in iris and choroid; nystagmus and myopic astigmatism; in blacks, may be limited to nystagmus, foveal hypoplasia, and tessellated fundus; mosaic pigment pattern in fundi *Autosomal recessive form:* Ocular signs as above, females as severely affected as males, and obligate heterozygotes have normal fundi	Normal pigmentation elsewhere; occasional hypopigmented cutaneous macules; giant melanosomes in normal skin; patients appear more lightly pigmented than their relatives May be the same as brown albinism	X-linked recessive, Xp22.3 Autosomal recessive
Chédiak-Higashi syndrome	Partial albinism; diminished uveal and retinal pigmentation with photophobia and nystagmus. On histologic examination: papilledema; lymphocytic infiltration of the optic nerve; leukocytes containing the typical metachromatic inclusion granules in the limbal area, iris, and choroid	Early death from recurrent infections; silver tinge to hair; neutropenia with tendency toward lymphocytosis, anemia, and thrombocytopenia, hepatosplenomegaly, lymphadenopathy; leukemia, lymphoma	Autosomal recessive, chromosome 1q42–43
Temperature-sensitive (OCA1TS)	Similar to findings for OCA1A	White hair on warmer parts of body including scalp, darker hair on extremities	Autosomal recessive, allelic with OCA1A form due to a temperature-sensitive tyrosinase
Minimal pigment (OCAMP)	Vision 20/50–20/200; some iris pigment develops; foveal hypoplasia and nystagmus	Minimal hair and skin pigment; low tyrosinase levels	Autosomal recessive
With deafness	Typical ocular changes	Typical albinism with nerve deafness	X-linked recessive
Dominant oculocutaneous	Fine diffuse pattern of depigmentation on irides	Hypomelanism of skin, hair	Autosomal dominant, very rare

Table adapted and updated from Nelson LB, Calhoun JH, Harley RD, eds. *Pediatric Ophthalmology,* 3rd ed. Philadelphia: Saunders; 1991.

Gangliosidoses

In *GM₁ type I* gangliosidosis all three β-galactosidase isoenzymes (hexosaminidase A, B, and C) are absent. This severe disease often occurs with congenital edema and hepatosplenomegaly. A cherry-red spot is present in 50% of patients. Acuity is greatly diminished and pendular nystagmus is present. Tortuous conjunctival vessels with saccular microaneurysms, optic atrophy, occasional corneal clouding, papilledema, and high myopia may be present. Other features of this disease include psychomotor retardation, hypotonia, Hurler-like facial features, kyphosis, and congestive heart failure. Affected children usually die by 2 years of age.

In *GM₁ type II* gangliosidosis (Derry disease) β-galactosidase isoenzymes B and C are lacking. There is no cherry-red spot, but nystagmus, esotropia, pigmentary retinopathy, and optic atrophy have been observed. The first sign is locomotor ataxia followed by progressive psychomotor deterioration and seizures. Affected children are decerebrate and rigid by the end of their second year of life. Death occurs between the ages of 3 and 10.

GM₂ type I gangliosidosis (Tay-Sachs disease) is caused by a deficiency in isoenzyme hexosaminidase A. A foveal cherry-red spot is characteristic by 6 months of age, and vision is reduced by 12–18 months of age. The pathologic finding is the white ring resulting from accumulation of storage material in the ganglion cells around the normally pigmented macula. Nystagmus, optic atrophy, and narrowing of the retinal vessels develop. As the ganglion cells of the retina die, the white ring can disappear. Affected children become apathetic, hypotonic, and abnormally sensitive to sound. Seizures and progressive neurologic deterioration ensue, and patients usually die by 24–30 months of age.

This disease is the most common of the gangliosidoses. It used to occur most often in individuals of eastern European Jewish (Ashkenazi) descent. A very effective genetic screening and counseling program in that population has reduced the number of cases of Tay-Sachs disease by 90% in the United States. Other groups such as French Canadians can also be affected more often than the general population. The heterozygous condition can be identified so that carriers can be counseled, and the homozygous state can be diagnosed in utero by amniocentesis.

In *GM₂ type II* gangliosidosis (Sandhoff disease) hexosaminidase A and B are absent. Ocular findings include decreased visual acuity, strabismus, inconspicuous corneal clouding, a prominent cherry-red spot, and normal-appearing optic nerves. This disorder has an ocular and systemic course similar to that of Tay-Sachs disease. Hepatosplenomegaly is not a conspicuous feature. Most affected children die as a result of progressive psychomotor deterioration by the age of 2–12 years.

In *GM₂ type III* gangliosidosis (Bernheimer-Seitelberger disease) there is partial deficiency of hexosaminidase A. The eye findings include late-onset visual loss, optic atrophy, and pigmentary retinopathy. No cherry-red spot appears. The disorder begins in early childhood with progressive psychomotor retardation, locomotor ataxia, speech loss, and spasticity. It leads to death before the age of 15 years.

Many other subtypes of gangliosidoses, with differing genetic defects, occur. Most present later with motor problems, and few have cherry-red spots.

Giugliani R, Dutra JC, Pereira ML, et al. GM₁ gangliosidosis: clinical and laboratory findings in eight families. *Hum Genet.* 1985;70:347–354.

SCREENING EXAMINATION OF PREMATURE INFANTS FOR RETINOPATHY OF PREMATURITY

A Joint Statement of the American Academy of Pediatrics, the American Association for Pediatric Ophthalmology and Strabismus, and the American Academy of Ophthalmology

Progressive retinopathy of prematurity (ROP) was once considered an untreatable condition leading to blindness. The results of the Cryotherapy for Retinopathy of Prematurity Trial indicated that treatment was associated with an approximately 50% reduction in the occurrence of posterior retinal traction folds and/or detachments.[1] An accompanying editorial stated that "a new standard of care is evolving [requiring] careful retinal examination beginning four to six weeks after birth by an ophthalmologist experienced in looking at retinas in premature infants."[2]

This statement outlines the principles upon which a screening program to detect ROP in Infants at risk might be based. It is emphasized at the outset that any screening program set up to implement an evolving standard of care suffers from inherent defects such as over- or under-referral and cannot, by its nature, duplicate the precision and rigor of a scientifically-based, randomized, prospective clinical trial. With that in mind, and based on the information published thus far,[3-5] the sponsoring organizations suggest the following guidelines:

1. Infants with a birth weight of less than or equal to 1500 grams or with a gestational age of 28 weeks or under, as well as those infants over 1500 grams with an unstable clinical course felt to be at high risk by their attending pediatrician or neonatologist, should have a dilated indirect ophthalmoscopic examination to detect ROP.

2. This examination should be carried out by an ophthalmologist with experience in the examination of pre-term infants.

3. Examination should be done between 4 and 6 weeks of chronological age or between 31 and 33 weeks post-conceptional age* as determined by the infant's attending pediatrician or neonatologist.

4. Follow-up examinations are best determined by the findings at the first examination using the International Classification of Retinopathy of Prematurity (e.g., if the retinal vasculature is immature and in Zone II but no disease is present, follow-up examination should be planned at approximately 2 to 4 week intervals until vascularization proceeds into Zone III).

5. Infants with ROP or immature vessels detected in Zone I should be seen at least every 1 to 2 weeks until normal vascularization proceeds to Zone III or the risk of attaining threshold conditions is passed.

6. Infants with threshold disease (Stage 3 ROP, Zone I or II in 5 or more continuous clock hours or 8 cumulative clock hours with the presence of "plus disease") should be considered candidates for ablative therapy of at least one eye within 72 hours of diagnosis.

* Post-conceptional age = gestational age at birth plus chronological age.

7. The attending pediatrician or neonatologist should refer the infants who fit the criteria for initial examination to the ophthalmologist and indicate which infants are medically able to be examined. If an infant is transferred to another neonatal unit or hospital, the new primary care physician should ascertain the current ocular examination status of the baby from the record or communication with the transferring physician, so that any necessary ophthalmologic examinations can be arranged.

These recommendations are evolving and, as more long-term ROP outcomes are known, may have to be modified.

1. Cryotherapy for Retinopathy of Prematurity Cooperative Group. Multicenter trial of cryotherapy for retinopathy of prematurity: preliminary results. *Arch Ophthalmol.* 1988; 106:471–479.

2. Tasman W. Multicenter trial of cryotherapy for retinopathy of prematurity [editorial]. *Arch Ophthalmol.* 1988;106:463–464.

3. Cryotherapy for Retinopathy of Prematurity Cooperative Group. Multicenter trial of cryotherapy for retinopathy of prematurity: three-month outcome. *Arch Ophthalmol.* 1990; 108:195–204.

4. Cryotherapy for Retinopathy of Prematurity Cooperative Group. Multicenter trial of cryotherapy for retinopathy of prematurity: one-year outcome—structure and function. *Arch Ophthalmol.* 1990;108:1408–1416.

5. Palmer EA, Flynn JT, Hardy RJ, et al. Incidence and early course of retinopathy of prematurity. *Ophthalmology.* 1991;98:1628–1640.

Developed by
American Academy of Pediatrics, Approved 3/97
American Association for Pediatric Ophthalmology and Strabismus, Approved 10/96
American Academy of Ophthalmology, Quality of Care Secretariat, Approved 11/96

CHAPTER XXV

Optic Nerve Disorders

Developmental Anomalies

Morning glory disc anomaly   This congenital funnel-shaped excavation of the posterior fundus incorporates the optic disc, which is surrounded by an elevated annular zone of altered retinal pigment (Fig XXV-1). Blood vessels are increased in number and loop at the edges of the disc. A central core of white glial tissue occupies the position of the normal optic cup. Visual acuity can range anywhere from 20/20 to no light perception. Serous retinal detachments occur in approximately one third of affected patients, but the source of subretinal fluid is unknown. Morning glory disc anomaly has been associated with basal encephalocele in patients with midfacial anomalies. The precise embryologic defect is unknown, but either an abnormal closure of the embryonic fissure or abnormal development of the distal optic stalk at its junction with the primitive optic vesicle is probably responsible.

> Pollock S. The morning glory disc anomaly: contractile movement, classification, and embryogenesis. *Doc Ophthalmol.* 1987;65:439–460.

> Traboulsi EI, O'Neill JF. The spectrum in the morphology of the so-called "morning glory disc anomaly." *J Pediatr Ophthalmol Strabismus.* 1988;25:93–98.

Coloboma of the optic nerve   This condition may be part of a complete chorioretinal coloboma that involves the entire embryonic fissure, or it may involve only the proximal portion of the fissure, causing a deformity of the optic disc. Mild optic disc defects resemble deep physiologic cupping. More extensive disorders appear as an enlargement of the peripapillary area with a deep, central excavation lined by a glistening white tissue with blood vessels crossing over the edge of this deep cavity (Fig XXV-2). This defect usually extends inferonasally and is often associated with

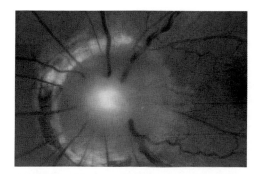

FIG XXV-1—Morning glory disc anomaly, left eye.

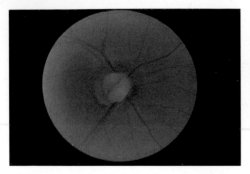 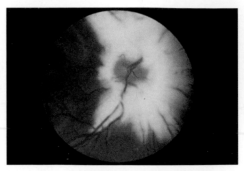

FIG XXV-2—Optic nerve coloboma, right eye.

FIG XXV-3—Myelinated nerve fibers of optic nerve and retina, right eye.

retinal defects in the periphery. Nonrhegmatogenous retinal detachments may occur. This condition may be unilateral or bilateral and can be very asymmetric. Visual acuity may be mildly or severely decreased, and it is difficult to predict from the optic disc appearance. Ocular colobomas may also be accompanied by multiple systemic abnormalities in a number of conditions such as the CHARGE association (see chapter XX).

Brodsky MC. Congenital optic disk anomalies. *Surv Ophthalmol.* 1994;39:89–112.

Pagon RA. Ocular coloboma. *Surv Ophthalmol.* 1981;25:223–236.

Myelinated (medullated) retinal nerve fibers   This condition is rarely bilateral and is more common in males. Myelination appears as a white superficial retinal area with frayed and feathered edges in a configuration coincident with the normal pattern seen for retinal nerve fibers (Fig XXV-3). Vessels that pass within the superficial layer of the nerve fibers are obscured. The myelinated fibers may occur in several isolated patches and commonly are found along the marginal disc. Myelination normally starts at the lateral geniculate ganglion and ceases at the lamina cribrosa. Occasionally, some of the fibers in the retina acquire a myelin sheath. Visual loss can occur if the macula is involved or from anisometropic amblyopia resulting from unilateral high myopia. Visual defects coincident with the areas of myelination are present.

Tilted disc syndrome (Fuchs coloboma)   In this condition the superior pole of the optic disc appears elevated, and the inferior nasal disc is posteriorly displaced, resulting in an oval-appearing optic disc with its long axis obliquely oriented (Fig XXV-4). This condition is accompanied by a scleral crescent located inferiorly or inferonasally, sinus inversus (a nasal detour of the temporal retinal vessels as they emerge from the disc before turning back temporally), and posterior ectasia of the inferior nasal fundus.

Because of the fundus abnormality, affected patients have myopic astigmatism with the plus axis oriented parallel to the ectasia. Patients may present with bitemporal hemianopia, which is typically incomplete and involves the superior quad-

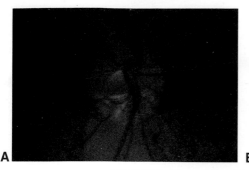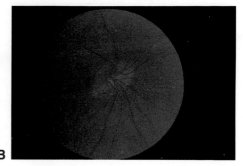

FIG XXV-4—Tilted disc syndrome. *A,* Right eye. *B,* Left eye.

rants. It can be distinguished from a chiasmal lesion as the defect does not respect the vertical midline. Large and small isopters are fairly normal, while medium-sized isopters are severely constricted. Appropriate refractive correction will often result in elimination of the visual field defect. Tilted discs, myopic astigmatism, bilateral decreased vision, and visual difficulty at night should suggest the possibility of X-linked congenital stationary night blindness, which is discussed in chapter XXIV.

Apple DJ, Rabb MF, Walsh PM. Congenital anomalies of the optic disc. *Surv Ophthalmol.* 1982;27:3–41.

Bergmeister's papillae (persistent hyaloid system) This condition results when the hyaloid artery is not resorbed before birth. The entire artery may remain as a fine thread or cord extending from the optic disc to the lens. In such situations it can be associated with persistent hyperplastic primary vitreous. The artery may be patent and contain blood where it was attached to the posterior lens capsule. In mild cases the attachment to the posterior lens capsule is located inferonasally (Mittendorf's dot) and is usually visually insignificant. Various amounts of glial tissue can occur on the disc in association with prepapillary veils and epipapillary membranes. When small and avascular, they are termed Bergmeister's papillae.

Megalopapillae This anomaly features an abnormally large optic disc diameter and is often associated with an increased cup/disc ratio that can be confused with normal-tension glaucoma. Visual acuity is usually normal or slightly decreased, and visual fields may demonstrate a slightly enlarged blind spot. Rarely, megalopapillae has been associated with optic nerve glioma. The condition can be unilateral or bilateral, and the etiology is unknown.

Optic nerve hypoplasia This is a common congenital optic disc anomaly. The disc is pale and smaller than normal. It may be associated with a yellow to white ring around the small disc, which may or may not have pigment hypoplasia at the inner or outer edge of the ring *(double ring sign)* (Fig XXV-5). Because the size of the surrounding ring often corresponds to the normal disc diameter, careful observation is necessary to avoid mistaking the entire hypoplastic disc/ring complex for a normal-

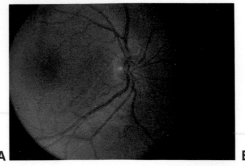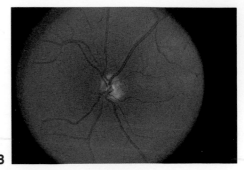

A   **B**

FIG XXV-5—Optic nerve hypoplasia. *A,* Normal right optic nerve. *B,* Hypoplastic left optic nerve.

sized disc. The vascular pattern is also abnormal and can be associated with too few or too many disc vessels. Retinal vascular tortuosity is commonly seen. Histologically, optic nerve hypoplasia is characterized by a decreased number of optic nerve axons of otherwise normal architecture.

Visual acuity ranges from normal to light perception, and visual field defects are invariably present. Visual acuity is related to the integrity of the macular fibers and often does not correlate with the overall size of the disc. Since patients with optic nerve hypoplasia also have strabismus and nystagmus, unilateral visual loss may be a result of amblyopia and may respond to patching therapy. This condition can be unilateral or bilateral and is often asymmetric in its severity. Segmental hypoplasia with an inferior visual defect occurs in some children of mothers with insulin-dependent diabetes. Intrauterine damage to the visual pathways can result in corresponding hypoplasia of each optic nerve.

Optic nerve hypoplasia has been associated with a wide variety of central nervous system and systemic anomalies. The most common, *septo-optic dysplasia (de Morsier syndrome),* combines optic nerve hypoplasia with associated midline central nervous system anomalies consisting of absence of the septum pellucidum and agenesis of the corpus callosum. Septo-optic dysplasia is often accompanied by manifestations of hypothalamic and pituitary dysfunction. The most common of these is growth hormone deficiency, but neonatal hypoglycemia, diabetes insipidus, panhypopituitarism, hyperprolactinemia, and hypothyroidism are also seen.

In an infant with optic nerve hypoplasia, history of neonatal jaundice suggests hypothyroidism, while neonatal hypoglycemia or seizures indicates panhypopituitarism. A T_4 level should be obtained in infants with optic nerve hypoplasia to rule out neonatal hypothyroidism. Because of difficulties measuring normal growth hormone levels, most patients with septo-optic dysplasia should be followed closely and only investigated for these normal levels if growth is retarded or MRI shows evidence of posterior pituitary ectopia.

MRI is the preferred neuroimaging technique for evaluating central nervous system abnormalities in patients with optic nerve hypoplasia. These abnormalities include small intracranial optic nerves; absent septum pellucidum; agenesis of the corpus callosum; and cerebral hemisphere abnormalities such as schizencephaly, leukomalacia, or encephalomalacia. Special attention should be directed to the pituitary infundibulum, where a posterior pituitary ectopia may be found. This abnormality is seen in approximately 15% of patients and suggests anterior pituitary hormone deficiency requiring further endocrinologic work-up. Posterior pituitary ectopia appears on MRI as an absence of the pituitary infundibulum with an abnormal bright spot located at the upper infundibulum area. Absence of the septum pellucidum or agenesis of the corpus callosum is not detectable by clinical evaluation. Neurodevelopmental defects, when present, are usually the result of the associated cerebral hemispheric abnormalities. Patients with optic nerve hypoplasia and diabetes insipidus have significant problems with thermal regulation and should be monitored carefully during febrile illnesses.

Brodsky MC, Glasier CM. Optic nerve hypoplasia. Clinical significance of associated central nervous system abnormalities on magnetic resonance imaging. *Arch Ophthalmol.* 1993;111:66–74.

Coston G, Murphree AL. Hypothalamic-pituitary function in children with optic nerve hypoplasia. *Am J Dis Child.* 1995;139:249–254.

Hoyt WF, Kaplan SL, Grumbach MM, et al. Septo-optic dysplasia and pituitary dwarfism. *Lancet.* 1970;1:893–894.

Optic nerve aplasia   This defect is rare. There is no optic nerve or retinal blood vessels, making the choroidal pattern clearly visible.

Optic pits or holes   These developmental defects can be considered similar to colobomas. Pits usually appear in the inferotemporal quadrant or central portion of the disc. A pit may be shallow or very deep, and it is usually unilateral and often covered with a gray veil of tissue. Optic pits have been associated with serous retinal detachments occurring mainly during the second and third decade of life (Fig XXV-6).

Peripapillary staphyloma   This condition is a posterior bulging of the sclera in which the optic disc occupies the bottom of the bowl. The disc may be normal but is surrounded by stretched choroid, thereby exposing the white sclera encircling the disc. Visual acuity is usually poor.

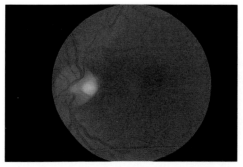

FIG XXV-6—Temporal optic nerve pit with serous retinal detachment, left eye.

TABLE XXV-1

ETIOLOGIES OF ACQUIRED OPTIC ATROPHY IN CHILDHOOD

Craniopharyngioma
Optic nerve/chiasmal glioma
Retinal degenerative disease
Hydrocephalus
Optic neuritis
Postpapilledema
Hereditary

Optic Atrophy

Optic atrophy in children is most frequently the result of anterior visual pathway disease (Table XXV-1). Other causes include inflammation (optic neuritis), hereditary optic atrophy, perinatal disease, and hydrocephalus. The work-up should include neuroimaging in all cases of uncertain etiology (negative family history, normal neurologic examination), since over 40% of these cases will have a tumor or hydrocephalus.

Hereditary Optic Atrophy

Any child with bilateral loss of central vision must be suspected of hereditary optic atrophy. This condition usually begins before the age of 10 years and is bilateral but can be asymmetric. Visual loss is mild, ranging from 20/40 to 20/100. Visual fields show central or cecocentral scotomata with normal peripheral isopters. Color vision testing is often diagnostic, revealing a generalized dyschromatopsia. Clinically, the temporal pallor of the optic disc is parallel with an area of triangular excavation. Inheritance is usually autosomal dominant, and family pedigrees are hard to elicit. Long-term prognosis is good with visual function rarely reduced to the 20/200 level. A recessive form of the disorder can occur with severe bilateral visual loss before the age of 5. Nystagmus is present in approximately half of the patients. Funduscopic exam reveals a pale optic disc with vascular attenuation of the type characteristically seen in retinal degeneration. ERG testing, however, is normal.

Behr optic atrophy This hereditary disorder occurs mainly in males with onset in childhood. It is associated with increased deep tendon reflexes, cerebellar ataxia, bladder dysfunction, mental retardation, hypotonia of the extremities, and external ophthalmoplegia.

Leber hereditary optic neuropathy (LHON) This maternally inherited disease is characterized by acute or subacute bilateral loss of central vision to the 20/200 level or worse, acquired red-green dyschromatopsia, and central or cecocentral scotomata in otherwise healthy patients (usually males) in their second to fourth decade of life. Progressive atrophy results in a flat, pale disc with dense central scotoma.

Clinically, this disorder presents as a low-grade optic neuritis with circumpapillary telangiectasia, pseudoedema of the disc, and absence of fluorescein staining. Pallor of the entire disc indistinguishable from primary atrophy generally develops within a few weeks after onset of visual disturbance. Final visual acuity is rarely better than 20/200. Associated neurologic abnormalities may include paraplegia, dementia, deafness, migraines, vertigo, spasticity, and a cardiac preexcitation arrhythmia syndrome (Wolff-Parkinson-White).

This condition is transmitted by female carriers and involves the mitochondrial DNA (mtDNA). Primary mtDNA point mutations have been located at nucleotide positions 11718, 3460, and 14484. Molecular genetic analysis of mtDNA from leukocytes is currently available and the finding of a primary mutation is pathognomonic for the disease. No effective treatment currently exists.

Nikoskelainen EK, Savontaus ML, Wanne OP, et al. Leber's hereditary optic neuropathy, a maternally inherited disease. A genealogic study in four pedigrees. *Arch Ophthalmol.* 1987;105:665–671.

Singh G, Lott MT, Wallace DC. A mitochondrial DNA mutation as a cause of Leber's hereditary optic neuropathy. *N Engl J Med.* 1989;320:1300–1305.

Optic Neuritis

Optic neuritis in childhood frequently presents with systemic infections such as measles, mumps, chickenpox, and viral illnesses (Fig XXV-7). It can also be associated with immunizations. Visual loss can be quite severe to 20/400 or worse, and it is often bilateral. Over half of the affected children have a history suggestive of intracranial involvement including headache, nausea, vomiting, lethargy, or malaise. Disc swelling, when present, can be extensive and may result in a macular star formation (*Leber idiopathic stellate neuroretinitis*, Fig XXV-8).

The cause of this "postinfectious" form of viral optic neuritis is unknown. It has been speculated that a presumed autoimmune process triggered by previous viral infection may result in a demyelinative injury. Spontaneous recovery can occur, but dramatic improvement in visual function can be achieved with intravenous corticosteroid treatment. This modality should be considered in patients with severe bilateral visual loss or in patients with optic neuritis in their only good eye.

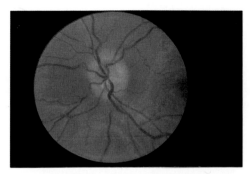

FIG XXV-7—Optic neuritis, left eye.

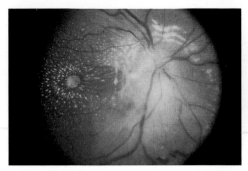

FIG XXV-8—Leber idiopathic stellate neuroretinitis.

The relationship between optic neuritis and the development of multiple sclerosis (MS), which is commonly seen in adults, is less clear in children. However, a subset of children does eventually develop signs and symptoms consistent with MS, usually within 1 year of the onset of optic neuritis. In a majority of these children the neurologic deficits are minor. Occasionally, however, severe disability can occur; while this is rare, it is important to realize that the immunologic events typical of MS can start in childhood. BCSC Section 5, *Neuro-Ophthalmology,* discusses the relationship between optic neuritis and MS at length.

Farris BK, Pickard DJ. Bilateral postinfectious optic neuritis and intravenous steroid therapy in children. *Ophthalmology.* 1990;97:339–345.

Good WV, Muci-Mendoza R, Berg BO, et al. Optic neuritis in children with poor recovery of vision. *Aust N Z J Ophthalmol.* 1992;20:319–323.

Riikonen R, Donner M, Erkkila H. Optic neuritis in children and its relationship to multiple sclerosis: a clinical study of 21 children. *Dev Med Child Neurol.* 1988; 30:349–359.

Steinlin MI, Blaser SI, MacGregor DL, et al. Eye problems in children with multiple sclerosis. *Pediatr Neurol.* 1995;12:207–212.

Papilledema

Increased intracranial pressure in children is caused by either hydrocephalus, a mass lesion, or pseudotumor cerebri. Patients should have a full evaluation including neuroimaging and lumbar puncture. In infants increased intracranial pressure results in firmness and distension of the open fontanelles. Significantly elevated pressures are usually accompanied by nausea, vomiting, and headaches. In the older child transient visual obscurations may be noted. Esotropia and diplopia may also occur as a result of injury to the sixth nerve. A sixth nerve palsy will usually resolve once intracranial pressure is reduced.

TABLE XXV-2

CONDITIONS ASSOCIATED WITH PEDIATRIC OPTIC DISC SWELLING

Papillitis

Optic neuritis (postinfectious)

Neuroretinitis (Leber)

Toxocara of disc

Papilledema
    Intracranial mass
    Pseudotumor cerebri
        Dural sinus thrombosis
    Hypertension
    Cranial synostosis
    Hydrocephalus
        Chiari malformation
        Aqueductal stenosis
        Dandy-Walker syndrome
        Infection

Astrocytoma of optic disc
    (tuberous sclerous)

Optic disc drusen

Hyperopia

Glial veils

Pseudotumor Cerebri

This benign condition consists of increased intracranial pressure of unknown etiology and duration. The presenting symptoms are headache and visual loss. It can occur in children of any age and has been associated with viral infections, drug use (tetracycline, corticosteroids, vitamin A, and nalidixic acid), and venous sinus thrombosis. Often the etiology is not determined. Ocular examination reveals excellent visual acuity with markedly swollen optic nerves bilaterally. The patient should be monitored closely for signs of visual loss and worsening headaches. Medical treatments include acetazolamide and corticosteroids. Repeated lumbar punctures have been used to control intracranial pressure, and optic nerve sheath fenestration has been shown to reduce the incidence of visual loss. The visual prognosis is excellent in most cases with spontaneous resolution within 12–18 months.

Pseudopapilledema

Pseudopapilledema refers to any elevated anomaly of the optic disc that resembles papilledema (Table XXV-2). Disc anomalies that are frequently confused with papilledema in children include drusen, hyperopia, and prominent glial tissue. Pseudopapilledema can be differentiated from true papilledema by the absence of associated venous dilation and retinal hemorrhages or exudates and by the lack of

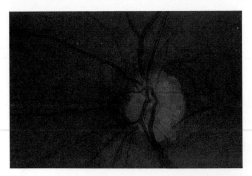

FIG XXV-9—Optic nerve drusen, right eye.

any systemic findings that are usually associated with increased intracranial pressure. Interpapillary *drusen*, which are the most common cause of pseudopapilledema in children, may appear within the first or second decade of life (Fig XXV-9). Drusen are frequently inherited, and examination of the parents is helpful in those children who are suspicious for having drusen.

The elevated disc does not obscure the retinal arterioles lying anteriorly, and the disc often has an irregular border suggesting the presence of drusen beneath the surface. There is no pallor, dilation of the papillary network, exudates, or hemorrhages. When drusen are not buried, they appear as shiny refractile bodies visible on the surface with a gray-yellow translucent appearance. Visual defects are frequently associated; lower nasal field defects are most common. However, central defects, arcuate scotoma, and concentric narrowing can also occur. These defects can be slowly progressive, and central visual acuity is rarely affected.

CHAPTER XXVI

Ocular Tumors in Childhood

Ocular and orbital tumors, both benign and malignant, occur relatively frequently in infants and children. Benign masses are much more common than malignant tumors in the orbital region. *Hamartomas,* defined as focal overgrowth of mature cells identical to those normally found at the site of origin but lacking normal tissue architecture and organization, are also found frequently. Hamartomas are present at birth and enlarge only in relation to growth of the child.

Many tumors of childhood show variable qualities and are sometimes difficult to categorize. The overall incidence of ophthalmic malignancy is greater during the first 5 years of life than during any subsequent age interval until the sixth decade. In comparison with other forms of childhood cancer, however, tumors with significant ocular involvement are uncommon, representing only about 4% of the total. See also BCSC Section 4, *Ophthalmic Pathology and Intraocular Tumors.*

Differential Diagnosis

The diagnosis of space-occupying lesions in the orbit is a particular challenge for the ophthalmologist because their clinical manifestations are relatively limited in variety and nonspecific:

☐ Proptosis or other displacement of the globe

☐ Swelling or discoloration of the eyelids

☐ Palpable subcutaneous mass

☐ Ptosis

☐ Strabismus

This list constitutes the presenting signs of most orbital tumors and of numerous other disorders as well (Table XXVI-1).

The problem of differential diagnosis in childhood is compounded by the fact that both benign and malignant tumors in young patients often enlarge very rapidly, making them difficult to distinguish from one another; from infectious and inflammatory disorders such as orbital cellulitis; and from the effects of trauma, which of course occurs with high frequency and often without a reliable history. Furthermore, proptosis of mild to moderate degree can be difficult to detect in an uncooperative child when there is associated eyelid swelling.

Fortunately, typical presentations of the common benign orbital and periorbital masses in infants and children (capillary hemangioma, dermoid cyst) are sufficiently distinctive to permit clinical diagnosis with confidence in a large majority of cases. Suspicion of a malignant process should arise when proptosis and eyelid swelling suggestive of cellulitis are *not* accompanied by warmth of the overlying skin, or when periorbital ecchymosis or hematoma develops in the absence of an unequivocal trauma history.

TABLE XXVI-1

DIFFERENTIAL DIAGNOSIS OF PROPTOSIS IN CHILDHOOD

Malignant neoplastic

Rhabdomyosarcoma
Other primary sarcoma
Metastatic neuroblastoma
Extraocular retinoblastoma
Other secondary tumor
Leukemic infiltration
Burkitt lymphoma
Malignant histiocytosis

Benign proliferative

Capillary hemangioma
Lymphangioma
Optic glioma
Meningioma
Fibrous dysplasia
Ossifying fibroma
Juvenile fibromatosis
Eosinophilic granuloma

Infectious/inflammatory

Cellulitis
Sinus mucocele
Echinococcal cyst
Idiopathic pseudotumor

Traumatic

Hematoma
Foreign body
Carotid cavernous fistula
Encephalocele

Endocrine/metabolic

Graves disease
Osteopetrosis
Infantile cortical hyperostosis

Developmental

Infantile glaucoma
Axial high myopia
Craniofacial dysostosis
Encephalocele
Colobomatous cyst
Dermoid cyst
Teratoma

The current widespread availability of high-quality imaging studies permits orbital masses to be noninvasively differentiated with confidence in a majority of cases. For initial diagnostic evaluation of the orbit CT scanning has advantages over MRI because of its high sensitivity to disturbances of bony architecture, its avoidance of interference from the high MRI signal intensity of orbital fat, and the greater ease of its use (although sedation is still generally required for young children). Dermoid cysts, teratomas, colobomatous cysts, and encephaloceles have highly distinctive appearances in CT images, as do the blood-filled cavities found in acutely deteriorated lymphangiomas. The superior ability of MRI to differentiate various tissue types makes it a valuable adjunctive study in many cases, and its lack of radiation exposure is an advantage when repeated imaging is required. In experienced hands ultrasonography may also provide important diagnostic information about the orbit.

Making a definitive diagnosis still often requires biopsy. Consultation should be obtained from a pediatric oncologist, and an appropriate metastatic work-up should be completed before resorting to orbital surgery; sometimes other, more easily accessible, sites can be found to use as tissue sources.

Pseudoproptosis can result from a mismatch between the volume of the globe and the capacity of the orbit. Examples include the elongation of the eyeball from infantile glaucoma or high myopia, and the shallowness of the orbit in craniofacial syndromes with midfacial hypoplasia (sometimes referred to as *exorbitism*). Confusion with orbital space-occupying lesions is unlikely to be a problem in such cases.

Musarella MA, Chan HSL, Gallie BL. Malignant pediatric ocular tumors: a sixty-year review from the Hospital for Sick Children. *Ophthalmol Clin North Am.* 1990; 3:177–193.

Nicholson DH, Green WR. *Pediatric Ocular Tumors.* New York: Masson; 1981.

Orbital Tumors

A wide variety of space-occupying lesions can develop in the region of the orbit during childhood. Several of the most important pediatric malignancies show a predilection for orbital involvement. Benign adnexal masses are common and, in many cases, represent a threat to vision. BCSC Section 7, *Orbit, Eyelids, and Lacrimal System,* and Section 4, *Ophthalmic Pathology and Intraocular Tumors,* also discuss and illustrate orbital tumors.

Shields JA. *Diagnosis and Management of Orbital Tumors.* Philadelphia: Saunders; 1989.

Stefanyszyn MA. Orbital tumors in children. In: *Focal Points: Clinical Modules for Ophthalmologists.* San Francisco: American Academy of Ophthalmology; 1990;8:9.

Primary Malignant Neoplasms

Malignant diseases of the orbit include primary tumors arising from orbital tissue elements, secondary growth of solid tumors originating elsewhere in the body (metastasis), and abnormally proliferating cells of the hematopoietic or lymphoreticular systems. A large majority of primary malignant tumors of the orbit in childhood are sarcomas. Tumors of epithelial origin (e.g., carcinoma of the lacrimal gland) are extremely rare.

Rhabdomyosarcoma The most common primary pediatric orbital malignancy is rhabdomyosarcoma. The incidence of this disease (about 5% of orbital biopsies in children and adolescents) exceeds that of all other sarcomas combined. The orbit is the origin of 10% of rhabdomyosarcomas; an additional 25% develop elsewhere in

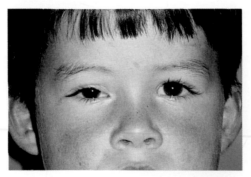

FIG XXVI-1—Rhabdomyosarcoma in a 4-year-old boy presenting with right upper eyelid ptosis of 3 weeks' duration and a palpable subcutaneous mass.

the head and neck, occasionally involving the orbit secondarily. The average age of onset is about 5–7 years. Roughly 5% of cases manifest before age 1 year and 15% after 10 years; 90% have occurred before age 16 years.

Proptosis, which can develop quite rapidly (within a few days), is the usual presenting sign of orbital rhabdomyosarcoma. Ptosis and strabismus are also common signs (Fig XXVI-1). The tumor can also arise as a localized mass in the eyelid or conjunctiva. CT or MRI demonstrates an irregular but well-circumscribed mass of uniform density.

A biopsy is required for confirmation of the diagnosis whenever suspicion of rhabdomyosarcoma arises. The most common histopathologic type is *embryonal,* which shows few cells containing characteristic cross-striations. Second in frequency is the prognostically unfavorable *alveolar* pattern, showing poorly differentiated tumor cells compartmentalized by orderly connective tissue septa. Rarely, *botryoid* ("grapelike") or well-differentiated *pleomorphic* tumors are found in the orbit, but the botryoid type may originate from conjunctiva.

Small encapsulated or otherwise well-localized rhabdomyosarcomas should be totally excised when possible. For larger or more extensive tumors chemotherapy and radiation are now the mainstays of treatment; exenteration of the orbit is seldom indicated. Primary orbital rhabdomyosarcoma has the best prognosis of any site, with a long-term survival rate of nearly 90% in a large multicenter study.

Wharam M, Beltangady M, Hays D, et al. Localized orbital rhabdomyosarcoma. An interim report of the Intergroup Rhabdomyosarcoma Study Committee. *Ophthalmology.* 1987;94:251–254.

Other sarcomas *Osteosarcoma, chondrosarcoma,* and *fibrosarcoma* can also develop in the orbit during childhood. The risk for these tumors increases in children with a history of bilateral retinoblastoma, particularly when external-beam radiation treatment has been given.

Metastatic Tumors

In contrast to adults, children with secondary ocular malignancy are much more likely to show involvement of the orbit than the globe.

Neuroblastoma   One of the most common childhood cancers is neuroblastoma, the most frequent source of orbital metastasis. It usually originates in either the adrenal gland or the sympathetic ganglion chain in the retroperitoneum or mediastinum. Approximately 20% of all neuroblastoma patients show clinical evidence of ocular involvement, which is sometimes the initial manifestation of the tumor.

Ipsilateral *Horner syndrome* manifesting with ptosis, pupillary miosis, and sometimes iris heterochromia is occasionally the initial indication of localized neuroblastoma arising in the neck or chest (Fig XXVI-2). Infants with suspected Horner syndrome should have a chest CT and urine catecholamines to exclude the possibility of neuroblastoma.

Opsoclonus, characterized by rapid multidirectional saccadic eye movements, is associated with some cases of neuroblastoma and may be the presenting sign. The mechanism of this very interesting phenomenon is unknown; a humoral factor produced by the tumor is probably responsible.

Metastatic neuroblastoma in the orbit typically produces proptosis associated with periorbital ecchymosis; occasionally ecchymosis alone is apparent externally (Fig XXVI-3). CT usually shows evidence of bone destruction. Bilateral involvement is present in roughly half of cases. The mean age at diagnosis of patients with orbital neuroblastoma metastasis is about 2 years. Even with intensive treatment including radiation and chemotherapy, only about 10%–25% of affected patients survive. The prognosis for disseminated neuroblastoma is considerably better in infants under age 1 year than in older children.

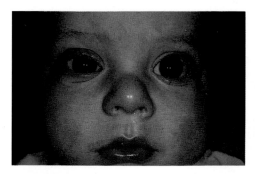

FIG XXVI-2—Right Horner syndrome, the presenting sign of localized intrathoracic neuroblastoma in a 6-month-old boy.

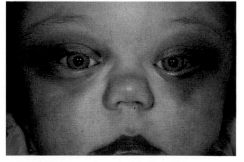

FIG XXVI-3—Bilateral orbital metastasis of neuroblastoma, presenting with periorbital ecchymosis in a 2-year-old girl.

Nonorbital neuroblastoma has a relatively good prognosis. In a recent series, long-term survival was documented in 11 of 14 cases of neuroblastoma with Horner syndrome and in all cases with opsoclonus.

Musarella MA, Chan HS, DeBoer G, et al. Ocular involvement in neuroblastoma: Prognostic implications. *Ophthalmology.* 1984;91:936–940.

Ewing sarcoma This tumor composed of small, round cells usually originates in the long bones of the extremities or the axial skeleton. It is the second most frequent solid tumor source of orbital metastasis. Contemporary treatment regimens involving surgery, radiation, and chemotherapy permit long-term survival in many cases with disseminated disease.

Wilms tumor One of the most common childhood cancers, Wilms tumor rarely metastasizes from the kidney to the orbit.

Leukemia By far the most common malignancy of childhood, leukemia is acute in 95% of cases, more often lymphocytic than myelocytic. Aside from retinal hemorrhage, orbital infiltration causing proptosis, eyelid swelling, and ecchymosis is its most frequent clinically evident ocular manifestation, occurring in 1%–2% of patients. Infiltration of the optic nerve by leukemic cells may cause loss of vision and papilledema, requiring prompt treatment with low-dose radiation.

Granulocytic sarcoma, or *chloroma* (in reference to the greenish color of involved tissue), is a localized accumulation of leukemic cells in the orbit more characteristic of myelocytic than of lymphocytic disease in childhood. This lesion typically develops several months before hematologic evidence of leukemia is present.

Davis JL, Parke DW 2nd, Font RL. Granulocytic sarcoma of the orbit. A clinicopathologic study. *Ophthalmology.* 1985;92:1758–1762.

Lymphoma In contrast to adults, lymphoma in children very rarely involves the orbit. Burkitt lymphoma, endemic to east Africa and uncommonly seen in North America, is the most likely form to involve the orbit.

Histiocytosis X (Langerhans cell histiocytosis) This is the collective term for a group of disorders involving abnormal proliferation of histiocytes, usually within bone. *Eosinophilic granuloma,* the most localized and benign form of histiocytosis, produces bone lesions that involve the orbit, skull, ribs, and long bones in childhood or adolescence. Symptoms may include proptosis, ptosis, and periorbital swelling, and localized pain and tenderness are relatively common. X-rays and CT characteristically demonstrate sharply demarcated osteolytic lesions without surrounding sclerosis (Fig XXVI-4). Treatment consists of excision, systemic corticosteroid administration, or low-dose radiation; all modalities have a high rate of success.

Hand-Schüller-Christian disease is a more disseminated and aggressive form of histiocytosis X that is likely to produce proptosis caused by involvement of the bony orbit in childhood. Diabetes insipidus is common. Chemotherapy is often required, but prognosis is generally good.

Letterer-Siwe disease is the most severe and malignant variety in infants and young children. It is characterized by soft-tissue lesions of multiple viscera (liver, spleen) but rarely involving the eye.

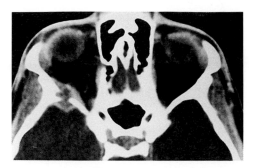

FIG XXVI-4—Axial CT image showing eosinophilic granuloma with partial destruction of the right posterior lateral orbital wall in a 15-year-old boy, who presented with retrobulbar pain and mild edema and erythema of right upper eyelid.

Moore AT, Pritchard J, Taylor DS. Histiocytosis X: an ophthalmological review. *Br J Ophthalmol.* 1985;69:7–14.

Benign Tumors

Capillary hemangioma This is the most common benign orbital tumor in childhood, with a female-to-male predominance of at least 2:1. Pathologic examination shows proliferated endothelial cells and small vascular channels, contrasting with the large blood-filled spaces found in adult-onset cavernous hemangioma of the orbit. Most periocular capillary hemangiomas involve primarily the upper eyelid, with variable extension into the orbit and surrounding tissues. Usually, the skin has a characteristic raised, red, dimpled appearance (strawberry nevus), but some lesions are entirely subcutaneous, appearing as a smooth, firm swelling or fullness with dark red to bluish discoloration of the overlying skin (Fig XXVI-5). Axial proptosis or other displacement of the globe indicates a significant intraorbital component. The mass may swell when the baby cries as a result of venous congestion from increased intrathoracic pressure. Many affected children show similar lesions elsewhere on the skin.

About 30% of capillary hemangiomas are evident at birth, and 95% are recognized by 6 months of age. Typically, they appear quite small and insignificant at first but then undergo a period of alarmingly rapid growth during the first few months of life. Maximum size is usually reached between 6 and 12 months of age. Spontaneous involution begins during the second year of life, initially manifested as lightening or graying of color in the central portion of the lesion. This process leads to complete regression in about 40% of cases by age 4 years, and 80% by age 8 years.

Approximately half of the children with eyelid or orbital hemangiomas develop some degree of amblyopia, usually resulting from anisometropic astigmatism oriented toward the lesion (i.e., a superonasal lesion of the right eye would require plus cylinder correction with an axis in the neighborhood of 45°). Ptosis is common and

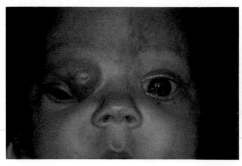

FIG XXVI-5—Capillary hemangioma in a 2-month-old girl involving the right upper eyelid and orbit with displacement of the globe and induction of 8 D of astigmatic refractive error.

can cause deprivation amblyopia. Strabismus develops in approximately one third of cases. Optic atrophy, exposure keratitis, and ulceration of the skin with bleeding and secondary infection are relatively rare complications in severe cases. Massive capillary hemangiomas may be associated with thrombocytopenia as a result of platelet sequestration within the lesion (Kasabach-Merritt syndrome).

Early treatment is indicated for capillary hemangioma when amblyopia is a serious concern and conventional measures (refractive correction, patching) are judged inadequate. The therapeutic approach currently preferred by most pediatric ophthalmologists is intralesional injection of corticosteroids. A total volume of about 1–2 cc of short- and longer-acting agents (usually betamethasone 6 mg/cc and triamcinolone 40 mg/cc) combined in 1:1 mixture is injected percutaneously with a fine needle deep into the lesion.

Shrinkage of the tumor after corticosteroid injection proceeds most rapidly during the first 2 weeks, but it can continue at a slower rate for several months. Sometimes the response is dramatic, leading to almost complete disappearance of the lesion, but more often reduction in size is moderate, and occasionally little or no improvement occurs. Injection may be repeated up to three or four times at intervals of 6 weeks or longer if initial treatment produces a partial but inadequate effect. No definite correlation between responsiveness to treatment and any characteristic of the lesion or patient has been recognized.

Infrequent but potentially serious reported complications of intralesional corticosteroid injection include depigmentation of the overlying skin and subcutaneous fat atrophy (both of which may be temporary), eyelid necrosis, and central retinal artery occlusion by particles of the drug. Subcutaneous whitish crystalline deposits are often observed to persist for months at the injection site. The possibility of pituitary-adrenal suppression that may retard growth must be kept in mind, especially with small infants.

Oral corticosteroid administration (prednisone 2 mg/kg/day or equivalent) is an alternative to injection that deserves consideration, particularly if the lesion is very extensive; however, rebound enlargement when medication is withdrawn may occur. Complete excision of the tumor as a primary treatment has been accomplished in selected patients. Hemangiomas that are small, well circumscribed, and not superficial are the best candidates for surgical removal. Because of the highly vascular nature of these tumors, excision is often difficult and meticulous dissection is necessary. Excision of residual tumor tissue with reconstructive surgery after steroid treatment may be necessary if significant disfigurement persists. This intervention should be delayed until school age to take advantage of the natural regression that occurs with these tumors.

Haik BG, Jakobiec FA, Ellsworth RM, et al. Capillary hemangioma of the lids and orbit: an analysis of the clinical features and therapeutic results in 101 cases. *Ophthalmology.* 1979;86:760–792.

Kushner BJ. Intralesional corticosteroid injection for infantile adnexal hemangioma. *Am J Ophthalmol.* 1982;93:496–506.

Lymphangioma   The second most common orbital tumor of vascular origin in childhood is lymphangioma. This lesion consists largely of lymph-filled channels lined by endothelium and separated by thin, delicate walls containing small blood vessels that are easily disrupted and have a tendency to hemorrhage spontaneously or after minor trauma. Lymphangiomas tend to infiltrate orbital tissues extensively, but occasionally they are localized to the eyelids or conjunctiva (Fig XXVI-6). In most cases orbital lymphangioma initially manifests with gradual development of mild proptosis during the first few years of life. Episodes of rapid enlargement with markedly increased proptosis can occur as a result of either hyperplasia of lymphoid tissue within the mass (typically induced by upper respiratory infection) or intralesional bleeding; such a development occurring between 5 and 15 years of age may in fact be the first indication of a problem.

Complete excision of an orbital lymphangioma is difficult. No treatment is indicated when the only symptom is mild proptosis, and biopsy should be avoided if possible because of the risk of inducing hemorrhage. Surgical evacuation of the hematoma should be considered when CT or MRI shows large, blood-filled cavities, indicating acute hemorrhagic deterioration, if it is accompanied by intractable pain, nausea, and vomiting or if development of an afferent pupillary defect indicates that the optic nerve is threatened. Otherwise, conservative management such as activity restriction, cold compresses, or lubricating ointment for corneal exposure is recommended.

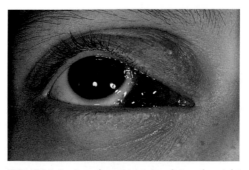

FIG XXVI-6—Lymphangioma involving the right orbit, upper eyelid, and conjunctiva in a 15-year-old girl.

Wilson ME, Parker PL, Chavis RM. Conservative management of childhood orbital lymphangioma. *Ophthalmology.* 1989;96:484–490.

Other vascular tumors   Other orbital tumors composed of vascular elements are rarely seen in childhood. *Hemangiopericytoma* is a generally benign lesion with a tendency to become locally invasive that makes its long-term prognosis guarded. *Orbital varix* is a venous malformation that usually does not become clinically evident until early adulthood, although it may cause intermittent proptosis in childhood, typically associated with prone position or Valsalva maneuver.

Tumors of bony origin   A variety of uncommon benign orbital tumors of bony origin may present during the early years of life with gradually increasing proptosis. *Fibrous dysplasia* and *ossifying fibroma* are similar disorders characterized by destruction of normal bone and its replacement by fibro-osseous tissue. Orbital x-rays and CT in both conditions show varying degrees of lucency and sclerosis.

Fibrous dysplasia has a slow progression that ceases when skeletal maturation is complete. Its most serious complication is visual loss caused by optic nerve compression, which may occur acutely. Affected individuals should have periodic assessment of vision, pupil function, and optic disc appearance. Surgical treatment is indicated for functional deterioration or significant disfigurement.

Histopathologically, ossifying fibroma is distinguished by the presence of osteoblasts. Ossifying fibroma tends to be a more locally invasive lesion than fibrous dysplasia; some authorities recommend early excision.

Brown tumor of bone is an osteoclastic giant cell reaction occurring as a result of hyperparathyroidism. *Aneurysmal bone cyst* is a degenerative process in which normal bone is replaced by cystic cavities containing fibrous tissue, inflammatory cells, and blood, producing a characteristic appearance in x-rays.

Tumors of connective tissue origin   Benign orbital tumors originating from connective tissue are rare in childhood. *Juvenile fibromatosis* may present as a mass in the inferior anterior portion of the orbit. These tumors, sometimes called *myofibromas* or *desmoid tumors,* are composed of relatively mature fibroblasts. They have a tendency to recur locally after excision and can be difficult to control, but they do not metastasize.

Tumors of neural origin   *Optic glioma* is the most important orbital tumor of neural origin in childhood. About 50% of these cases are associated with type 1 neurofibromatosis. *Plexiform neurofibroma* nearly always occurs in the context of neurofibromatosis and not infrequently involves the eyelid and orbit. (These tumors are discussed fully in the following chapter, Phakomatoses.) Orbital *meningioma* and *schwannoma* (neurilemoma, neurinoma) are rarely seen prior to adulthood and also usually appear in patients with neurofibromatosis. Meningioma typically presents with progressive visual loss, mild proptosis, and restriction of ocular motility; a large majority of patients are female. Childhood meningiomas tend to be locally aggressive and should be totally excised if possible, unless the involved eye retains good vision.

Hidayat AA, Font RL. Juvenile fibromatosis of the periorbital region and eyelid. A clinicopathologic study of six cases. *Arch Ophthalmol.* 1980;98:280–285.

Karp LA, Zimmerman LE, Borit A, et al. Primary intraorbital meningiomas. *Arch Ophthalmol.* 1974;91:24–28.

Moore AT, Buncic JR, Munro IR. Fibrous dysplasia of the orbit in childhood. Clinical features and management. *Ophthalmology.* 1985;92:12–20.

Shields JA, Nelson LB, Brown JF, et al. Clinical, computed tomographic, and histopathologic characteristics of juvenile ossifying fibroma with orbital involvement. *Am J Ophthalmol.* 1983;96:650–653.

Wright JE, McDonald WI, Call NB. Management of optic nerve gliomas. *Br J Ophthalmol.* 1980;64:545–552.

Ectopic Tissue Masses

The term *choristoma* is applied to growths consisting of normal cells and tissues appearing at a site other than normal. They may result from abnormal sequestration of germ layer tissue during embryonic development or from faulty differentiation of pluripotential cells. Masses composed of such ectopic tissue growing in the orbit can also be a consequence of herniation or outpouching of tissue from adjacent structures.

Epidermoid cysts   A capsule composed of epidermis-like tissue (keratinizing stratified squamous epithelium) faces a cavity containing keratin and fatty material with high cholesterol content (responsible for the alternative designation *cholesteatoma*) in the choristomas known as *epidermoid cysts.* Often a surrounding condensation of connective tissue resembling normal dermis gives rise to inward-directed hairs and sebaceous glands, creating a *dermoid cyst.* Dermoid and epidermoid cysts both result from abnormal sequestration of surface ectoderm beneath the skin during embryonic development. The cysts enlarge as desquamated material accumulates. Secondary deformation of adjacent bone is occasionally seen.

The suture connections of the orbital bones are common sites for dermoid cysts. Typically, the cysts arise just external to the orbital rim in the superotemporal quadrant (frontal/zygomatic) or just inside the orbital rim superonasally (frontal/nasal) (Fig XXVI-7). A small minority develop deep within the orbit, but these generally do not become clinically detectable until adulthood, when gradually increasing proptosis reveals their presence.

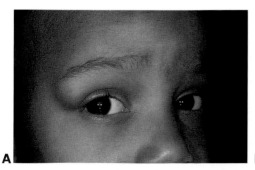
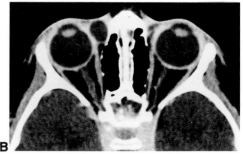

A

B

FIG XXVI-7—*A,* Periorbital dermoid cyst, right eye, with typical superotemporal location in a 3-year-old girl. *B,* Axial CT image showing a dermoid cyst of the superonasal anterior orbit, right eye, in a 6-year-old boy.

Periorbital dermoid cysts are usually noted during the first year of life and may continue to enlarge slowly during childhood. They are usually firm, about 1 cm in diameter, nontender, and fixed to underlying periosteum through a fibrous stalk that often permits some relative movement but not to overlying skin. A homogeneous low-density core surrounded by a thin wall is revealed by CT, which is not routinely necessary but helpful for ruling out extension into the orbit in selected cases.

Surgical excision of a dermoid cyst is indicated to treat progressive enlargement or to prevent the severe inflammation that can result from traumatic rupture releasing the irritating cyst contents into surrounding tissue. Care must be taken to avoid intraoperative penetration of the capsule, which may have similar inflammatory consequences. If rupture occurs, all released material should be removed with forceps or suction and the site thoroughly irrigated with saline. Postoperative systemic administration of corticosteroids may be necessary. Incomplete excision of the cyst wall may lead to recurrence or development of a draining fistula. With incision parallel to the eyebrow or eyelid crease and careful two-layer closure, scarring is minimal after removal of a lesion in the typical superotemporal location. Superonasal lesions, which tend to be partially intraorbital, are more difficult to excise and more likely to heal with visible scarring. Surgery for dermoid cysts situated deep within the orbit should be undertaken only by the experienced orbital surgeon.

Teratomas   Choristomatous tumors that contain multiple tissues derived from all three germinal layers (ectoderm, mesoderm, and endoderm) are known as *teratomas*. Skin and dermal appendages, neural tissue, muscle, and bone are typically present; endodermal elements such as respiratory and intestinal tract epithelium are less consistently found. Most teratomas are partially cystic with variable fluid content. Orbital teratomas represent a very small fraction of both orbital tumors and teratomas in general, which usually arise in the gonads or sacrococcygeal region. The clinical presentation of orbital teratomas is particularly dramatic, however, with massive proptosis evident at birth (Fig XXVI-8). In contrast to teratomas in other locations, which tend to show malignant growth, most orbital lesions are benign. Surgical excision, facilitated by prior aspiration of fluid, can often be accomplished without sacrificing the globe. Permanent optic nerve damage from stretching and compression usually results in poor vision in the involved eye.

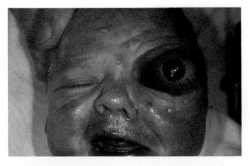

FIG XXVI-8—Congenital cystic teratoma originating in the left orbit of a 1-day-old girl.

Mamalis N, Garland PE, Argyle JC, et al. Congenital orbital teratoma: a review and report of two cases. *Surv Ophthalmol.* 1985;30:41–46.

Ectopic lacrimal gland This rare choristomatous lesion may present with proptosis in childhood. Cystic enlargement and chronic inflammation sometimes aggravate the problem.

Sudoriferous cyst Originating from ectopic apocrine gland tissue resembling that found in the eyelid glands of Moll, the sudoriferous cyst is a rare lesion of the eyelid or anterior orbit in childhood.

Colobomatous cyst Also known as *microphthalmos with cyst,* this mass is composed of tissues that originate from the eye wall of a malformed globe with posterior segment coloboma. Most fundus colobomas show some degree of scleral ectasia, resulting from a deficiency of tissue in the region where apposing edges of the embryonic neuroectodermal fissure have failed to fuse properly. In extreme cases a bulging globular appendage grows to become as large as or larger than the globe itself, which is invariably microphthalmic, sometimes to a marked degree.

Like other colobomatous malformations, microphthalmos with cyst may occur either as an isolated congenital defect or in association with a variety of intracranial or systemic anomalies. Frequently, evidence of coloboma appears in the other eye as well. The wall of a colobomatous cyst consists of thin sclera lined by rudimentary tissue of neuroectodermal origin, occasionally incorporating hyperplastic glial tissue accumulations; the cyst contains aqueous fluid with a few suspended cells. The usual location is inferior or posterior to the globe, with which it is always in contact. The cyst interior communicates with the vitreous cavity, sometimes through a channel so small it is undetectable even with high-resolution imaging.

Posteriorly located colobomatous cysts may or may not cause proptosis, depending on the sizes of the globe and the cyst. Inferiorly located cysts present as a bulging of the lower eyelid or a bluish subconjunctival mass (Fig XXVI-9). Occasionally, the globe is pushed so far superiorly that it disappears behind the upper eyelid. If the diagnosis is not obvious based on fundus examination, demonstration with CT, MRI, or ultrasonography of a cystic lesion with the uniform internal density of vitreous attached to the globe excludes other possibilities. No treatment is necessary unless disfigurement is a problem. Aspiration of cyst fluid provides relief of variable duration; reaccumulation may be retarded or prevented by placement of a cosmetic shell behind the eyelids. For more definitive treatment surgical excision is indicated. Preservation of the globe is possible in some cases; in others the globe must be removed with the cyst.

Weiss A, Martinez C, Greenwald M. Microphthalmos with cyst: Clinical presentations and computed tomographic findings. *J Pediatr Ophthalmol Strabismus.* 1985; 22:6–12.

Encephalocele or meningocele These masses in the orbital region may result from a congenital bony defect that permits herniation of intracranial tissue or may develop after trauma that disrupts the bone and dura mater of the anterior cranial fossa. Intraorbital location leads to proptosis or downward displacement of the globe. Anterior presentation takes the form of a subcutaneous mass, typically located above the medial canthal ligament. Pulsation of the globe or the mass from the transmission of intracranial pulse pressure is characteristic. Neuroimaging readily confirms the diagnosis of this rare condition.

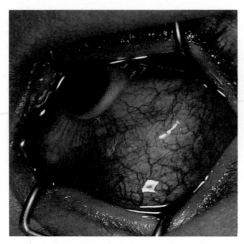

FIG XXVI-9—Microphthalmos with cyst, left eye.

Rothstein TB, Romano PE, Shoch D. Meningomyelocele. *Am J Ophthalmol.* 1974; 77:690–693.

Childhood Orbital Inflammations

Several noninfectious, nontraumatic disorders that may simulate an orbital mass lesion deserve brief mention. *Graves disease,* the most common cause of proptosis in adults, rarely occurs in prepubescent children but is seen occasionally in adolescents (Fig XXVI-10). See also chapter XI, Special Forms of Strabismus.

Orbital pseudotumor This idiopathic inflammatory cause of proptosis in childhood differs significantly from the adult form. Its typical pediatric presentation is acute and painful, resembling orbital cellulitis more than tumor or Graves ophthalmopathy (Fig XXVI-11). Bilaterality and episodic recurrence are common, as are associated systemic complaints such as headache, fever, nausea and vomiting, and lethargy. Evidence of uveitis is frequently present and occasionally constitutes the dominant manifestation. Imaging studies may show increased density of orbital fat, thickening of posterior sclera and Tenon's layer, or enlargement of extraocular muscles. Treatment with systemic corticosteroid usually provides prompt and dramatic relief.

Orbital myositis This idiopathic inflammatory infiltration of the extraocular muscles can involve only one muscle or multiple muscles in both eyes. The clinical presentation depends on the amount of inflammation. Diplopia, conjunctival chemosis, and orbital pain are common. Symptoms can be subacute for weeks or can progress quite rapidly. Visual function is rarely involved unless massive muscle enlargement is present. CT or MRI findings consist of diffusely enlarged muscles with the enlarge-

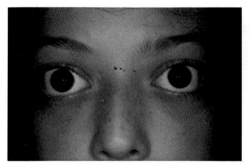

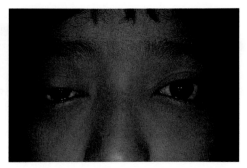

FIG XXVI-10—Graves disease with bilateral exophthalmos in a 15-year-old girl.

FIG XXVI-11—Bilateral orbital pseudotumor in an 11-year-old boy with a 1-week history of eye pain. Ocular rotation was markedly limited in all directions. CT confirmed proptosis and also showed enlargement of all extraocular muscles. Laboratory work-up was negative for thyroid disease and rheumatologic disorders. Complete resolution occurred after 1 month of corticosteroid treatment.

ment extending all the way to the insertion (unlike thyroid myopathy, which involves mainly the muscle belly). Corticosteroid treatment usually results in prompt resolution of symptoms, but prolonged treatment (4–6 weeks) is often necessary to avoid reccurrence.

Mottow LS, Jakobiec FA. Idiopathic inflammatory orbital pseudotumor in childhood. I. Clinical characteristics. *Arch Ophthalmol.* 1978;96:1410–1417.

Young LA. Dysthyroid ophthalmopathy in children. *J Pediatr Ophthalmol Strabismus.* 1979;16:105–107.

Eyelid and Epibulbar Tumors

Malignant tumors arising from eyelid skin or conjunctiva (*basal cell carcinoma, squamous cell carcinoma, melanoma*) are relatively common in adults, but they are extremely rare in childhood. These tumors are discussed elsewhere in the BCSC: Section 4, *Ophthalmic Pathology and Intraocular Tumors;* Section 7, *Orbit, Eyelids, and Lacrimal System;* and Section 8, *External Disease and Cornea.* Pediatric cases are likely to be associated with underlying systemic disorders that predispose to malignancy, such as basal cell nevus syndrome or xeroderma pigmentosum. In addition, rhabdomyosarcoma may present atypically as an eyelid or conjunctival mass.

Benign lesions of the ocular surface and surrounding skin are frequent, and these may be classified as originating from epithelium, melanocytes, or vascular tissue.

Papillomas These benign epithelial proliferations usually appear as sessile masses at the limbus or as pedunculated lesions of the caruncle, fornix, or palpebral conjunctiva. They may be transparent, pale yellow, or salmon colored, sometimes speckled with red dots. Papillomas in children usually result from viral infection, similar to verrucae, and are likely to disappear spontaneously. Surgical excision is indicated if there is persistent associated conjunctivitis or keratitis or if new lesions continue to appear.

Conjunctival epithelial inclusion cysts   Usually resulting from surgery or trauma, these cysts are filled with clear fluid. Excision is indicated only if they are a source of bothersome symptoms.

Epibulbar dermoid tumors   Although both are classified as choristomas, dermoid tumors represent an entity completely distinct from dermoid cysts. Limbal dermoids are evident at birth as whitish dome-shaped masses, straddling the limbus in the inferotemporal quadrant in about three quarters of cases, with diameter of about 2–10 mm and thickness of 1–3 mm. They are composed of keratinizing surface epithelium with an underlying dermislike layer that frequently contains a few hair follicles and a small amount of fatty tissue. Little if any postnatal growth is seen. Apart from their undesirable appearance, limbal dermoids may cause ocular irritation and interfere with vision by inducing astigmatism or haziness of adjacent clear cornea.

There is no urgency in removing epibulbar dermoids unless irritating symptoms persist. Epibulbar limbal dermoids are removed by shelling out the lesion from the corneal side along its readily identifiable cleavage plane and excising the episcleral portion flush with the plane of surrounding tissue. In general, the surgeon need not remove underlying clear corneal tissue or mobilize surrounding tissue or apply a patch graft over the resulting surface defect. Cornea and conjunctiva heal within a few days to several weeks, generally with some scarring and imperfect corneal transparency but nevertheless showing considerably improved appearance.

Lipodermoid (dermolipoma)   This conjunctival lesion, usually located near the temporal fornix, is composed of adipose tissue and dense connective tissue. The overlying conjunctival epithelium is normal and hair follicles are absent. Lipodermoids may be quite extensive, involving orbital tissue, lacrimal gland, and extraocular muscle in some cases. Both limbal dermoids and conjunctival lipodermoids are frequently associated with Goldenhar syndrome (Fig XXVI-12). In these patients they are accompanied by a variety of other anomalies including ear deformities (preauricular appendages, aural fistulas), maxillary or mandibular hypoplasia (hemifacial microsomia), vertebral deformities, notching of the upper eyelid, and Duane syndrome.

Since lipodermoids rarely need to be excised, the surgeon should attempt to remove only the portion of the lesion visible within the palpebral fissure, disturbing forniceal conjunctiva and Tenon's layer as little as possible to minimize scarring. Even with a conservative operative approach, cicatrization may be a problem that requires surgical revision.

Conjunctival nevi   These lesions are relatively common in childhood, occurring mainly in light-skinned persons. They may be flat or elevated. Most show compound histopathology (nevus cells found in both epithelium and substantia propria), while others are junctional (nevus cells confined to the interface between epithelium and substantia propria). Color is typically brown, but approximately one third are nonpigmented, having a pinkish appearance. The lesions are occasionally noted at birth but more commonly develop during later childhood or adolescence (Fig XXVI-13).

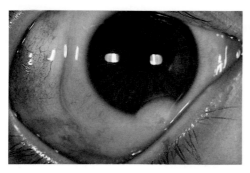 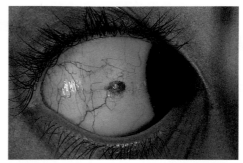

FIG XXVI-12—Small inferior limbal dermoid and larger lipodermoid involving the temporal conjunctival fornix, right eye, in a child with Goldenhar syndrome.

FIG XXVI-13—Pigmented nevus of the bulbar conjunctiva, right eye, recently developed in a 4-year-old girl.

No well-documented cases of malignant transformation of a conjunctival nevus have occurred in a patient under age 20 years. Malignant melanoma of the conjunctiva and primary acquired melanosis (PAM), a premalignant nevoid lesion of adulthood, are extremely rare in childhood.

Ocular melanocytosis (melanosis oculi)   This congenital pigmentary lesion is characterized by unilateral patchy but extensive slate gray or bluish discoloration of the sclera (not conjunctiva). Intraocular pigmentation is also increased, which contributes to a higher incidence of glaucoma and possibly increases the risk of malignant melanoma. Some patients, particularly persons of Asian ancestry, may have associated involvement of eyelid and adjacent skin with dermal hyperpigmentation that produces brown, bluish, or black discoloration without thickening or other abnormality (oculodermal melanocytosis, nevus of Ota). Small patches of slate gray scleral pigmentation, typically bilateral and without clinical significance, are commonly seen in black children. Melanosis of skin and sclera is occasionally associated with Sturge-Weber syndrome and Klippel-Trénaunay-Weber syndrome.

Port-wine stain (nevus flammeus)   This congenital vascular nevus typically involves the eyelid skin and episclera in Sturge-Weber syndrome (see discussion of this condition in chapter XXVII), but it is seen more often as an isolated cutaneous anomaly on the eyelids or elsewhere.

Capillary hemangioma   The section on orbital tumors above describes this condition, the most common vascular lesion of the eyelids in childhood.

Elsas FJ, Green WR. Epibulbar tumors in childhood. *Am J Ophthalmol.* 1975; 79:1001–1007.

McDonnell JM, Carpenter JD, Jacobs P, et al. Conjunctival melanocytic lesions in children. *Ophthalmology.* 1989;96:986–993.

Panton RW, Sugar J. Excision of limbal dermoids. *Ophthalmic Surg.* 1991;22:85–89.

Inflammatory Conditions

Inflammatory masses of the eyelids and ocular surface are much more common than tumors. Although *chalazia* occur less frequently in children than in adults, the pediatric ophthalmologist must be prepared to encounter them. Because surgical treatment usually requires a trip to the operating room and general anesthesia, conservative management is worth an extended trial. Most lesions resolve spontaneously over a period of weeks to months with frequent application of warm compresses. *Pyogenic granuloma* is a typically pedunculated fleshy pink growth of granulation tissue that develops, sometimes rapidly and exuberantly, from the conjunctiva overlying a chalazion.

Phlyctenular keratoconjunctivitis and *ligneous conjunctivitis* are two uncommon inflammatory disorders of the conjunctiva that typically occur in young patients and may result in formation of ocular surface masses. *Nodular episcleritis* occasionally is seen in childhood. Eyelid and epibulbar lesions can develop in *juvenile xanthogranuloma,* which is discussed below. See also BCSC Section 8, *External Disease and Cornea.*

Intraocular Tumors

Iris and Ciliary Body Lesions

Both primary and secondary malignant tumors of the iris are very rare in children. Approximately 1% of *malignant uveal melanomas* occur in patients younger than 20 years old. *Leukemic infiltration* of iris tissue may create a mass lesion, which is one of the less common ocular manifestations of pediatric leukemia. Metastasis of solid tumors to the uveal tract virtually never occurs in childhood.

A number of relatively common and entirely benign iris lesions may generate concern about the possibility of malignancy in childhood. Pigmented *iris nevi* and *freckles* large enough to be noticed by family members or primary care physicians sometimes require repeated observation to provide reassurance concerning their harmless nature. Children with type 1 neurofibromatosis occasionally develop melanocytic lesions similar to the common Lisch nodule that are large enough to be considered benign tumors. *Nodules of iris pigmented epithelium* at the pupillary margin may be present as an insignificant congenital anomaly or may develop after prolonged use of miotic drops (e.g., echothiophate for treatment of strabismus).

Juvenile xanthogranuloma (JXG)   Also known as *nevoxanthoendothelioma,* this condition is a non-neoplastic histiocytic proliferation that develops in infants under 2 years of age. It is characterized by the presence of Touton giant cells. Skin involvement is typically but not invariably present in the form of one or more small round papules, orange or tan in color. Iris lesions are relatively rare and virtually always unilateral. The fleshy, yellow-brown mass may be small and localized or diffusely infiltrative of the entire iris, with resulting heterochromia. Spontaneous bleeding with hyphema is a characteristic clinical presentation. Secondary glaucoma may cause acute pain and photophobia and ultimately significant visual loss (Fig XXVI-14).

JXG is a self-limited condition that usually regresses spontaneously by age 5 years, but treatment is indicated for ocular involvement to avoid complications. Topical corticosteroids and IOP-lowering agents as necessary are generally sufficient

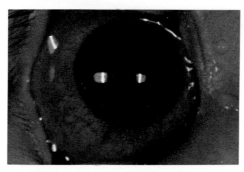

FIG XXVI-14—Juvenile xanthogranuloma of iris, right eye, in a 1-year-old boy with a 3-day history of redness and light sensitivity. Note small hyphema layered superonasally adjacent to the tan-colored iris lesion. Intraocular pressure was 30 mm Hg. The lesion regressed without further complications over 6 months with topical corticosteroid treatment.

to control the problem; surgical excision or radiation should be considered if intractable glaucoma is present.

Medulloepithelioma (diktyoma) This tumor originates from the nonpigmented epithelium of the ciliary body and most often presents as an iris mass during the first decade of life. Secondary glaucoma and hyphema are less frequent initial manifestations. A spectrum of clinical and pathologic characteristics is seen in patients with this rare lesion, ranging from benign to malignant. Although metastasis is rare, local invasiveness can lead to death. Teratoid elements are often present. Enucleation is usually required and is curative in a large majority of cases.

> Broughton WL, Zimmerman LE. A clinicopathologic study of 56 cases of intraocular medulloepitheliomas. *Am J Ophthalmol.* 1978;85:407–418.

> Shields CL, Shields JA, Milite J, et al. Uveal melanoma in teenagers and children. A report of 40 cases. *Ophthalmology.* 1991;98:1662–1666.

Choroidal and Retinal Pigment Epithelial Lesions

A pigmented fundus lesion in a child is usually benign. Flat *choroidal nevi* are common as an incidental fundus finding in children and need not be viewed as a particular cause for concern. Patients with type 1 neurofibromatosis often have flat tan-colored spots in the choroid.

Congenital hypertrophy of the retinal pigment epithelium (CHRPE) is a sharply demarcated flat hyperpigmented lesion that may be isolated or multifocal. Such lesions are also known as *bear tracks.* These lesions have been associated with familial adenomatous polyposis (Gardner syndrome), which has a very high risk for developing adenocarcinoma of the colon by age 50 years. These patients may also have skeletal hamartomas and various other soft-tissue tumors. Either the presence of four or more CHRPE lesions not restricted to one sector of the fundus or bilateral involvement should raise suspicion of familial polyposis syndrome.

Combined hamartoma of the retina and retinal pigment epithelium is an ill-defined, elevated, variably pigmented tumor that may be located either juxtapapillary or in the retinal periphery. In the peripheral location, dragging of the retinal vessels is a prominent feature. Visual tumors have a variable composition of glial tissue and retinal pigment epithelium. This condition can be associated with neurofibromatosis, incontinentia pigmenti, X-linked retinoschisis, and facial hemangiomas.

Melanocytoma is a darkly pigmented tumor with little or no growth potential that usually involves the optic disc and adjacent retina. Malignant melanoma of the choroid is extremely rare in children.

Choroidal osteoma is a benign bony tumor of the uveal tract that may occur in childhood, usually presenting with decreased visual acuity. Isolated localized *choroidal hemangioma* is extremely rare in childhood. Diffuse hemangioma of the choroid associated with Sturge-Weber syndrome is discussed in chapter XXVII.

Retinoblastoma

Retinoblastoma (RB) is the most common malignant ocular tumor of childhood and one of the most common of all pediatric solid tumors with an incidence of about 1 in 15,000. It is typically diagnosed during the first year of life in familial and bilateral cases and between 1 and 3 years of age in sporadic unilateral cases. Onset later than 5 years of age is rare but primary retinoblastoma can present in adulthood. The most common initial sign is leukocoria (white pupil), which is usually first noticed by the family and described as a glow, glint, or cat's-eye appearance (Fig XXVI-15A). In approximately 25% of cases strabismus (esotropia or exotropia) is the first sign. Less common presentations include vitreous hemorrhage, hyphema, ocular or periocular inflammation, glaucoma, proptosis, and hypopyon. BCSC Section 4, *Ophthalmic Pathology and Intraocular Tumors,* also discusses retinoblastoma in depth.

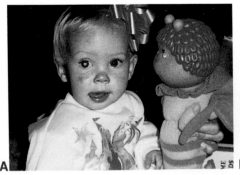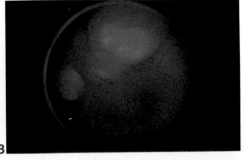

FIG XXVI-15—*A,* Leukocoria of the right eye shown in family photograph of a 1-year-old girl with retinoblastoma. *B,* Wide-angle fundus photograph showing multiple retinoblastoma lesions, left eye. (Photograph courtesy of A. Linn Murphree, MD.)

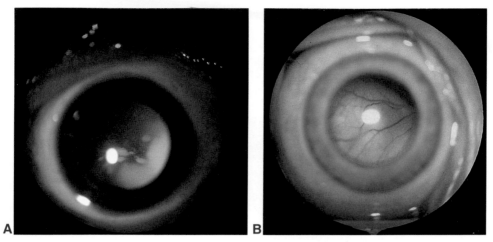

FIG XXVI-16—*A*, Endophytic retinoblastoma with vitreous seeding. *B*, Exophytic retinoblastoma with overlying detached retina.

Retinoblastoma is a neuroblastic tumor, biologically similar to neuroblastoma and medulloblastoma. It can usually be diagnosed on the basis of its ophthalmoscopic appearance. Intraocular retinoblastoma can exhibit a variety of growth patterns. With *endophytic* growth it appears as a white- to cream-colored mass that breaks through the internal limiting membrane and has either no surface vessels or small, irregular tumor vessels (Fig XXVI-15B). *Exophytic* tumors are usually yellow-white and occur in the subretinal space so that the overlying retinal vessels are commonly increased in caliber and tortuosity (Fig XXVI-16). Large tumors often show signs of both endophytic and exophytic growth. Small retinoblastoma lesions appear as a grayish mass and are frequently confined between the internal and external limiting membranes. In rare cases extensive tumor spread may occur within the retina to produce a diffuse infiltrating growth pattern.

Endophytic retinoblastoma is sometimes associated with *vitreous seeding,* in which individual cells or fragments of tumor tissue become separated from the main mass, as shown in Figure XXVI-16A. Vitreous seeds may be few in number and localized or so extensive that the clinical picture resembles endophthalmitis. Occasionally, malignant cells can find their way into the anterior chamber and form a pseudohypopyon.

Exophytic retinoblastoma growth is often associated with subretinal fluid accumulation that can obscure the tumor and closely mimic the appearance of an exudative retinal detachment suggestive of advanced Coats disease. Retinoblastoma cells and subretinal fluid and vitreous have the potential to implant on previously uninvolved retinal tissue and grow, thereby creating an impression of multicentricity in an eye with only a single primary lesion.

Pretreatment evaluation of a patient with presumed retinoblastoma should include a CT scan, bone marrow aspirate, and lumbar puncture. The demonstration of typical intraocular calcification by CT usually confirms the diagnosis and can

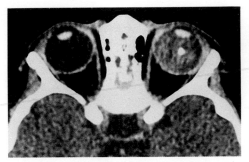

FIG XXVI-17—Axial CT image showing retinoblastoma filling most of the posterior segment of left eye, with localized calcification.

assist in evaluating possible extraocular extension and potential intracranial disease (Fig XXVI-17). Aspiration of ocular fluids for diagnostic testing should be performed only under the most unusual circumstances, since such procedures have the potential to disseminate malignant cells.

Both of the patient's parents and all siblings should also be examined (Table XXVI-2). In about 1% of cases a parent may be found to have an unsuspected fundus lesion that represents either spontaneously regressed retinoblastoma or a benign growth known as *retinoma,* or *retinocytoma,* that can be an expression of the retinoblastoma gene.

The differential diagnosis of leukocoria is shown in Table XXVI-3. The most common retinal lesion simulating retinoblastoma is Coats disease. The presence of crystalline material, extensive subretinal fluid, and peripheral vascular abnormalities combined with lack of calcium on CT would suggest Coats disease. *Astrocytic hamartoma* and *hemangioblastoma* are benign retinal tumors that may simulate the appearance of small retinoblastomas. Both are usually seen as parts of the neurocutaneous syndromes discussed in chapter XXVII along with other features that aid in differential diagnosis.

The characteristic histopathologic features of retinoblastoma include *Flexner-Wintersteiner rosettes,* which are usually present, and *fleurettes,* which are rarely seen. Both represent limited degrees of retinal differentiation. Calcification of variable extent is usually present. In some patients with bilateral retinoblastoma a third primary tumor, *pineoblastoma,* can be found in the pineal gland. Trilateral retinoblastoma can be seen at initial presentation or can occur years after successful ocular treatment.

Management of retinoblastoma   The treatment of retinoblastoma has undergone significant changes over the last 10 years. Although enucleation is still the most commonly used intervention, early recognition has promoted the use of more conservative eye-preserving methods. Enucleation is still indicated for all eyes in which little hope of vision exists, and the technique used for retinoblastoma differs from standard enucleation. Gentle manipulation of the eye during the procedure and the prevention of perforation of the globe are both very important. The surgeon should

TABLE XXVI-2

GENETIC COUNSELING FOR RETINOBLASTOMA

IF PARENT:	HAS BILATERAL RETINOBLASTOMA		HAS UNILATERAL RETINOBLASTOMA		IS UNAFFECTED	
Chance of offspring having retinoblastoma	45% affected	55% unaffected	7%–15% affected	85%–93% unaffected	<<1% affected	99% unaffected
Laterality	85% bilateral / 15% unilateral	0%	85% bilateral / 15% unilateral	0%	33% bilateral / 67% unilateral	0%
Focality	100% multifocal / 96% multifocal / 4% unifocal	0%	100% multifocal / 96% multifocal / 4% unifocal	0%	100% multifocal / 15% multifocal / 85% unifocal	0%
Chance of next sibling having retinoblastoma	45% 45% 45%	45%	45% 45% 45%	7%–15%	5%* <1%* <1%*	<1%

*If parent is a carrier, then 45%

Table created by David H. Abramson, MD.

TABLE XXVI-3

DIFFERENTIAL DIAGNOSIS OF LEUKOCORIA

CLINICAL DIAGNOSIS IN PSEUDORETINOBLASTOMA

Retinoblastoma
Persistent hyperplastic primary vitreous
Retinopathy of prematurity
Cataract
Coloboma of choroid or optic disc
Uveitis
Larval granulomatosis (toxocariasis)
Congenital retinal fold
Coats disease
Organizing vitreous hemorrhage
Retinal dysplasia
Corneal opacity
Familial exudative vitreoretinopathy (FEVR)
High myopia/anisometropia
Myelinated nerve fibers
Norrie disease
Retinal detachment

obtain the longest possible section of the optic nerve. Clamps on the optic nerve should be avoided, as damage can lead to difficulty in distinguishing meningothelial cells from crushed retinoblastoma cells. The results of enucleation for retinoblastoma are excellent with a cure rate greater than 95%. Survival decreases if the cut end of the nerve contains tumor cells.

In many cases of retinoblastoma it is possible to preserve the eye and salvage some vision. Treatment may include

- External-beam radiation for larger, posterior tumors
- Scleral plaque brachytherapy for some tumors of intermediate size
- Cryotherapy for small, anterior tumors
- Photocoagulation for small, posterior tumors in nonirradiated eyes

Chemotherapy has recently taken on an expanded role. Traditionally, chemotherapy had been reserved for those patients with a high risk for or known metastatic disease. Chemotherapy has recently been introduced as a primary treatment to reduce tumor bulk in an attempt to avoid external-beam radiation (chemoreduction). Cytotoxic drugs are given initially for 2–3 months to decrease tumor size. This method is effective even when a total retinal detachment is present.

Follow-up treatment with cryotherapy, laser therapy, or scleral plaque may be necessary for resistant tumors. A combination of chemotherapy and diode laser hyperthermia has also been effective in eradicating small and medium-sized endophytic tumors without vitreous seeds (thermochemotherapy). Several different modalities are sometimes necessary for eyes with large or multiple tumors. Decisions regarding whether and how to treat retinoblastoma are complex and best approached by a team of experienced specialists.

Treated retinoblastoma sometimes disappears altogether, but more often it persists as a calcified mass (type 1, or "cottage cheese" pattern) or a translucent grayish lesion (type 2, or "fish flesh" pattern, difficult to distinguish from untreated tumor). The child with treated retinoblastoma must be followed extremely closely with frequent examinations under anesthesia for several years to watch for renewed growth. Intraocular recurrence is particularly a concern in cases with vitreous seeding.

Intraocular spread or recurrence of retinoblastoma is usually associated with optic nerve or transscleral extension or with massive invasion of the choroid. The most common extraocular sites for disseminated retinoblastoma are the orbit, central nervous system, and skull bones. The prognosis for survival with recurrent retinoblastoma is poor, but if diagnosed early the disease can occasionally be cured with chemotherapy and/or radiation. Periodic repeated imaging of the head and orbits is advisable for several years after initial treatment.

Retinoblastoma patients who carry the germinal mutation, including those who present with unilateral involvement, are at risk for developing additional ocular and nonocular tumors. New retinoblastoma lesions may be discovered as late as 4–6 years of age, and the clinician must watch for them with repeated examinations under anesthesia. These children are also at risk for developing secondary nonocular tumors later in life. Osteosarcomas and various soft-tissue sarcomas may develop up to 30 years after treatment of retinoblastoma, particularly in the orbital region after external-beam radiation therapy but also elsewhere in the body with or without a history of radiation exposure. Primary extraocular tumors associated with retinoblastoma have a very poor prognosis for survival.

Albert DM, Dryja TP. Recent studies of the retinoblastoma gene. What it means to the ophthalmologist. *Arch Ophthalmol.* 1988;106:181–182.

Gallie BL, Budning A, DeBoer G, et al. Chemotherapy with focal therapy can cure intraocular retinoblastoma without radiotherapy. *Arch Ophthalmol.* 1996;114: 1321–1328.

Lueder GT, Goyal R. Visual function after laser hyperthermia and chemotherapy for macular retinoblastoma. *Am J Ophthalmol.* 1996;121:582–584.

Magramm I, Abramson DH, Ellsworth RM. Optic nerve involvement in retinoblastoma. *Ophthalmology.* 1989;96:217–222.

Murphree AL, Villablanca JG, Deegan WF 3rd, et al. Chemotherapy plus local treatment in the management of intraocular retinoblastoma. *Arch Ophthalmol.* 1996;114: 1348–1356.

Shields CL, De Potter P, Himelstein BP, et al. Chemoreduction in the initial management of intraocular retinoblastoma. *Arch Ophthalmol.* 1996;114:1330–1338.

Shields JA, Pesin SR. Seven cases of trilateral retinoblastoma. *Am J Ophthalmol.* 1989; 107:121–126.

Smith BJ, O'Brien JM. The genetics of retinoblastoma and current diagnostic testing. *J Pediatr Ophthalmol Strabismus.* 1996;33:120–123.

CHAPTER XXVII

Phakomatoses

The phakomatoses, or neurocutaneous syndromes, are a group of disorders featuring multiple discrete lesions of one or a few histologic types that are found in two or more organ systems, including the skin or central nervous system or both. In general, it is not the characteristics of the individual lesions but rather their multiplicity or association with one another that defines each syndrome. Eye involvement is frequent, and it may constitute an important source of morbidity or provide information of critical importance to diagnosis. Four major disorders have traditionally been designated phakomatoses:

☐ Neurofibromatosis (also known as von Recklinghausen disease)

☐ Tuberous sclerosis (Bourneville disease)

☐ Angiomatosis of the retina and cerebellum (von Hippel–Lindau disease)

☐ Encephalofacial or encephalotrigeminal angiomatosis (Sturge-Weber syndrome)

Other conditions sometimes classified as phakomatoses include

☐ Incontinentia pigmenti (Bloch-Sulzberger syndrome)

☐ Ataxia-telangiectasia (Louis-Bar syndrome)

☐ Racemose angioma (Wyburn-Mason syndrome)

Table XXVII-1 lists the phakomatoses.

Neurofibromatosis

Persons with neurofibromatosis (NF) manifest characteristic lesions composed of melanocytes or neuroglial cells, which are both primarily derivatives of neural crest mesenchyme. Although these melanocytic and glial lesions in NF are often referred to as *hamartomas,* this designation is questionable in that most do not become evident until years after birth, and many have histology indistinguishable from that of low-grade neoplasms originating in the same tissues.

At least two genetically distinct forms of neurofibromatosis are recognized. Type 1 (*NF-1*), sometimes referred to as *peripheral neurofibromatosis,* is by far the more common, with a prevalence of 1 in 3000–5000. Its clinical and pathological manifestations are described in detail below.

Type 2 (*NF-2*), or *central neurofibromatosis,* is defined by the presence of bilateral acoustic neuromas that are frequently accompanied by multiple other nervous system tumors including meningiomas, schwannomas (neurilemomas), and ependymomas, typically involving cranial nerves (though not the optic pathways) and spinal cord or nerve roots. Melanocytic lesions and cutaneous neurofibromas are relatively infrequent in NF-2. The principal ophthalmic manifestation of NF-2 is the development of lens opacities (posterior capsular cataracts) in a majority of cases during adolescence or young adulthood, approximately the same age that nervous system lesions become clinically evident.

TABLE XXVII-1

THE PHAKOMATOSES

CONDITION	DESCRIPTION	ASSOCIATED OCULAR CONDITION	ASSOCIATED CONDITIONS AND RISKS	TRANSMISSION
von Hippel–Lindau disease (retinal angiomatosis)	Retinal angioma supplied by dilated tortuous arteriole and venule; may be multiple	Retinal exudates, hemorrhages, retinal detachment, glaucoma	Cerebellar capillary hemangiomas, malformation of visceral organs	Autosomal dominant, chromosome 3p25
Sturge-Weber syndrome (encephalofacial angiomatosis)	Capillary hamartia (nevus flammeus) of skin, conjunctiva, episclera, and/or uveal tract, and of meninges	Glaucoma (especially with upper eyelid involvement by nevus flammeus)	Diffuse meningeal hemangioma with seizure disorder, hemiplegia or hemianopia, or mental retardation	Sporadic
Neurofibromatosis (von Recklinghausen disease)	Occasionally congenital, widespread hamartomas of peripheral nerves and tissue of neural crest derivation	Neurofibromas of eyelid and orbit, uveal melanocytic nevi, retinal glial hamartomas, congenital glaucoma, optic nerve glioma, absence of greater wing of sphenoid with pulsating exophthalmos	Similar hamartomas of central nervous system, peripheral and cranial nerves, gastrointestinal tract; malignant transformation possible	Autosomal dominant NF-I: chromosome 17q11.2
Tuberous sclerosis (Bourneville disease)	Mental deficiency, seizures, and adenoma sebaceum	Angiofibromas of eyelid skin; glial hamartomas of retina and optic disc	Adenoma sebaceum (angiofibromas), cerebral glial hamartomas	Autosomal dominant, chromosome 9q34
Ataxia-telangiectasia (Louis-Bar syndrome)	Progressive cerebellar ataxia, ocular and cutaneous telangiectasis, pulmonary infections	Conjunctival telangiectasis, anomalous ocular movements, and nystagmus	Dysarthria, coarse hair and skin, immunologic deficiency, and mental and growth retardation	Autosomal recessive, chromosome 11q22
Wyburn-Mason syndrome (racemose angioma)	Retinal and midbrain arteriovenous (AV) communication (aneurysms and angiomas) and facial nevi	AV communication (racemose angioma) of retina, with vision loss depending on location of AV communication	AV aneurysm at midbrain; intracranial calcification	Sporadic
Incontinentia pigmenti (Bloch-Sulzberger syndrome)	Cutaneous, dental, central nervous system, and ocular changes	ROP-like vasculopathy may progress to retinal detachment and retrolental membrane	"Splashed paint" hyperpigmented maculas, microcephaly, seizures, and mental deficiency	X-linked dominant

Modified from Isselbacher KJ, Braunwald E, Wilson JD, eds. *Harrison's Principles of Internal Medicine.* 13th ed. New York: McGraw-Hill Inc; 1994:2207–2210.

Both NF-1 and NF-2 are familial disorders that show autosomal dominant inheritance with very high penetrance (virtually 100% in NF-1). However, a large percentage of cases (nearly half in NF-1) are sporadic, presumably reflecting the high rate of mutation known to be true for the responsible gene. The genetic locus of NF-1 is on the long arm of chromosome 17 and that of NF-2 is on the long arm of chromosome 22. Recently, the NF-1 gene was isolated and cloned. The function of this gene is still poorly understood, but it is believed to code for a protein involved in regulation of cellular proliferation.

Melanocytic Lesions

Almost all adults with NF-1 have melanocytic lesions involving both skin and eye. The most common cutaneous expression, *café-au-lait spots,* have the clinical appearance of perfectly flat, sharply demarcated, uniformly hyperpigmented macules of variable size and shape. At least a few are usually present at birth, but their number and size increase during the first decade of life. Clusters of small café-au-lait spots, or *freckling,* in the axillary or inguinal regions are particularly characteristic of NF-1, occurring in a majority of affected individuals over 10 years old.

Many unaffected individuals have one to three café-au-lait spots, but greater numbers are rarely seen except in association with neurofibromatosis. In the past, neurofibromatosis was often diagnosed solely on the basis of multiple café-au-lait spots, but it is now recognized that a few individuals with this finding never develop other stigmata of the disease and may have offspring with a similarly limited condition, suggesting the existence of a genetic disorder distinct from NF-1. Currently, NF-1 is diagnosed only when two or more criteria from the following group of seven are met:

□ Six or more café-au-lait spots >5 mm in diameter in prepubescent or >15 mm in diameter in postpubescent individuals

□ Two or more neurofibromas of any type, or one plexiform neurofibroma

□ Freckling of axillary, inguinal, or other intertriginous areas

□ Optic nerve glioma

□ Two or more iris Lisch nodules

□ A distinctive osseous lesion, such as sphenoid bone dysplasia or thinning of the long-bone cortex, with or without pseudarthrosis

□ A first-degree relative with NF-1 according to the above criteria

Neurofibromatosis. Conference Statement. National Institutes of Health Consensus Development Conference. *Arch Neurol.* 1988;45:575–580.

Occasionally, hyperpigmentation of eyelid skin or conjunctiva is seen in NF-1, but melanocytic lesions of the uveal tract are far more common ocular manifestations. In the iris these take the form of small (usually no larger than 1 mm), sharply demarcated, dome-shaped excrescences known as *Lisch nodules* (Fig XXVII-1). Clinically, Lisch nodules usually appear to have smooth surfaces and a translucent interior suggesting a gelatinous consistency, but in some individuals they look solid and wartlike. Color varies but can be described as tan in most cases. In heavily pigmented brown irides they tend to stand out against the smooth, dark anterior surface and are often visible to the unaided eye. When overall iris stromal pigmentation is

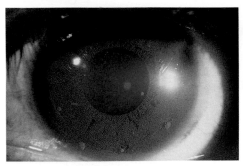

FIG XXVII-1—Lisch nodules of iris, left eye in child with type 1 neurofibromatosis.

lighter, Lisch nodules can be partly hidden within recesses in the lacy stromal tissue and may be overlooked unless a slit lamp is used to search for them. They may be difficult to differentiate from small clumps of normal pigmented tissue, especially when they are few in number and the patient is less than fully cooperative. Histopathologically, the lesions consist primarily of uniform spindle-shaped melanin-containing cells, indistinguishable from those found in iris nevi and low-grade spindle-cell melanomas.

Most Lisch nodules develop during childhood or adolescence. They are seen infrequently before age 3 years, appear in a majority of cases of NF-1 between 5 and 10 years of age, and are present in nearly 100% of affected adults. The finding of two or more Lisch nodules is a diagnostic criterion for NF-1, but an affected adult's eye typically has dozens, and occasionally 100 or more (see also chapter XX, Iris Abnormalities).

Choroidal lesions have been reported to occur in one third to one half of adults with NF-1. These lesions are described as flat with indistinct borders, hyperpigmented in relation to the surrounding fundus but ranging from yellow-white to dark brown in color. Their number varies from 1 to 20 per eye, with each lesion typically one to two times the size of the optic disc. Direct histopathologic correlation for this clinical finding is lacking, but it is presumed to represent localized concentration of melanocytes similar to a choroidal nevus.

Like café-au-lait spots, none of the common ocular melanocytic lesions of NF-1 has any clinical significance beyond establishing the diagnosis. Neither the vision nor the health of the eye is affected by these lesions, regardless of their extent. Persons with NF-1 are believed to be predisposed to developing uveal melanoma, as well as a number of other malignant neoplasms. However, the incidence of iris, and especially choroidal, tumors is still quite low.

Glial Cell Lesions

Nodular neurofibromas   Among lesions of neuroglial origin in NF-1, *nodular cutaneous* and *subcutaneous neurofibromas,* or *fibroma molluscum,* are by far the most common. These are soft papulonodules, often pedunculated, with color ranging from that of normal skin to violescent. They typically begin to appear in late childhood and increase in number throughout adolescence and adulthood; nearly all adults with NF-1 have at least a few. In some cases hundreds of these lesions are present, causing considerable disfigurement.

Plexiform neurofibromas   Of much greater clinical significance than nodular neurofibromas are the less common *plexiform neurofibromas,* which are seen in approximately 30% of individuals with NF-1. They are very rarely seen in other contexts. These lesions appear clinically as extensive subcutaneous swellings with indistinct margins. Hyperpigmentation or hypertrichosis of the overlying skin is often present, and hypertrophy of underlying soft tissue and bone (regional gigantism) is common. The consistency of plexiform neurofibromas is typically soft and not easily distinguished from that of normal tissue; the often-repeated statement that they feel like a "bag of worms" applies in only a minority of cases.

Plexiform neurofibromas develop earlier than nodular lesions, frequently becoming evident in infancy or childhood. They often show considerable enlargement over time, resulting in severe disfigurement and functional impairment. Rarely, malignant degeneration occurs within the lesion, producing a neurofibrosarcoma capable of widespread metastasis.

Approximately 10% of plexiform neurofibromas involve the face, commonly the upper eyelid and orbit. At onset the involved upper eyelid is thicker than normal and usually appears mildly ptotic (Fig XXVII-2). Its inner surface may override the lower eyelid margin and lashes when the eye is closed. Characteristically, the greater involvement of its temporal portion gives the eyelid margin an S-shaped configuration and an overall appearance of an eyelid that is "too big for the eye." Considerable and sometimes massive growth of the lesion occurs during childhood and adolescence, although extension across the facial midline is rare. Complete ptosis may eventually result from the increasing bulk and weight of the upper eyelid. Irritation of the upper palpebral conjunctiva caused by rubbing against the lower lashes can create significant discomfort. Glaucoma in the ipsilateral eye is found in as many as half of cases.

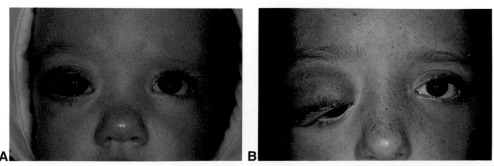

FIG XXVII-2—Plexiform neurofibroma involving the right upper eyelid, associated with ipsilateral buphthalmos, in girl with NF-1. *A,* Age 8 months. *B,* Age 8 years.

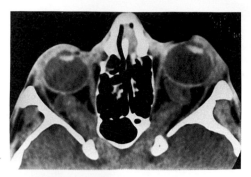

FIG XXVII-3—Axial CT image showing bilateral optic glioma with chiasmal involvement, associated with severe bilateral visual loss, in an adolescent boy with NF-1. Note relatively low density of tissue surrounding the central core of the enlarged optic nerve.

Complete excision of a plexiform neurofibroma involving the eyelid is generally not possible. Treatment is directed toward the relief of specific symptoms and is likely to be partially successful at best. Topical ointment is helpful in reducing conjunctival irritation. Resection of distorted and chronically inflamed conjunctiva is sometimes necessary. Surgical debulking and frontalis suspension procedures can reduce ptosis sufficiently to permit binocular vision, but the resulting benefit is often only temporary.

Optic glioma   Low-grade pilocytic astrocytoma involving the optic nerve and/or chiasm (*optic glioma*) is among the most characteristic and potentially serious complications of NF-1. Symptomatic optic gliomas (i.e., tumors producing significant visual loss, proptosis, or other complications) occur in 1%–5% of persons with NF-1. When CT or MRI is performed prospectively on unselected NF-1 patients, abnormalities of the optic nerve (often bilateral) or chiasm indicating the presence of glioma are found in approximately 15% of cases.

Typically, the entire orbital portion of an involved optic nerve shows cylindrical or fusiform enlargement (Fig XXVII-3). A relatively narrow central core usually differs from surrounding tissue because of the characteristic growth pattern of optic nerve glioma in NF-1: most cellular proliferation occurs in the perineural intradural space (arachnoidal gliomatosis) associated with production of abundant mucinous material that gives this tissue the signal characteristics of water. This core shows higher density in CT imaging; with MRI the core shows higher density on T1-weighted images and lower density on T2-weighted images.

Increased length of the intraorbital nerve segment results in exaggerated sinuousness or "kinking" that often creates an appearance of discontinuity or localized constriction on axial images. These appearances distinguish optic glioma reliably from the principal differential diagnostic alternative, *optic nerve sheath meningioma,* which also occurs with increased frequency in neurofibromatosis. However, it occurs much less commonly than optic glioma and rarely in childhood.

Gliomas involving the intracranial optic nerve or chiasm in NF-1 produce enlargement of these structures on both CT and MRI and, frequently, abnormal signal intensity on MRI, which is now the preferred means of diagnosis. Associated contiguous involvement of the orbital portion of one or both optic nerves usually occurs, and extension into the optic tracts and posterior visual pathways is often evident, especially on MRI.

Optic gliomas that become symptomatic in NF-1 patients nearly always do so before age 10 years, often apparently following a brief period of rapid enlargement. Even without treatment many then appear to enter a phase of stability or much slower growth, and spontaneous improvement has been documented in a few cases.

Tumors confined to the optic nerve at the time of clinical presentation infrequently extend into the chiasm subsequently and very rarely develop extradural extension or distant metastasis; mortality is virtually nil. Treatment remains controversial. Complete excision through a transfrontal approach that preserves the globe but sacrifices any remaining vision on the involved side is recommended for such cases by many authorities, but it has not been convincingly demonstrated that this approach improves the prognosis for sight in the other eye. Most patients treated with subtotal orbital excision for relief of proptosis also do well.

In addition to bilateral visual loss, tumors primarily involving the chiasm may produce significant morbidity, including hydrocephalus and hypothalamic dysfunction leading to precocious puberty or hypopituitarism. Mortality of 50% or higher has been reported for glioma of the chiasm. In the past most deaths occurred within months of diagnosis, but recent series show longer survival, reflecting earlier detection and improved management of complications in addition to treatment of the tumor itself that may be more effective. Megavoltage radiation therapy appears to retard or reverse progression in many cases, but it is not firmly established that this therapy can substantially reduce the ultimate rate of tumor-related blindness and death, which may occur as late as 20 years after presentation. In an effort to avoid complications of brain irradiation in early childhood, chemotherapy has been investigated as an alternative treatment modality with encouraging preliminary results.

Other neuroglial abnormalities   Abnormal proliferation of peripheral neuroglial or other neural crest–derived cells may occur in relation to deeper tissues and visceral organs as well as skin (spinal and gastrointestinal neurofibromas, pheochromocytoma). Prominence of corneal nerves, believed to represent glial hypertrophy, may be noted on slit-lamp examination in as many as 20% of cases. A frequent histopathological finding in the choroid is the presence of so-called ovoid bodies, onion-like formations that appear to consist of hyperplastic Schwann cells surrounding peripheral nerve axons. Rarely, a localized neurofibroma may develop within the orbit in association with neurofibromatosis. Retinal hamartomas indistinguishable from those seen in tuberous sclerosis have also been found in patients with NF-1.

Other Manifestations

NF-1 is associated with increased, but still generally low, incidence of a number of conditions that cannot be explained on the basis of abnormal proliferation of neural crest–derived cells. These conditions include a variety of benign tumors that may involve skin or eye (juvenile xanthogranuloma, capillary hemangioma) and several forms of malignancy (leukemia, rhabdomyosarcoma, Wilms tumor). Also relatively common are bony defects (scoliosis, pseudarthrosis of the tibia, and hypoplasia of the sphenoid bone, which may result in ocular pulsation) and a number of ill-defined abnormalities of the central nervous system (macrocephaly, aqueductal stenosis, seizures, and usually minor intellectual deficits).

The most significant ophthalmic disorder in this category is glaucoma, virtually always unilateral, which occurs in 1%–2% of individuals with NF-1. It is associated in most cases with ipsilateral plexiform neurofibroma of the upper eyelid or with the iris abnormality known as congenital iris ectropion (see Figure XX-9 and discussion in chapter XX). Buphthalmos, or enlargement of the cornea and the globe as a whole, is seen if IOP is elevated during the first 2 years of life. Excessive growth of the eyeball may also, at least in part, be a manifestation of regional hypertrophy in some cases. Corneal edema and high myopia can result from high pressure in early or later childhood.

The pathogenesis of glaucoma in NF-1 is unknown. Abnormal trabecular meshwork development in some patients can lead to an early-onset childhood or congenital glaucoma. In others synechial closure of the angle may result from neurofibromatous tissue posterior to the iris or neurofibromatous infiltration of the angle directly. Treatment is surgical in most cases. A variety of procedures have been employed with moderate success; achievement of adequate pressure control often requires several operations. Useful vision is seldom retained in the involved eye. Contributing to this poor prognosis are frequently associated, significant orbital and optic nerve abnormalities as well as refractory amblyopia (anisometropic or deprivation).

A child or adult who appears to have any one of the abnormalities typically associated with NF-1 should have an eye examination that includes the following:

□ Assessment of vision (acuity and color discrimination)

□ Pupillary light reaction, including careful scrutiny for relative afferent defect

□ Slit-lamp examination with particular attention to the iris

□ Ophthalmoscopy to identify disc pallor or edema and choroidal lesions

□ Measurement of IOP, when indicated by other findings

The discovery of Lisch nodules has been used to confirm the presence of NF-1 in a patient with café-au-lait spots, and their absence in an adult patient has been said to virtually rule out the diagnosis. However, the use of iris changes as a diagnostic marker for NF-1 has recently been questioned. Iris changes in known NF-1 patients are more diverse than the classic descriptions of Lisch nodules, and interobserver reliability for the diagnosis of NF-1 based on iris findings is often poor.

Although the role of routine screening with MRI remains controversial, abnormalities of vision, pupil function, or optic disc appearance indicate a need for neuroimaging studies to look for optic glioma. An appropriate interval for periodic ophthalmologic reassessment in childhood is 1–2 years, unless a significant abnormality requires closer observation. New onset of significant eye involvement is very unlikely in adults, but blood pressure should be regularly monitored because of the risk of pheochromocytoma.

Beauchamp GR. Neurofibromatosis type 1 in children. *Trans Am Ophthalmol Soc.* 1995; 93:445–472.

Kaiser-Kupfer MI, Freidlin V, Datiles MB, et al. The association of posterior capsular lens opacities with bilateral acoustic neuromas in patients with neurofibromatosis type 2. *Arch Ophthalmol.* 1989;107:541–544.

Lewis RA, Riccardi VM. von Recklinghausen neurofibromatosis. Incidence of iris hamar-tomata. *Ophthalmology*. 1981;88:348–354.

Listernick R, Charrow J, Greenwald MJ, et al. Natural history of optic pathway tumors in children with neurofibromatosis type 1: a longitudinal study. *J Pediatr*. 1994; 125:63–66.

Mulvihill JJ, Parry DM, Sherman JL, et al. Neurofibromatosis 1 (Recklinghausen disease) and neurofibromatosis 2 (bilateral acoustic neurofibromatosis). An update. *Ann Intern Med*. 1990;113:39–52.

Stern J, Jakobiec FA, Housepian EM. The architecture of optic nerve gliomas with and without neurofibromatosis. *Arch Ophthalmol*. 1980;98:505–511.

Tuberous Sclerosis (Bourneville Disease)

Tuberous sclerosis (TS) is a familial disorder associated with a variety of abnormalities involving the skin, eye, central nervous system, and other organs. Estimates of the prevalence of TS range from as high as 1 in 10,000 to 1 in 100,000 or lower. The responsible gene has been localized to the long arm of chromosome 9. Transmission as an autosomal dominant trait has been documented in numerous pedigrees, but new mutations account for as many as 80% of cases.

Several distinct skin lesions are characteristic of TS (Fig XXVII-4). The earliest cutaneous sign to appear is the "white spot," or *hypopigmented macule,* which is present in almost all cases at birth or in infancy. These lesions are sharply demarcated with a shape that often resembles an ash leaf. Ultraviolet light from a Wood's lamp increases the visibility of white spots in light-skinned individuals. Histopathologically, these spots have decreased melanin but normal numbers of melanocytes.

Facial angiofibromas often called *adenoma sebaceum* begin to appear in childhood and increase progressively in number; they are present in three quarters of adolescents and adults with TS. These lesions are often mistaken for common acne. Subungual and periungual fibromas are also common after puberty; gingival fibromas may occur as well. A thickened plaque of skin known as a *shagreen patch,* or

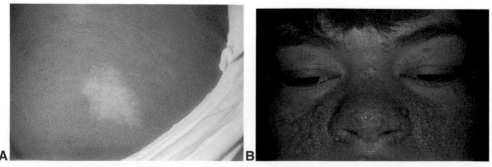

A   B

FIG XXVII-4—Cutaneous lesions of tuberous sclerosis. *A,* Hypopigmented macule. *B,* Adenoma sebaceum of the face.

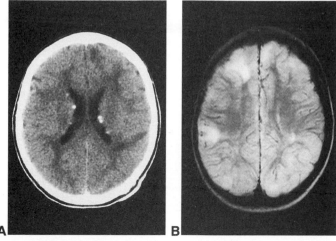

FIG XXVII-5—Brain lesions of tuberous sclerosis. *A,* Axial CT image showing small periventricular calcifications in the basal ganglia bilaterally. *B,* Axial T2-weighted MRI showing two tuberous malformations of the right hemisphere cortex.

collagenoma, is seen in approximately one quarter of cases, typically in the lumbosacral area. Plaques involving the forehead that sometimes extend into the eyelids may be present at birth.

Seizures occur in 80% of patients with TS, and they may be very difficult to control. Severe mental retardation is present in 50% of patients, but intelligence is normal in many of those affected. Characteristic findings in neuroimaging studies include nodular periventricular or basal ganglion calcifications (representing benign astrocytomas) and tuberous malformations of the cortex (Fig XXVII-5). Malignant astrocytomas occur infrequently. Obstruction of the foramen of Monro by tumor may produce hydrocephalus, and cardiac tumors (rhabdomyomas) can lead to early death or severe disability. Lesions of bone and kidney are common but usually produce no significant disturbance of function.

Hypopigmented lesions analogous to white spots of the skin are occasionally seen in the iris or choroid, but the most frequent and characteristic ocular manifestation of TS is the *retinal phakoma* (Fig XXVII-6). Pathologically, this growth arises from the innermost layer of the retina and is composed of nerve fibers and relatively undifferentiated cells that appear to be of glial origin; it is frequently referred to as an *astrocytic hamartoma.* Phakomas can develop anywhere in the fundus but are usually found near the posterior pole, involving the retina, the optic disc, or both. They vary in size from about half to twice the diameter of the disc. Vision is rarely affected to a significant degree.

Phakomas usually have one of two distinct appearances, although intermediate forms can occur. The first type is relatively flat with a smooth surface, indistinct margins, and gray-white color. These lesions are translucent to a degree that at times makes them difficult to detect ophthalmoscopically. The examiner can most easily

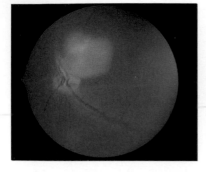

FIG XXVII-6—Fundus lesions of tuberous sclerosis, left eye. In addition to the large phakoma partially overlying the optic disc, a small hypopigmented lesion appears in the temporal macula and a barely visible second phakoma partially obscures a retinal blood vessel near the edge of the photograph directly below the disc.

locate them by tracing retinal vessels from the disc peripherally and scrutinizing points at which a vessel is partially obscured by overlying tissue. The examiner can then perceive domelike elevations with the binocular indirect ophthalmoscope by carefully observing the surface light reflection while shifting viewing direction slightly. The second type of phakoma is sharply demarcated and more elevated than the first type with an irregular surface that has been compared to a mulberry or cluster of tapioca grains or fish eggs. These lesions are opaque, glistening, and yellow-white in color as a result of calcification. They are found relatively more often in older patients and on or adjacent to the optic disc. The term *giant drusen* has been applied to disc involvement by a mulberry phakoma because of its resemblance to the common but unrelated condition known as drusen (or hyaline bodies) of the optic nerve head.

The reported frequency of phakomas in persons with tuberous sclerosis varies greatly, but data from recent series suggest that they are present in from one third to more than one half of cases. One to several may be found in a single eye, and bilateral involvement is noted in about 40% of those affected. There is no evidence that the number of lesions increases with age, although the increasing size of individual tumors over time has been documented. Phakomas are not pathognomonic of TS: they occur occasionally in association with neurofibromatosis and in the eyes of unaffected persons.

Gomez MR, ed. *Tuberous Sclerosis.* 2nd ed. New York: Raven; 1988.

Osborne JP. Diagnosis of tuberous sclerosis. *Arch Dis Child.* 1988;63:1423–1425.

Williams R, Taylor D. Tuberous sclerosis. *Surv Ophthalmol.* 1985;30:143–154.

von Hippel–Lindau Disease (Retinal Angiomatosis)

von Hippel–Lindau disease (VHL) is an autosomal dominantly inherited disorder characterized by vascular tumors (hemangioblastomas) of the retina and central nervous system, most often the cerebellum. These tumors have only limited proliferative capacity, but exudation across thin vessel walls in the lesions leads to the formation of fluid accumulations that may attain considerable size and compromise vital structures. Cysts and tumors, malignant as well as benign, occur frequently in numerous other organs, including the kidneys (renal cell carcinoma), pancreas, liver, epididymis, and adrenal glands (pheochromocytoma). Despite its well-accepted classification as a neurocutaneous syndrome, VHL disease rarely has significant cutaneous manifestations, although café-au-lait spots and port-wine stains are seen occasionally. Mental deficiency is not a feature of the disease. The von Hippel–Lindau gene is now known to occupy a locus on chromosome 3.

Pedigree studies suggest that ocular involvement occurs in a majority of individuals with VHL disease. (Identical eye disease without familial transmission or systemic involvement is three to four times more common than the complete syndrome.) The retinal lesions originally described by von Hippel usually become visible ophthalmoscopically between ages 10 and 35 years, with an average age of onset of 25 years, about a decade before the peak clinical incidence of cerebellar disease. Tumors are multiple in the same eye in about one third of cases and bilateral in as many as half of cases. They typically occur in the peripheral fundus, but lesions adjacent to the optic disc have also been described.

The incipient retinal lesion appears as a minor nonspecific vascular anomaly or a small reddish dot in the fundus that gradually enlarges into a flat or slightly elevated grayish disc. It ultimately acquires the fully developed appearance of a pink globular mass one to three or more disc diameters in size. The hallmark of the mature tumor is a pair of markedly dilated vessels (artery and vein) running between the lesion and the optic disc, indicating significant arteriovenous shunting (Fig XXVII-7). Recent observations suggest that characteristic paired or twin retinal vessels of normal caliber may be present before the development of a visible tumor.

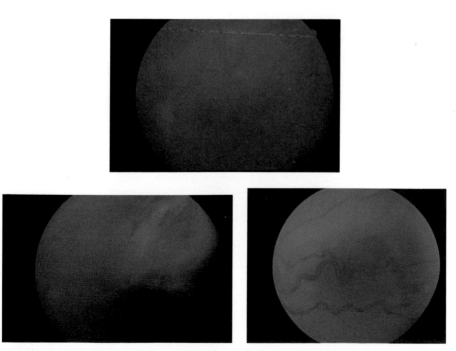

FIG XXVII-7—von Hippel retinal angiomatosis, left eye.

Histopathologically, retinal angiomas consist of relatively well formed capillaries; however, fluorescein angiography shows these vessels to be leaky. Transudation of fluid into the subretinal space causes lipid accumulation, retinal detachment, and consequent loss of vision in many involved eyes. Secondary degenerative changes, including cataract and glaucoma, often occur in blind eyes with long-standing retinal detachment; ultimately, enucleation may become necessary.

Retinal angiomas can be effectively treated with cryotherapy or laser photocoagulation in two thirds or more of cases, particularly when the lesions are still small. Multiple treatment sessions may be necessary to achieve complete success. Early diagnosis increases the likelihood of successful treatment, yet the ocular lesions of VHL are asymptomatic prior to the occurrence of retinal detachment. Therefore, children known to be at risk for the disease should have periodic ophthalmologic evaluation beginning at about age 5 years.

Blodi CF, Russell SR, Pulido JS, et al. Direct and feeder vessel photocoagulation of retinal angiomas with dye yellow laser. *Ophthalmology.* 1990;97:791–797.

de Jong PT, Verkaart RJ, van de Vooren MJ, et al. Twin vessels in von Hippel–Lindau disease. *Am J Ophthalmol.* 1988;105:165–169.

Filling-Katz MR, Choyke PL, Oldfield E, et al. Central nervous system involvement in von Hippel–Lindau disease. *Neurology.* 1991;41:41–46.

Welch RB. von Hippel–Lindau disease: the recognition and treatment of early angiomatosis retinae and the use of cryosurgery as an adjunct to therapy. *Trans Am Ophthalmol Soc.* 1970;68:367–424.

Sturge-Weber Syndrome (Encephalofacial Angiomatosis)

Sturge-Weber syndrome (SWS) consists of a facial cutaneous angioma (nevus flammeus, or port-wine stain) with an ipsilateral leptomeningeal vascular malformation that typically results in the following:

□ Cerebral calcification

□ Seizures, which may show a Jacksonian pattern, progressing from focal to grand mal

□ Focal neurologic deficits (hemianopia, hemiparesis)

□ A highly variable degree of mental deficiency (with normal intelligence in many affected individuals)

SWS is unique among the four major neurocutaneous syndromes in that it is not a genetically transmitted disorder. Lesions are always present at birth, however. The distribution of cutaneous and cerebral involvement suggests a disturbance very early in embryonic development (4–8 weeks gestation), when primitive facial structures overlie the future occipital lobes of the developing brain. The prevalence of SWS is not reliably known.

Calcium deposits characteristic of Sturge-Weber syndrome form after birth in brain parenchyma, usually involving the occipital lobe and variable portions of the parietal, temporal, and occasionally frontal lobes. Curvilinear densities, paralleling cerebral convolutions to produce the so-called railroad-track sign, can be demonstrated by means of CT earlier and more consistently than by conventional radiographs, but they are often not detectable before age 2 years. MRI is less sensitive than CT for identifying calcification but may provide better delineation of other abnormalities associated with the angiomatous malformation that can confirm the

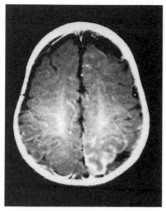

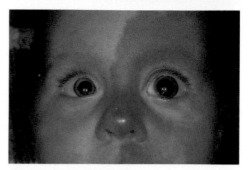

FIG XXVII-8—Axial gadolinium-enhanced T1-weighted MRI shows vascular malformation with underlying cortical atrophy in the left occipital lobe of a 4-month-old girl with Sturge-Weber syndrome.

FIG XXVII-9—Facial port-wine nevus involving the left eyelids, associated with ipsilateral buphthalmos in an infant girl with Sturge-Weber syndrome.

diagnosis in very young children (Fig XXVII-8). These abnormalities include cerebral volume reduction, abnormal signal intensity in cortex and white matter, prominent deep venous system, and enlarged choroid plexus.

The Sturge-Weber skin lesion, which can be quite disfiguring, consists of dilated and excessively numerous but well-formed capillaries in the dermis. It usually involves the forehead and upper eyelid on the same side as the cerebral vascular malformation, with variable extension to the ipsilateral lower eyelid and maxillary and mandibular regions (Fig XXVII-9). The sharply demarcated area of the port-wine nevus frequently does not conform to the distribution of the trigeminal divisions, and involvement of the contralateral face, the scalp, and the trunk and extremities is common. (The designation *Klippel-Trénaunay-Weber syndrome* is sometimes applied to cases with extensive lesions of the extremities.) Hypertrophy of soft tissue and bone underlying the angioma is often seen in childhood, and thickening of the involved skin (sometimes with a nodular pattern) may develop later in life. Recently, treatment of affected skin with the pulsed dye laser has been shown to markedly reduce vascularity, considerably improving appearance without causing significant damage to dermal tissue.

Ocular Involvement

Any portion of the ocular circulation may be anomalous in SWS when the skin lesion involves the eyelids. Increased conjunctival vascularity commonly produces a pinkish discoloration. Frequently, an abnormal plexus of episcleral vessels appears, although it may be hidden by the overlying tissue of Tenon's layer. Tortuous vessels and arteriovenous communications are sometimes seen in the retina.

The choroid is the site of the most significant purely vascular anomaly of the eye associated with SWS. In a majority of cases of SWS with ocular involvement,

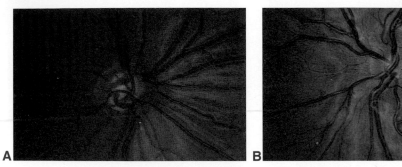

FIG XXVII-10—Fundus appearance in an adolescent boy with Sturge-Weber syndrome. *A,* Right eye. Note glaucomatous disc cupping and deeper red color of surrounding choroid, compared with normal fellow eye. *B,* Left eye.

increased numbers of well-formed choroidal vessels give the fundus a uniform bright red or red-orange color that has been compared to tomato catsup (Fig XXVII-10). Typically, the region of the posterior pole is involved; in some cases there is gradual transition to a normal vascular pattern in the periphery, while in others the entire fundus seems to be affected. Choroidal angiomatosis usually remains asymptomatic in childhood. During adolescence or adulthood, however, marked thickening of the choroid sometimes becomes evident. Degeneration or detachment of the overlying retina with severe visual loss may follow, but the frequency of this progression is not established. No treatment is known to be effective in preventing or reversing such deterioration, although scattered application of laser photocoagulation, which has proved useful in the management of circumscribed choroidal angiomas not associated with SWS, may help.

Glaucoma is the most serious ocular complication seen in children with SWS. It occurs in about one third of cases, including some that lack intracranial lesions. Involvement of the skin of both eyelids of the affected eye is usually but not invariably present. Bilateral glaucoma may be seen in association with bilateral cutaneous involvement. Corneal enlargement is present in about two thirds of cases. Anomalies of the anterior chamber angle similar to those seen in primary developmental glaucoma appear to be responsible for increased resistance to aqueous fluid outflow and consequent IOP elevation in most cases. An additional factor may be elevated pressure in the episcleral veins that receive the aqueous flow as a result of abnormal arteriovenous communication.

Management

When SWS is first documented or suspected, a complete ophthalmological evaluation is essential, including measurement of IOP. Sedation or general anesthesia may be necessary for uncooperative children. Examination should be repeated periodically throughout childhood even if no ocular abnormality is initially detected. Sturge-Weber glaucoma usually requires surgical treatment. Adequate long-term pressure control can frequently be achieved, although multiple operations are typically necessary. Aqueous shunting devices or setons have shown promise in the management of otherwise intractable glaucoma in Sturge-Weber patients (see BCSC Section 10, *Glaucoma*). A particular hazard of glaucoma surgery in SWS is the risk of massive intraoperative or postoperative exudation or hemorrhage from anomalous choroidal vessels as a result of rapid ocular decompression. Special care must be taken with implanted drainage devices to prevent excessive early postoperative hypotony. Choroidal or subretinal fluid accumulation after surgery may be dramatic, but spontaneous resorption usually occurs within 1–2 weeks.

Garden JM, Polla LL, Tan OT. The treatment of port-wine stains by the pulsed dye laser. Analysis of pulse duration and long-term therapy. *Arch Dermatol.* 1988;124: 889–896.

Iwach AG, Hoskins HD Jr, Hetherington J Jr, et al. Analysis of surgical and medical management of glaucoma in Sturge-Weber syndrome. *Ophthalmology.* 1990;97: 904–909.

Sujansky E, Conradi S. Outcome of Sturge-Weber syndrome in 52 adults. *Am J Med Genet.* 1995;57:35–45.

Sullivan TJ, Clarke MP, Morin JD. The ocular manifestations of the Sturge-Weber syndrome. *J Pediatr Ophthalmol Strabismus.* 1992;29:349–356.

Susac JO, Smith JL, Scelfo RJ. The "tomato-catsup" fundus in Sturge-Weber syndrome. *Arch Ophthalmol.* 1974;92:69–70.

Ataxia-Telangiectasia (Louis-Bar Syndrome)

Ataxia-telangiectasia (AT) is an autosomal recessive disorder that involves primarily the central nervous system (particularly the cerebellum), the ocular surface, the skin, and the immune system. Although rare (about 1 in 40,000 prevalence), it is believed to be the most common cause of progressive ataxia in early childhood. Truncal ataxia is usually noted during the second year of life, with subsequent development of dysarthria, dystonia, and choreoathetosis. Progressive deterioration of motor function leads to serious disability by age 10 years. Intellectual impairment, if present, is usually mild.

Recognition of ocular features is often the key to diagnosis of AT. Ocular motor abnormalities are found in nearly all patients with AT, and they are frequently among the earliest manifestations. Characteristically, the ability to initiate saccades with preservation of vestibulo-ocular movements is poor, very similar to the findings of congenital ocular motor apraxia. Strabismus and nystagmus may also be present.

Telangiectasia of the conjunctiva develops in all cases beginning between the ages of 3 and 5 years. Involvement is initially interpalpebral but away from the limbus, eventually becoming generalized (Fig XXVII-11). Similar, though less obvious, vessel changes can appear in the skin of the eyelids and other sun-exposed areas. A variety of skin changes that suggest accelerated aging are common in older children and adults with AT.

Individuals with AT show greatly increased sensitivity to the tissue-damaging side effects of therapeutic radiation and many chemotherapeutic agents. Defective T-cell function in AT patients is associated with hypoplasia of the thymus and decreased levels of circulating immunoglobulin in a majority of cases. Recurrent respiratory tract infections are a serious problem, frequently causing death in adolescence or young adulthood even with optimal antimicrobial and supportive treatment. The increased susceptibility to the development of various malignancies,

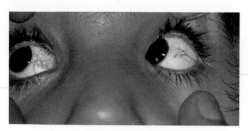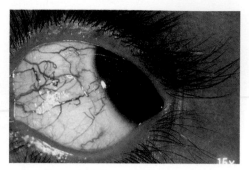

FIG XXVII-11—Abnormally dilated and tortuous conjunctival vessels, left eye, in a child with ataxia-telangiectasia.

particularly lymphomas and leukemias, contributes to early mortality in one third to one half of cases.

The function of the AT gene or genes, now localized to the long arm of chromosome 11, is unknown but probably relates to DNA repair. AT heterozygosity is present in an estimated 1%–3% of the population. Although gene carriers are generally healthy and cannot be identified except in the context of a known AT pedigree, they have significantly increased risk of developing common forms of malignancy and show greater than normal sensitivity to radiation. It has been estimated that breast cancer in women heterozygous for the AT gene is about seven times more frequent than in noncarriers and accounts for nearly 10% of all cases in the U.S. population.

Gatti RA, Boder E, Vinters HV, et al. Ataxia-telangiectasia: an interdisciplinary approach to pathogenesis. *Medicine.* 1991;70:99–117.

Harley RD, Baird HW, Craven EM. Ataxia telangiectasia. Report of seven cases. *Arch Ophthalmol.* 1967;77:582–592.

Incontinentia Pigmenti (Bloch-Sulzberger Syndrome)

Incontinentia pigmenti (IP) is a syndrome involving the skin, brain, and eye that shows the unusual inheritance pattern of X-linked dominance with a presumed lethal effect on the hemizygous male fetus. Nearly all affected individuals are female, with mother-to-daughter transmission in familial cases. BCSC Section 2, *Fundamentals and Principles of Ophthalmology,* discusses this inheritance pattern in detail in the chapters on Genetics.

The cutaneous manifestations of IP are very distinctive. Skin appearance is usually normal at birth, but erythema and bullae develop during the first few days of life, usually on the extremities, and persist for weeks to months. A second distinct phase characterized by verrucous changes begins at about 2 months of age, subsiding after a few more months. Finally, clusters of small hyperpigmented macules in a characteristic "splashed-paint" distribution make their appearance, most prominently on the trunk (Fig XXVII-12).

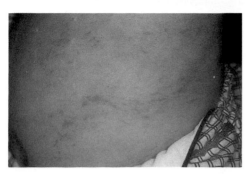

FIG XXVII-12—Pigmented skin lesions of incontinentia pigmenti.

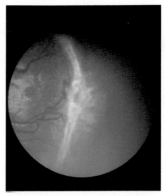

FIG XXVII-13—Vascular abnormalities of the temporal retina, right eye, in a 2-year-old child with incontinentia pigmenti. Note avascularity peripheral to the circumferential white vasoproliferative lesion, which showed profuse leakage on fluorescein angioscopy.

Histopathologically, the early vesicular lesions show local accumulation of unusual large macrophages and eosinophils accompanied by peripheral blood eosinophilia. In the lesions of the pigmentary stage, which persist for years before gradually fading, free melanin granules are found abnormally scattered in the dermis. Although present in all cases, skin involvement varies considerably in extent, occasionally being so limited that it is completely overlooked at one or more of its stages.

About one third of patients with IP have central nervous system problems that may include microcephaly, hydrocephalus, seizures, and varying degrees of mental deficiency. Dental abnormalities (missing and malformed teeth) are found in roughly two thirds of cases. Other, less common, findings include scoliosis, skull deformities, cleft palate, and dwarfism.

Ocular involvement occurs in at least one quarter to one third of cases, typically in the form of a proliferative retinal vasculopathy that closely resembles retinopathy of prematurity. At birth, the only detectable abnormality may be incomplete peripheral retinal vascularization. Abnormal arteriovenous connections, microvascular abnormalities, and neovascular membranes develop at or near the junction of vascular and avascular retina (Fig XXVII-13). Rapid progression leads in some cases to total retinal detachment and retrolental membrane formation (*pseudoglioma*) within the first few months of life. Other affected eyes show gradual deterioration over a period of several years, while still others have proliferative lesions of limited extent that may persist for decades. Microphthalmos, cataract, glaucoma, optic atrophy, strabismus, and nystagmus are occasionally seen, representing secondary consequences of endstage retinopathy in most if not all cases.

The retinopathy of incontinentia pigmenti has been treated using photocoagulation or cryotherapy in a small number of cases with varying degrees of reported success. No consensus exists as to whether treatment should be applied primarily to the avascular peripheral retina, as in the currently preferred approach to management of retinopathy of prematurity, or to the proliferative lesions themselves.

Carney RG, Carney RG Jr. Incontinentia pigmenti. *Arch Dermatol.* 1970;102:157–162.

Catalano RA. Incontinentia pigmenti. *Am J Ophthalmol.* 1990;110:696–702.

Wyburn-Mason Syndrome (Racemose Angioma)

Wyburn-Mason syndrome is a nonhereditary arteriovenous malformation of the eye and brain, typically involving the optic disc or retina and the midbrain. Skin lesions are present in a minority of cases. The complete syndrome is considerably less common than isolated occurrence of similar ocular or intracranial disease.

Seizures, mental changes, hemiparesis, and papilledema may result from the central nervous system lesions, which are frequently a source of hemorrhage, unlike the hemangioma of Sturge-Weber syndrome.

Ocular manifestations are unilateral and congenital but may show some degree of progression during childhood. The typical lesion consists of markedly dilated and tortuous vessels that shunt blood flow directly from arteries to veins; they do not leak fluid (Fig XXVII-14). Vision ranges from normal to markedly reduced in the involved eye, and intraocular hemorrhage and secondary neovascular glaucoma are possible complications. No treatment is indicated for primary lesions.

Augsburger JJ, Goldberg RE, Shields JA, et al. Changing appearance of retinal arteriovenous malformation. *Graefes Arch Klin Exp Ophthalmol.* 1980;215:65–70.

Font RL, Ferry AP. The phakomatoses. *Int Ophthalmol Clin.* 1972;12:1–50.

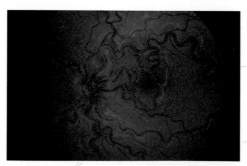

FIG XXVII-14—Racemose angioma of the retina, left eye.

CHAPTER XXVIII

Craniofacial Malformations

Approach to the Child with Craniofacial and Ocular Malformations

Children with congenital malformations and syndromes involving craniofacial structures are at a significant risk for ocular anomalies. The number of syndromes and isolated malformations is enormous, and the spectrum of eye problems vast. Therefore, the reader will find it more productive to develop an approach to the dysmorphic child than to attempt to memorize all ocular pathologic changes reported in the literature. It is useful to consider these findings in two large categories: *intrinsic ocular pathology* and *secondary ocular complications.*

Intrinsic Ocular Pathology

In this group the ocular findings are primary, not secondary, and they are related to the basic defect. The underlying insult, genetic or environmental, results in damage to the developing ocular tissues or their failure to form. Examples include

☐ Myopia and retinal pathologic changes in Stickler syndrome

☐ Anterior segment developmental anomalies associated with systemic anomalies, fetal alcohol syndrome, chromosomal anomalies

☐ Ocular colobomas in many syndromes

☐ Ocular muscle anomalies of position or size in craniosynostosis syndrome

☐ Cranial nerve/ocular motility involvement in Möbius syndrome, thalidomide embryopathy, Duane syndrome with systemic abnormalities

Secondary Ocular Complications

Complications secondary to changes in size, shape, or position of bony and soft-tissue orbital structures may occur as disruption or deformation during development, or they may be acquired after birth. These complications are derived changes that can be anticipated from the malformations present in the surrounding tissues. They are not necessarily specific to a syndrome but the result of a type of deformity or mechanical factors. Thus, the same anomaly may occur in various types of syndromes. Prototypes in this group are

☐ Corneal exposure resulting from extreme proptosis or eyelid defects (in craniosynostosis syndromes, corneal ulceration would be caused by shallow orbits that lead to proptosis)

☐ Refractive errors associated with soft-tissue anomalies of eyelid and adnexa (astigmatism appears in patients with eyelid coloboma or dermoids)

☐ Ocular motility deviations associated with abnormal position or shape of the orbits (exotropia with hypertelorism)

□ Papilledema or optic atrophy secondary to increased intracranial pressure (ICP) or local factors (craniosynostosis); optic atrophy secondary to fibrous dysplasia involving the optic canal

□ Ocular anomalies that are caused by environmental factors during embryogenesis (corneal opacities and eyelid colobomas in some patients with amniotic band syndrome)

Cohen MM Jr. *The Child with Multiple Birth Defects.* 2nd ed. New York: Oxford University Press; 1997.

Leppig KA, Werler MM, Cann CI, et al. Predictive value of minor anomalies. I. Association with major malformations. *J Pediatr.* 1987;110:531–537.

Spranger J, Benirschke K, Hall JG, et al. Errors of morphogenesis: concepts and terms. Recommendations of an international working group. *J Pediatr.* 1982;100:160–165.

Selected Craniofacial Syndromes

Craniosynostosis

Craniosynostosis is the premature closure of the cranial sutures in the embryonic period or early childhood. Normally, most cranial sutures do not close until adulthood. The involved synostosed suture(s) determines the shape of the skull, since growth is inhibited perpendicular to the closed suture. Compensatory growth occurs not only at the open sutures but also in weakened areas of the cranial vault. Variable patterns of suture closure may result in a wide spectrum of skull shapes. Mental retardation may occur, but many patients show normal intellectual capacity.

Craniosynostosis can occur as a primary isolated anomaly, or it can be associated with systemic malformations resulting from a variety of etiologic conditions (e.g., metabolic diseases, chromosomal anomalies, nutritional factors, or mendelian genetic syndromes). The most frequently encountered group, the *craniosynostosis syndromes,* usually show an autosomal dominant transmission (e.g., Apert, Crouzon, Pfeiffer, Saethre-Chotzen), although a few show autosomal recessive inheritance (e.g., Marshall syndrome). Mutations in the fibroblast growth factor receptors (FGFR-1–3) have been found in several of the syndromes.

Common systemic features of this syndrome group include abnormally shaped skull, midfacial hypoplasia, hypertelorism, oral and dental problems, and respiratory difficulties (Fig XXVIII-1). Syndactyly is seen in a number of the syndromes, including Apert, Saethre-Chotzen, and Pfeiffer.

Ocular complications Poor vision in one or both eyes is frequently seen in patients with craniosynostosis. It may be present at birth, develop slowly or rapidly (usually in childhood), or occur as a complication of reconstructive orbital surgery. Several low-frequency anomalies (e.g., cataracts, retinal pigmentary changes, keratoconus, ptosis) have also been reported.

Proptosis in craniosynostosis results from a reduced volume of the bony orbital space secondary to a variety of anatomic factors and differs from proptosis secondary to orbital masses. Although the ophthalmic complaints and complications are similar in both etiologies, the definitive treatment may be different. The severity of the proptosis in craniosynostosis patients is not uniform and frequently increases with age as a result of the impaired growth of the bony orbit.

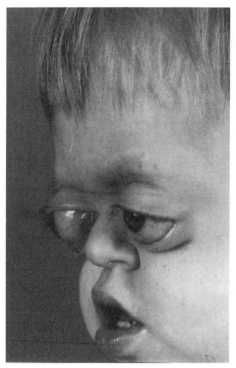

FIG XXVIII-1—Side view of patient with Crouzon syndrome showing midfacial hypoplasia, very prominent eyes that developed severe corneal exposure and ulceration, and "parrot beak." (Reproduced by permission from Miller MT. Ocular malformations in craniofacial malformations. *Int Ophthalmol Clin.* 1984;24:148.)

Because the eyelids may not afford adequate protection for the globe, the most serious complication of severe proptosis is corneal exposure. Exposure keratitis results, and if inadequately managed, perforation of the globe and irreversible damage to the eye may occur in some patients. The progression of proptosis caused by craniosynostosis syndromes may be slow, permitting conservative treatment such as use of lubricating ointment. However, if the exorbitism is severe or rapidly progressive, an emergency tarsorrhaphy may be indicated. This procedure is still not a definitive treatment because the underlying cause of shallow orbit has not been eliminated.

Rarely, the eye may be completely dislocated because of the extremely shallow orbit, constituting a medical emergency because of the problems of corneal exposure and possible compromise of the blood supply to the eye and/or conjunctiva. The clinician can sometimes retroplace the eye by gently bringing the upper eyelid over the globe with a finger. If conjunctival prolapse occurs, treatment must be aimed at keeping the exposed conjunctiva moist.

Closure of certain crucial cranial sutures, especially the coronal, frequently results in increased intracranial pressure and papilledema. If this is not reversed, optic atrophy occurs. Some authors suggest that optic atrophy is always secondary to high ICP, while others believe that local changes in the optic canal can also cause damage to the optic nerve in some cases. Optic atrophy is infrequent if the sagittal suture is the only one involved or if suture closure is unilateral. The latter results in an asymmetric skull, or *plagiocephaly.*

A mild, chronic type of papilledema without retinal hemorrhages has also been described. This form of papilledema is difficult to differentiate from pseudo-papilledema, a condition in which the optic disc gives the false appearance of papilledema. Papilledema may also disappear without residual signs. The apparent increased frequency of tortuous vasculature reported in craniosynostosis has been suggested as evidence of previous papilledema. Chapter XXV, Optic Nerve Disorders, also discusses papilledema and pseudopapilledema.

Strabismus and amblyopia Patients with craniosynostosis demonstrate a variety of horizontal deviations in primary position, with exotropia the most frequent. The most consistent finding, however, is a marked V pattern, most commonly with a large exotropia on upgaze and a small exotropia, orthophoria, or esotropia on downgaze. Often this V pattern is accompanied by a marked, apparent overaction or pseudo-overaction of the inferior oblique muscles, frequently caused by abnormal insertions of the rectus muscles. Some patients show a definite limitation of movement on testing of ocular movements in various fields of action, especially in connection with the superior rectus muscle. Ocular muscles in a number of patients have been shown on CT or MRI or seen at the time of surgery to be abnormally inserted or unusually small. Amblyopia is common secondary to strabismus or refractive differences between the two eyes. Recognition of the risk factors aids in prevention or reversal with treatment.

Management Major advances in reconstructive surgery for severe craniofacial malformation have occurred in the last 25 years. This surgery is frequently extensive in nature and involves en bloc movement of the facial structures. The status of the visual system should be documented preoperatively, and certain relationships such as intercanthal and interpupillary distance as well as palpebral fissure should be measured. Postoperatively, the function of the visual system should be reevaluated and appropriate treatment instituted.

The medical team determines the timing of the reconstructive surgery by prioritizing the child's multiple problems. However, vision-threatening corneal exposure and ulceration may precipitate a decision by the team to intervene earlier than they would otherwise have chosen. Postoperative corneal damage, which may go unnoticed because of transient or permanent decrease in corneal sensation, may be caused by bandage abrasion of the cornea or exposure from incomplete protection by the eyelids as a result of postoperative edema. Changes in the position of the eye or the canthi may also occur, and ptosis and new symptoms of lacrimal system obstruction may ensue.

Additionally, reconstructive surgery that involves moving the orbits may significantly change the degree or type of strabismus, thereby modifying the strabismus surgery indicated. Another consideration is that improved binocular function may not be attainable in these patients because of their unusual and incomitant form of ocular muscle imbalance. Thus, early surgery is of no particular advantage, and deferring treatment may be appropriate.

Cohen MM. *The Child with Multiple Birth Defects.* 2nd ed. New York: Oxford University Press; 1997:178–196.

Other Craniofacial Anomalies

Hypertelorism   This descriptive term indicates increased separation (>2 standard deviation) between the bony orbits; it is not a diagnostic entity. It may be the result of morphokinetic arrest during embryogenesis and is usually sporadic. Mild to moderate hypertelorism is found in many syndromes but occurs most frequently in the *median facial cleft syndrome (frontonasal dysplasia).* Characteristic findings in this syndrome are medial cleft nose, lip, and palate; a widow's peak; and cranium bifidum occultum. It usually occurs sporadically. The most common abnormality is a nonparetic form of exotropia. Occasionally, epibulbar dermoids, palpebral fissure changes, Duane syndrome, and optic atrophy have been reported. Lacrimal system anomalies are frequent, with symptomatic tearing and infection. In reconstructive repair of hypertelorism the anterior part of the orbits is rotated inward, thus reducing the pupillary distance and frequently decreasing the exotropia.

Waardenburg syndrome   Affected patients with this autosomal dominant disorder may have any of the following:

□ Lateral displacement of the inner canthi and lacrimal puncta

□ Confluent eyebrows

□ Heterochromia iridis (complete or partial)

□ Congenital bilateral sensorineural deafness

□ White forelocks

□ Fundus hypopigmentation

Hemifacial microsomia   Other terms for this condition are *hemifacial hypoplasia, oculoauriculovertebral dysplasia, first and second arch syndrome,* and *Goldenhar syndrome.* They describe a group of patients with microtia, macrostomia, and mandibular anomalies (Fig XXVIII-2). Ear tags frequently appear, as do inner ear anomalies in some cases. Vertebral anomalies are common; the central nervous system occasionally is affected. Most, but not all, patients show unilateral involvement (70%–80%). Ocular manifestations may range from clinical anophthalmos to minor fissure asymmetry.

Goldenhar syndrome   Also known as *oculoauriculovertebral dysplasia,* this condition is proposed to represent a variant of the above group, with characteristic epibulbar dermoids or lipodermoids, usually in the inferotemporal quadrant. Limbal dermoids are reported more frequently than lipodermoids, and they may occasionally be bilateral (25%). They occasionally impinge on the visual axis but more commonly interfere with visual acuity by causing astigmatism and predisposing to secondary strabismus from anisometropic amblyopia. Another common finding is an upper eyelid coloboma, almost always on the most affected side. Duane syndrome has been reported in some patients with Goldenhar syndrome. Low-incidence anomalies include decreased corneal sensitivity, cataract, and iris abnormalities.

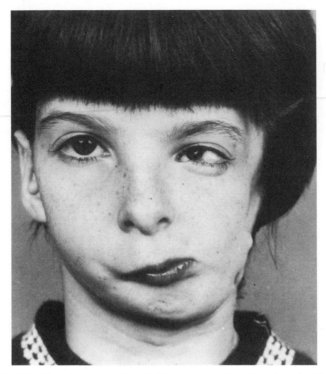

FIG XXVIII-2—Hemifacial microsomia, Goldenhar variant. Patient has facial asymmetry, hypoplastic left ear, ear tag near right ear, conjunctival lipodermoid in left eye, and esotropia. Patient also has a left Duane syndrome.

Hallermann-Streiff syndrome   Also known as *oculomandibulofacial dyscephaly*, this condition is characterized by mandibular hypoplasia, beaked nose, and bilateral cataracts often associated with microphthalmos or microcornea or both. Spontaneous resorption of the lens has been reported frequently; occasionally, patients present with apparent congenital aphakia. Glaucoma may complicate the ocular findings. Additional anomalies may include atrophy of the facial skin, hypotrichosis, and marked dwarfism with dental and nasal abnormalities. All cases have been sporadic, and the causative factors are unknown.

Pierre Robin sequence (anomaly, deformity)   This condition is characterized by micrognathia, glossoptosis, and cleft palate. These abnormalities occur in a variety of syndromes, and associated ocular anomalies include retinal detachment, microphthalmos, congenital glaucoma, cataracts, and high myopia. The Pierre Robin sequence is a frequent finding in *Stickler syndrome.*

Mandibulofacial dysostosis (Treacher Collins–Franceschetti syndrome)   This disorder is characterized by bilateral involvement of facial structures, including malar and

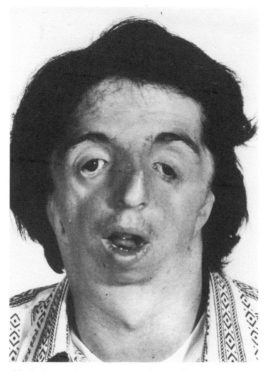

FIG XXVIII-3—Mandibulofacial dysostosis (Treacher Collins–Franceschetti syndrome). Note downward slant of palpebral fissure, low-set abnormal ears, notch or curving of inferotemporal eyelid margin, and maxillary and mandibular hypoplasia. (Reproduced by permission from Peyman GA, Sanders DR, Goldberg MF. *Principles and Practice of Ophthalmology.* Philadelphia: Saunders; 1980:2411.)

mandibular hypoplasia, microstomia, coloboma in the outer third of the lower lid, and external and middle ear anomalies (Fig XXVIII-3).

In the severe form the zygomatic bone is underdeveloped and may be absent. A fissure in the maxilla and a defect in the lower margin of the orbit are often present. Hypoplasia of the supraorbital rim has also been observed.

In about 50% of the patients the lateral canthus is displaced downward, producing the characteristic antimongoloid slant. At times the lower eyelid coloboma produces the illusion of a slant. Deficiency in the cilia medial to the eyelid coloboma may also occur, as may a number of low-incidence anomalies such as iris coloboma and absence of lower lacrimal puncta and meibomian glands. The syndrome is inherited as an autosomal dominant trait with incomplete penetrance and variable expressivity.

Dixon MJ. Treacher Collins syndrome. *J Med Genet.* 1995;32:806–808.

Gorlin RJ, Cohen MM, Levin LS. *Syndromes of the Head and Neck.* 3rd ed. New York: Oxford University Press; 1990.

Hertle RW, Ziylan S, Katowitz JA. Ophthalmic features and visual prognosis in the Treacher-Collins syndrome. *Br J Ophthalmol.* 1993;77:642–645.

Fetal Alcohol Syndrome

A pattern of malformations has been observed in children born to women with a history of heavy alcohol use during pregnancy. Alcohol and other teratogens can produce a wide range of effects on the developing fetus depending on consumption or dose, timing of intake, genetic background, and so on. The presence of certain dysmorphic features along with other symptoms and signs has been designated *fetal alcohol syndrome* (FAS) (Fig XXVIII-4). The more consistent characteristics of FAS include

- Facial abnormalities with short palpebral fissures, thin vermilion border of upper lip, and epicanthal folds
- Mental retardation varying in degree from mild to severe
- Small weight and height at birth that persist in the postnatal period
- Abnormalities of cardiovascular and skeletal systems

The most frequently reported ocular finding in FAS is a small palpebral fissure with increased distance between the medial canthi. The increased distance is caused by a soft-tissue disturbance, *primary telecanthus,* and does not reflect an increase in bony interorbital distance, or hypertelorism. A high incidence of ptosis, often asymmetric, has also been noted. A comitant type of strabismus is a frequent finding, occurring in about 50% of patients with complete FAS.

Visual acuity is often reduced as a result of a variety of causes, both refractive and organic. High myopia is present in some patients. Anterior segment anomalies, including microphthalmos and forms of mesenchymal dysgenesis (e.g., Peters anomaly), have been noted in a number of patients, although this finding cannot be classified as characteristic. It has been proposed that the anterior segment anomalies may represent a teratogenic action of alcohol during a very narrow critical period of development.

The most serious eye problems are retinal and optic nerve anomalies that range from hypoplasia of the optic nerve head to increased tortuosity of retinal vasculature. Optic disc anomalies are the most common malformations of the fundus (up to 48%). Frequently, the disc is small with sharp and often irregular margins; the condition may be unilateral or bilateral. A combination of anomalies of the optic disc and the retinal vessels is a typical finding in the fundus of an FAS child.

Clarren SK, Smith DW. The fetal alcohol syndrome. *N Engl J Med.* 1978;298:1063–1067.

Miller MT, Epstein RJ, Sugar J, et al. Anterior segment anomalies associated with the fetal alcohol syndrome. *J Pediatr Ophthalmol Strabismus.* 1984;21:8–18.

Stromland K. Ocular involvement in the fetal alcohol syndrome. *Surv Ophthalmol.* 1987;31:277–284.

Stromland K, Hellstrom A. Fetal alcohol syndrome—an ophthalmological and socioeducational prospective study. *Pediatrics.* 1996;97:845–850.

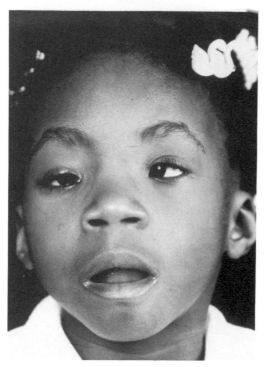

FIG XXVIII-4—Fetal alcohol syndrome. Asymmetric ptosis; telecanthus; strabismus; long, flat philtrum; anteverted nostrils. This child also had a Peters anomaly of the left cornea and myopia of the right eye. (Reproduced by permission from Miller MT. Fetal alcohol syndrome. *J Pediatr Ophthalmol Strabismus.* 1981;18:6–15.)

Fetal Hydantoin Syndrome (FHS)

Offspring of women treated with hydantoins for convulsive disorders show a variable pattern of altered growth, decreased mental performance, unusual facies, and systemic malformations. Although severe ocular abnormalities are rare, strabismus, ptosis, hypertelorism, and epicanthal folds have been reported. These children also frequently have a broad and/or depressed nasal bridge and microcephaly. Although congenital anomalies occur in 4%–5% of children born to epileptic mothers not taking anticonvulsants (compared with a normal incidence of 2%–3%), the rate increases to 6%–11% if the mother is taking anticonvulsants.

Davies SM. Epilepsy and pregnancy. *Am Fam Physician.* 1986;34:179–183.

Jones KL. Fetal hydantoin effects. In: Jones KL, ed. *Smith's Recognizable Patterns of Human Malformation.* 5th ed. Philadelphia: Saunders; 1997:559.

CHAPTER XXIX

Ocular Findings in Inborn Errors of Metabolism

With advances in ophthalmology and medicine over the past 50 years, and the elimination of infectious diseases and cataract as major causes of blindness in the United States and other industrialized countries, genetic and metabolic disorders affecting the eye have assumed a much larger role in visual impairment and blindness. Ophthalmologists must therefore be increasingly knowledgeable concerning the ophthalmic manifestations of genetic and metabolic disorders. Genetic disorders are also discussed in detail in BCSC Section 2, *Fundamentals and Principles of Ophthalmology.*

Inborn errors of metabolism are a group of disorders characterized by the genetic absence, either physically or functionally, of one or more enzymes. This enzyme deficiency creates a block in one of the many metabolic or biochemical pathways critical to the normal growth, development, or functioning of the organism. Clinically, the enzyme deficiency may produce the observed ocular changes in one of three ways, as shown in Figure XXIX-1.

Inborn errors of metabolism are generally inherited as recessive disorders. The presence of half the normal quantity of an enzyme, as expected in patients with one normal gene and one defective one, results in adequate metabolic function. Carrier detection is generally possible by measurement of enzyme activity in suspected carriers, where documentation of enzyme levels that are half of normal is frequently diagnostic of the carrier state. Furthermore, measurement of enzyme levels in fetal cells obtained through amniocentesis has made prenatal detection of many of these metabolic conditions possible. Different clinical pictures can be caused by different but allelic mutations or compound mutations where each of the pair of chromosomes has a different mutation in the same gene. In some disorders the control of an enzyme is defective rather than the enzyme itself.

Ophthalmologists must be aware of the ophthalmic manifestations of inborn errors of metabolism, both in carriers and in affected individuals. Eye findings may be the earliest signs in a number of systemic disorders such as the phakomatoses, connective tissue disorders, metabolic disorders, and albinism. Early diagnosis of these conditions permits genetic counseling regarding the risk of recurrence of a particular disorder in the family, as well as aids in determining the prognosis and clinical expectations for affected individuals. In addition, through genetic counseling, services such as prenatal testing using amniocentesis can be made available to an affected family.

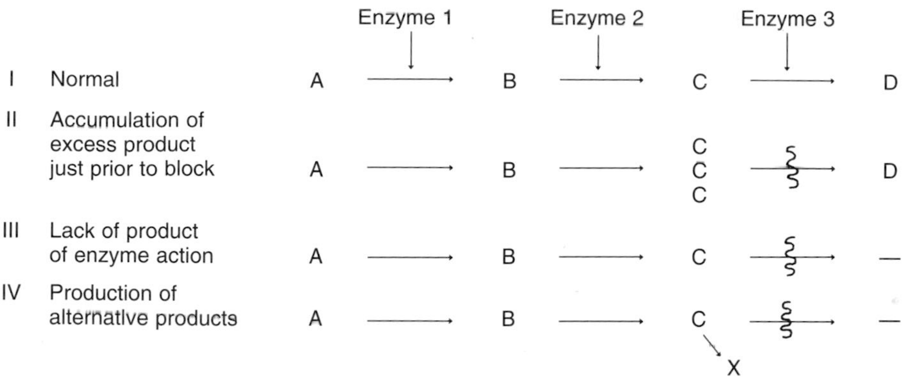

		Enzyme 1		Enzyme 2		Enzyme 3	
I	Normal	A ———→	B	———→	C	———→	D
II	Accumulation of excess product just prior to block	A ———→	B	———→	C C C	—‖→	D
III	Lack of product of enzyme action	A ———→	B	———→	C	—‖→	—
IV	Production of alternative products	A ———→	B	———→	C↘X	—‖→	—

FIG XXIX-1—In the normal state, substance A is converted by enzyme 1 to substance B, which is converted by enzyme 2 to substance C, etc. The absence of functional enzyme 3 may result in an accumulation of excess product C just prior to the block, as is clinically observed in alkaptonuria. Alternatively, deficiency of enzyme 3 may result in a lack of the product of this enzyme's action, as in albinism. Finally, a deficiency of enzyme 3 may block the normal conversion of product C to product D and result in the up-regulation of alternative pathways, which produce abnormal products or products normally present in very low quantity. These abnormal products may be toxic and produce disease manifestations as in phenylketonuria.

Table XXIX-1 summarizes the common ophthalmic manifestations of the major inborn errors of metabolism that affect the eye. Evaluation of suspected patients should include

☐ Complete ocular and family history

☐ Examination of other family members for additional evidence or findings that confirm the carrier state

☐ Complete ocular examination focusing on the expected findings

☐ Appropriate, directed laboratory testing

Scriver CR, Beaudet AL, Sly WS, et al, eds. *The Metabolic and Molecular Bases of Inherited Disease.* 7th ed. New York: McGraw-Hill; 1995.

Table XXIX-1

Ocular Findings in Mucopolysaccharidoses, Mucolipidoses, Lipidoses, Gangliosidoses, and Miscellaneous Disorders

DISEASE	ENZYME DEFICIENCY	CORNEAL CLOUDING	MOTILITY DISORDERS	CHERRY-RED SPOT	RPE DEGENERATION	OPTIC ATROPHY	OTHER	INHERITANCE
Mucopolysaccharidoses								
MPS IH, IS Hurler (25280)* Scheie	alpha iduronidase	+++	–	–	+++	+	glaucoma papilledema	AR
MPS II Hunter (30990)	iduronate sulfatase	–	–	–	++	+	–	XR
MPS III Sanfilippo (25290)	A: heparan N-sulfatase B: N-acetyl-α-D-glucosaminidase	+	–	–	++	rare	late blindness	AR
MPS IV Morquio (25300)	A: N-acetyl-galactosamine-6-sulfatase B: β-galactosidase	++	–	–	rare	rare	–	AR
MPS VI Maroteaux-Lamy (25320)	arylsulfatase B	++	–	–	–	+	papilledema glaucoma	AR
MPS VII Sly (25322)	β-glucuronidase	+	–	–	–	–	–	AR
Mucolipidoses								
Type I (25240) sialidosis (type 2) cherry-red spot myoclonus syndrome	neuraminidase	–	+	+	+	–	hearing loss	AR
Type II I-cell disease (25250)	multiple lysosomal enzymes	++	–	–	–	–	Hurler-like	AR
Type III pseudo-Hurler polydystrophy (25260)	multiple lysosomal enzymes	+++	–	–	–	–	Hurler-like puffy eyelids (25260)	AR
Type IV (25265)	partial ganglioside sialidase	+++	–	–	++	+	photophobia	AR
Lipidoses								
Niemann-Pick disease (25720)	sphingomyelinase	+	nystagmus	+	–	+	eventual vision loss	AR
Fabry disease (30150)	α-galactosidase A	whorl-like	–	–	–	–	angiokeratoma, spokelike cataract, aneurysmal conjunctival vessels	XR
Gaucher disease (Type 1 23080) (Type II 23090) (Type III 23100)	glucocerebrosidase	–	paralytic strabismus, looped saccades	–	+	–	pinguecula, conjunctival pigmentation	AR
Metachromatic leukodystrophy (25010)	arylsulfatase A	–	nystagmus	+	–	+	blindness, decreased pupil reaction	AR
Krabbe disease (24520)	galactocerebrosidase	–	nystagmus	rare	–	+	cortical blindness	AR
Fucosidosis (23000)	α-L-fucosidase	–	–	–	+	–	Hurler-like features, angiokeratoma tortuous conjunctival vessels	AR

Gangliosidoses

DISEASE	ENZYME DEFICIENCY	CONJUNCT. TORTUOSITY	CORNEAL CLOUDING	MOTILITY DISORDERS	CHERRY-RED SPOT	RPE DEGENERATION	OPTIC ATROPHY	HIGH MYOPIA	BLINDNESS	INHERITANCE
Generalized (GM_1) gangliosidosis										
(1) Type I (23050)	β-galactosidase A, B, and C	+	±	ET, nystagmus	50% of patients	-	+	+	+	AR
(2) Type II (23060) Derry disease juvenile GM_1	β-galactosidase B and C	-	-	ET, nystagmus	-	+	±	-	late	AR
(3) Type III (23065) adult GM_1	β-galactosidase (partial)	±	rare	-	-	-	-	-	-	AR
GM_2 gangliosidosis										
(1) Type I (27280) Tay-Sachs disease	hexosaminidase A	-	-	nystagmus, ophthalmoplegia	+	-	+	-	+	AR
(2) Type II (26880) Sandhoff disease	hexosaminidase A and B	-	rare	ET	+	-	±	-	+	AR
(3) Type III (23065) juvenile GM_2 Bernheimer-Seitelberger disease	hexosaminidase A (partial)	-	-	-	-	+	+	-	late	AR

Miscellaneous Disorders

DISEASE	ENZYME DEFICIENCY	CORNEAL CLOUDING	MOTILITY DISORDERS	CHERRY-RED SPOT	RPE DEGENERATION	OPTIC ATROPHY	OTHER	INHERITANCE
Galactosialidosis	β-galactosidase neuraminidase	+	-	+	-	+	dwarfism, seizures, coarse facies	AR
Ceroid lipofuscinosis (20420)								
Hagberg-Santavuori disease	unknown	-	+	Macular	+	+	blindness	AR
Jansky-Bielschowsky disease	unknown	-	+	bull's	+	+	blindness	AR
Spielmeyer-Vogt disease	unknown	-	+	eye	+	+	blindness	AR
Kufs disease	unknown	-	-	-	-	-		AR
Cystinosis (21980)	unknown	crystals	-	-	++	-	conjunctival crystals, renal problems	AR
Galactosemia (23040)	gal-1-PO_4 uridyl transferase	-	-	-	-	-	cataracts if not treated	AR
Mannosidosis (24850)	α-mannosidase	++	-	-	-	pallor, blurred margin	Hurler-like, spokelike cataract	AR
Homocystinuria (23620)	cystathionine β-synthase	-	-	-	+	-	dislocated lens, cataract	AR
Refsum disease (26650)	phytanic acid α-hydrolase	-	-	-	++	-	cataract, night blindness	AR

*These code numbers refer to the system developed by Victor McKusick (McKusick VA, Francomano CA, Antonarakis SE. *Mendelian Inheritance in Man: Catalogs of Autosomal Dominant, Autosomal Recessive, and X-linked Phenotypes*. 10th ed. Baltimore: The Johns Hopkins University Press; 1992).
Plus (+) and minus (–) signs indicate the relative likelihood of occurrence of ocular findings in these systemic disorders.

CHAPTER XXX

Ocular Trauma in Childhood

Trauma is one of the most important causes of ocular morbidity in childhood. Only strabismus ranks higher in frequency among reasons for pediatric eye surgery, and only amblyopia is responsible for more early acquired monocular vision loss. Children 11–15 years old have a particularly high incidence of severe eye injury in comparison with other age groups. Injured boys outnumber girls by a factor of 3 or 4 to 1.

Most ocular trauma in younger children occurs during casual play with age mates. Older children and adolescents are most likely to be injured while participating in sports. A majority of serious childhood eye injuries could thus in principle be prevented by appropriate adult supervision and by regular use of protective eyewear for sports. Fireworks and BB guns are among the less frequent causes of pediatric ocular trauma, but the severity of the injuries they are likely to produce is significant.

> Vinger PF. Athletic eye injuries and appropriate protection. In: *Focal Points: Clinical Modules for Ophthalmologists.* San Francisco: American Academy of Ophthalmology; 1997;15:8.

Several special considerations must be kept in mind while managing eye trauma in very young patients. First, the difficulty of evaluation and treatment is often considerably increased by inadequate cooperation. Even school-age children, stressed by the recent injury, may put up strong resistance against any approach to the eye. Overcoming the child's opposition by force creates a risk of exacerbating the damage caused by penetrating wounds or blunt impact. In a child more than 3 years old a forceful approach may make it exceedingly difficult to establish rapport needed for subsequent treatment. Examination in cases likely to involve minor injury can be facilitated by instilling topical anesthesia and by giving the child a chance to calm down in quiet surroundings. When assessment of the circumstances of injury or limited inspection indicates that prompt surgical treatment may be necessary, it is appropriate to defer detailed physical examination of the eye until the patient is in the operating room under general anesthesia.

A second issue in the care of children with eye trauma is the potential for the injury or its treatment to lead to visual loss from amblyopia. In children younger than age 5 years visual deprivation amblyopia associated with traumatic cataract or other media opacity may be more likely to result in severe long-term reduction of acuity than the original physical damage. Minimizing the interval between injury and restoration of optimal media clarity and optics, including adequate aphakic refractive correction, must be a high priority. Monocular occlusion following injury should be kept to a minimum as well; the expected benefit from an occlusive dressing must be weighed against the risk of disturbing binocular function or inducing amblyopia.

Child Abuse

While most eye injuries in childhood are accidental or innocently caused by other children, a significant portion result from physical abuse by adults. Child abuse is a pervasive problem in our society, with an estimated 2 million victims per year in the United States. Abusive behavior in a parent or other care giver usually reflects temporary loss of control during a period of anger or stress rather than premeditated cruelty. Lack of knowledge of the proper way to care for or discipline a child is also a frequent contributing factor. In the relatively rare *Münchausen syndrome by proxy* the child is physically harmed by a psychopathic parent to create signs of illness in an effort to manipulate medical care providers.

A reliable history is often difficult to obtain when child abuse has occurred. Suspicion should be aroused when repeated accounts of the circumstances of injury or histories obtained from different individuals are inconsistent or when the events described seem to conflict with the extent of injuries (e.g., bruises on multiple aspects of the head after a fall) or with the child's developmental level (e.g., a 2-month-old rolling off a bed, or a 6-month-old climbing out of a high chair).

Any physician who *suspects* that child abuse might have occurred is required by law in every U.S. state and Canadian province to report the incident to a designated governmental agency. Once this obligation has been discharged, the ophthalmologist is probably best advised to leave full investigation of the situation to appropriate specialists or authorities.

The presenting sign of child abuse involves the eye in approximately 5% of cases, and ocular manifestations are detected in the course of evaluating many others. Blunt trauma inflicted with fingers, fists, or implements such as belts or straps is the usual mechanism of nonaccidental injury to the ocular adnexa or anterior segment. Periorbital ecchymosis, subconjunctival hemorrhage, and hyphema should raise suspicion of recent abuse if the explanation provided is less than completely plausible. Cataract and lens dislocation may be signs of repeated injury or trauma inflicted more remotely in the past. A majority of rhegmatogenous retinal detachments that occur in childhood have a traumatic origin; abuse should be suspected when such a finding is encountered in a child without a history of injury or an apparent predisposing factor such as high myopia. By far, the most common posterior segment manifestation of child abuse is retinal hemorrhage, usually a consequence of shaking injury.

Friendly DS. Ocular manifestations of physical child abuse. *Trans Am Acad Ophthalmol Otolaryngol.* 1971;75:318–332.

Levin AV. The ocular findings in child abuse. In: *Focal Points: Clinical Modules for Ophthalmologists.* San Francisco: American Academy of Ophthalmology; 1998;16:7.

Strahlman E, Elman M, Daub E, et al. Causes of pediatric eye injuries: A population-based study. *Arch Ophthalmol.* 1990;108:603–606.

Shaking Injury

A unique complex of ocular, intracranial, and sometimes other injuries is seen in infants who have been abused by violent shaking. The essential features of what is now generally known as *shaken baby syndrome* were first identified in the early 1970s, and the syndrome became widely recognized as one of the most important forms of child abuse during the 1980s.

Victims of shaking injury are always under 3 years old and usually under 12 months. When a reliable history is available, it typically involves a parent or other care giver who shook an inconsolably crying baby in anger and frustration. Often, however, the only information provided is that the child's mental status deteriorated or that seizures or respiratory difficulty developed. It may be related that an episode of relatively minor trauma occurred, such as a fall from a bed. Even without a supporting history, the diagnosis of shaken baby syndrome can still be made with confidence on the basis of characteristic clinical findings. It must be kept in mind, however, that answers to important questions concerning the timing and circumstances of injury and the identity of the perpetrator frequently cannot be inferred from medical evidence alone.

Intracranial injury in shaken infants almost always includes subdural hematoma, typically bilateral over the cerebral convexities or in the interhemispheric fissure. Evidence of subarachnoid bleeding is also often apparent. In many cases cerebral parenchymal damage is manifest on neuroimaging, acutely as edema, ischemia, or contusion, and in later stages as atrophy. These findings are believed to result from repetitive abrupt deceleration of the child's head as it whiplashes back and forth during the shaking episode. Some authorities, citing the frequency with which shaken baby syndrome victims also show evidence of having received blows to the head, believe that impact is an essential component of the condition's causation. Displacement of the brain in relation to the skull and dura mater ruptures bridging vessels, and compression against the cranial bones produces further damage. The infant's head is particularly vulnerable to such effects because of its relatively large mass in relation to the body and poor stabilization by neck muscles.

Ocular involvement   The most common ocular manifestation of shaking injury, present in a large majority of cases, is retinal hemorrhage. Preretinal, nerve fiber layer, deep retinal, or subretinal localization may be seen. Hemorrhages tend to be concentrated in or near the macular region but not uncommonly are so extensive that they occupy nearly the entire fundus (Fig XXX-1). Vitreous hemorrhage may also develop, usually as a secondary phenomenon resulting from migration of blood that was initially intraretinal. Occasionally, the vitreous becomes almost completely opacified by dispersed hemorrhage within a few days of injury. Retinal hemorrhages in shaken infants resolve over a period ranging from 1 or 2 weeks to several months, showing gradual reduction in volume and extent but no characteristic change in the appearance of extravasated blood. Vitreous hemorrhage may persist for many months or even years. Consideration should be given to vitrectomy if amblyopia is threatened.

Some eyes of shaken infants show evidence of retinal tissue disruption in addition to hemorrhage. Full-thickness folds in the neurosensory retina, typically with circumferential orientation around the macula that creates a craterlike appearance, are highly characteristic. Splitting of the retina (traumatic retinoschisis), either deep to the nerve fiber layer or superficial involving only the internal limiting membrane, may create partially blood-filled cavities of considerable extent, also usually in the macular region (Fig XXX-2). Full-thickness retinal breaks and detachment are rarely seen. Retinal folds usually flatten out within a few weeks of injury, but schisis cavities can persist indefinitely.

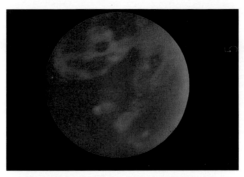

FIG XXX-1—Extensive retinal hemorrhages, left eye, in a 2-month-old infant believed to have been violently shaken. Temporal portion of the disc is visible near the left edge of the photograph.

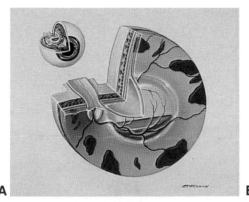
A

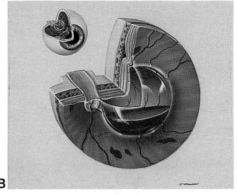
B

FIG XXX-2—Traumatic retinoschisis. A, Deep splitting of the retina, typically associated with severe permanent visual impairment and loss of ERG b-wave. B, Superficial splitting, with separation of the internal limiting membrane and a full-thickness perimacular fold. Recovery of good vision is frequently observed. (Reproduced by permission from Greenwald MJ. The shaken baby syndrome. *Semin Ophthalmol.* 1990;5:202–213. Illustrations by S. Gordon.)

The mechanism of ocular injury in shaken baby syndrome remains a matter of controversy. Some authorities believe that intraocular hemorrhages result from increased pressure in retinal veins, secondary either to increased intracranial pressure from bleeding or edema or to increased intrathoracic pressure from squeezing during the shaking episode. In this scheme retinal folds and schisis are viewed as consequences of blood extravasation. Others have postulated that repetitive vitreoretinal traction resulting from shaking trauma itself causes retinal tissue damage, to which hemorrhage may be secondary.

A striking feature of shaken baby syndrome is the typical lack of external evidence of trauma. The ocular adnexa and anterior segments have an entirely normal appearance. Occasionally, bruises representing the imprint of the perpetrator's hands are seen on the trunk or extremities. In a minority of cases broken ribs or characteristic metaphyseal fractures of the long bones result from forces generated during shaking. It must be kept in mind, however, that many shaken babies are also victims of other forms of abuse. In particular, signs of impact to the head must be carefully sought.

When extensive retinal hemorrhage accompanied by perimacular folds and schisis cavities is found in association with intracranial hemorrhage or other evidence of trauma to the brain in an infant, the diagnosis of shaking injury can be made with confidence regardless of other circumstances. Extensive retinal hemorrhage without other ocular findings strongly suggests that intracranial injury has been caused by shaking, but alternative possibilities such as the presence of a coagulation disorder must be considered as well. Severe accidental head trauma (e.g., sustained in a fall from second-story level or a motor vehicle collision) is infrequently accompanied by retinal hemorrhage, which is virtually never extensive. Retinal hemorrhage is very uncommon and has never been documented to be extensive following cardiopulmonary resuscitation by trained personnel. Spontaneous subarachnoid hemorrhage occurs rarely in young children and may be associated with some degree of intraocular bleeding. Retinal hemorrhages resulting from birth trauma are common in newborns but seldom persist beyond age 1 month.

Prognosis   Many shaken babies die from their injuries. Survivors may suffer permanent impairment ranging from severe retardation and quadriparesis to mild learning disability and motor disturbances. Visual loss from deep retinal splitting, optic nerve damage (from perineural hemorrhage), or cortical injury may be profound, but lesser degrees are typical, and complete or nearly complete recovery of vision is common. Dense vitreous hemorrhage, usually associated with deep traumatic retinoschisis, carries a poor visual prognosis. Vitrectomy should be considered only if bright flash electroretinography shows preservation of the b-wave.

Caffey J. The whiplash shaken infant syndrome: manual shaking by the extremities with whiplash-induced intracranial and intraocular bleeding, linked with residual permanent brain damage and mental retardation. *Pediatrics.* 1974;53:396–403.

Elner SG, Elner VM, Arnall M, et al. Ocular and associated systemic findings in suspected child abuse. A necropsy study. *Arch Ophthalmol.* 1990;108:1094–1101.

Greenwald MJ, Weiss A, Oesterle CS, et al. Traumatic retinoschisis in battered babies. *Ophthalmology.* 1986;93:618–625.

Ludwig S, Warman M. Shaken baby syndrome: a review of 20 cases. *Ann Emerg Med.* 1984;13:104–107.

Superficial Injury

Corneal abrasion is one of the most common ocular injuries among children, as it is among older individuals. Use of a pressure patch to keep the eyelids closed so that an abrasion will heal faster is of questionable value for the preschool child. Obtaining and maintaining the desired effect is difficult in this age group, and if the patch loosens, contact between the cotton eye pad and the ocular surface may actually aggravate the problem. Even moderately large traumatic corneal epithelial defects usually heal within 1–2 days in young children without patching. Use of topical cycloplegic drops and antibiotic ointment may help reduce discomfort and risk of infection.

Cigarette burns of the cornea are the most common thermal injuries to the ocular surface in childhood. Usually, these occur in the 2–4 year age range and are accidental, not manifestations of abuse. They result from the toddler's running into a cigarette held at eye level by an adult. Despite the alarming initial white appearance of coagulated corneal epithelium, cigarette burns typically heal very rapidly and without scarring. Treatment is the same as for mechanical abrasions.

Chemical burns in childhood are generally caused by organic solvents or soaps found in household cleaning agents. Even those involving almost total loss of corneal epithelium are likely to heal in a week or less with or without patching. Acid and alkali burns in children, as in adults, can be much more serious. The initial and most important step in management of all chemical injuries is copious irrigation and meticulous removal of any particulate matter from the conjunctival fornices. See also BCSC Section 8, *External Disease and Cornea.*

Corneal foreign bodies in children can usually be dislodged with a forceful stream of irrigating solution from a small bottle, thus avoiding the need for use of an instrument. When mechanical removal proves necessary, it is better to use a blunt-tipped spud or a battery-powered burr-tipped polishing device than a sharp needle.

Penetrating Injury

Unless an adult has witnessed a traumatic incident, history cannot be relied on to exclude the possibility of penetrating injury to the globe. Thorough inspection of the anterior segment and fundus must be made in suspicious circumstances, using general anesthesia if necessary. An area of subconjunctival hemorrhage or chemosis or a small break in the skin of the eyelid may be the only surface manifestation of scleral perforation by a sharp-pointed object such as a dart or scissors blade (Fig XXX-3). Distortion of the pupil may be the most evident sign of a small corneal or limbal perforation. CT scan of the orbits should be considered if there is any reason to suspect a deeply situated foreign body.

Corneoscleral lacerations in children are repaired according to the same principles as for adults. Corneal wounds heal relatively rapidly in very young patients, however, and sutures should be removed correspondingly early.

Fibrin clots often form quickly in the anterior chamber of a child's eye after a penetrating injury to the cornea, and these can simulate the appearance of fluffy cataractous lens cortex to a remarkable degree. To avoid unnecessarily rendering the eye aphakic (and thereby significantly diminishing the chance for optimal visual rehabilitation), lens removal should not be performed in the course of primary wound repair unless the clinician is absolutely certain that the anterior capsule has been ruptured. Even if lens cortex is exposed, waiting 1–2 weeks until severe post-traumatic inflammation has quieted down before undertaking cataract surgery may result in a smoother recovery and reduced risk of complications, without significantly compromising the visual prognosis. See also BCSC Section 11, *Lens and Cataract.*

Full-thickness eyelid lacerations should be repaired in the operating room under general anesthesia even in older children. Otherwise, working near the eyes with sharp instruments and draping the face to create a sterile field are likely to frighten the patient and add to the difficulty of accomplishing the task at hand. Clearly superficial wounds can be repaired in the emergency room. Use of 6-0 plain or artificial

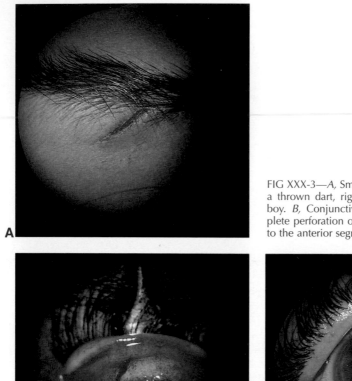

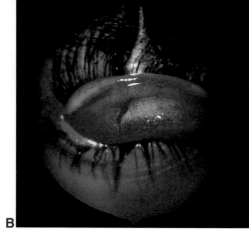

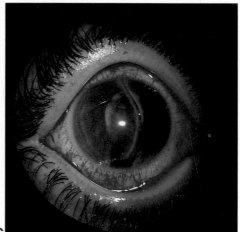

FIG XXX-3—*A,* Small skin entry wound created by a thrown dart, right brow region in a 7-year-old boy. *B,* Conjunctival exit wound indicates complete perforation of the eyelid. *C,* Extensive injury to the anterior segment of the same eye.

absorbable sutures is an acceptable alternative if the physician wishes to avoid the need for removal of nonabsorbable sutures.

Blunt Injury

Hyphema

The management of hyphema in infants and children requires special considerations. As with all forms of pediatric trauma, the precise occurrence that led to intraocular bleeding may be difficult to determine. The possibility of abuse must be considered, as well as the possibility of nontraumatic etiology: retinoblastoma, juvenile xanthogranuloma of the iris, and bleeding diathesis resulting from leukemia or other blood dyscrasia are relatively rare but important causes of spontaneous hyphema during the early years of life. Ultrasonography or CT should be performed to rule out intraocular tumor in suspicious cases where the iris and fundus cannot be adequately seen, and a complete blood count should be performed routinely, with coagulation studies if a bleeding disorder is suspected.

Intraocular pressure, an important parameter for therapeutic decision making with traumatic hyphema, is often very difficult to monitor in the pediatric patient. The risks of making inaccurate measurements and of further traumatizing the injured eye may outweigh the potential value of obtaining results in uncooperative children. With small blood collections, concern about pressure tends to be greatest in patients with sickle cell hemoglobin (Fig XXX-4). Such patients may develop sickling in the anterior chamber, elevating IOP and retarding resorption of blood, or in the retinal circulation, causing vascular occlusion.

It was once common practice to hospitalize all hyphema patients and place them on bed rest with bilateral patching of the eyes. Extreme activity restriction has never been shown to improve prognosis, however, and is particularly to be avoided with children. Hospitalization during the first 5 days after injury, the period of greatest risk for rebleeding, remains justifiable and is one way to ensure opportunity for daily follow-up evaluation and avoidance of running, jumping, or rough play with other children. Outpatient management with daily follow-up is an acceptable alternative.

Medical management of hyphema remains controversial in children as in adults. Cycloplegic and corticosteroid drops are used routinely by many ophthalmologists to facilitate fundus examination, improve comfort, and reduce the risk of inflammatory complications and possibly of rebleeding as well. The value of these topical agents is unproved, however, and some clinicians prefer to use them selectively for control of pain or obvious inflammation or avoid them altogether to minimize manipulation of the eye. Pressure-lowering medication is appropriate for eyes known or strongly suspected to be hypertensive. Aspirin-containing compounds should be scrupulously avoided because of their antiplatelet action.

Oral administration of an antifibrinolytic agent (ε-aminocaproic acid, 50 mg/kg every 4 hours to a maximum of 30 g daily; or tranexamic acid, 25 mg/kg every 8

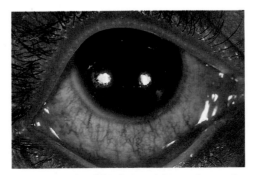

FIG XXX-4—Small hyphema, right eye, in an adolescent girl with sickle trait. Note corneal edema resulting from high intraocular pressure.

hours to a maximum of 4.5 g daily, for 5 days) has been shown in a number of controlled prospective studies to reduce significantly the incidence of rebleeding in traumatic hyphema. On the other hand, one such study limited to children without recent prior ingestion of aspirin-containing compounds showed similar low rates of rebleeding in both control and ε-aminocaproic acid–treated patients. Gastric upset and hypotension may be significant side effects of ε-aminocaproic acid. Recently, topical aminocaproic acid has been demonstrated to be an effective alternative.

Oral prednisone has also been advocated for prophylaxis against rebleeding, and a recent controlled prospective study showed no difference between this agent (at a dosage of 0.6 mg/kg/day to a maximum of 40 mg daily for 5 days) and ε-aminocaproic acid. No serious ocular or systemic side effects have been reported from the treatment of hyphema with any of these drugs.

Surgical evacuation of hyphema is usually performed in adults when early corneal blood staining is detected or when significant IOP elevation has persisted for 5–7 days. The difficulty of detecting early blood staining in a child and the risk that corneal staining may cause severe deprivation amblyopia coupled with the problems of accurately measuring IOP justify earlier surgical intervention whenever a total hyphema persists for 4–5 days. Varied operative techniques have been employed; none has been shown to offer particular advantages in childhood.

Crouch ER Jr, Williams PB, Gray MK, et al. Topical aminocaproic acid in the treatment of traumatic hyphema. *Arch Ophthalmol.* 1997;115:1106–1112.

Deans R, Noel LP, Clarke WN. Oral administration of tranexamic acid in the management of traumatic hyphema in children. *Can J Ophthalmol.* 1992;27:181–183.

Farber MD, Fiscella R, Goldberg MF. Aminocaproic acid versus prednisone for the treatment of traumatic hyphema. A randomized clinical trial. *Ophthalmology.* 1991; 98:279–286.

Kraft SP, Christianson MD, Crawford JS, et al. Traumatic hyphema in children. Treatment with ε-aminocaproic acid. *Ophthalmology.* 1987;94:1232–1237.

Fractures

Children, like adults, may sustain isolated fractures of orbital bone after blunt impact in the region of the eye. The most common such injury in early childhood is fracture of the orbital roof, a finding that is relatively rare at older ages. Isolated roof fractures typically result from impact to the brow region in a fall, often from a height of only a few feet or down a flight of stairs. The principal external manifestation is hematoma in the upper eyelid, usually appearing an hour or more after injury because of the time required for blood to extend to the eyelid from disrupted vessels in the superior orbit (Fig XXX-5). Coronal CT imaging is particularly sensitive for confirming the presence of isolated orbital roof fractures. Most are simple linear breaks that heal uneventfully, and persistent disturbance of ocular motility or eyelid function is unusual. When a fragment of bone is displaced inferiorly, or if evidence suggests a dural tear, neurosurgical repair should be considered because of the possibility of brain tissue herniation into the orbit.

Greenwald MJ, Boston D, Pensler JM, et al. Orbital roof fractures in childhood. *Ophthalmology.* 1989;96:491–497.

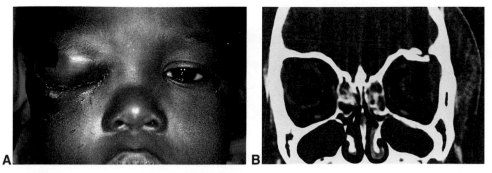

FIG XXX-5—Orbital roof fracture in infants who fell with frontal impact. *A,* Marked right upper eyelid swelling from hematoma originating in the superior orbit adjacent to a linear fracture. *B,* Coronal CT image of a different patient, showing a bone fragment displaced into left orbit.

CHAPTER XXXI

Decreased Vision in
Infants and Children

Visual Inattention in Infants

When the ophthalmologist is confronted with an infant several months of age who has not developed good visual attention or ability to fixate on and follow objects, many etiologies are possible. Most of them have been covered elsewhere in this book in the chapters on cataracts, glaucoma, retinal disorders, and malformations, and cross-references to the appropriate pages are included in the following discussions. Many of these conditions are relatively easily diagnosed by standard ophthalmic examinations. In some, however, the ocular abnormalities are subtle or difficult to detect.

Normal Visual Development

Visual development is a highly complex maturation process. Structural changes occur in both the eye and the central nervous system. Laboratory and clinical research has shown that normal vision develops as a result of both genetic coding and experience in a normal visual environment.

While it would be desirable to quantitate data regarding visual acuity in standard Snellen notation, vision in the newborn and the infant is usually assessed qualitatively. In addition to a clinical appraisal, visual acuity can be evaluated by psychophysical tests such as optokinetic nystagmus testing, visually evoked cortical potentials, and preferential looking techniques.

Several days after birth, a blink reflex to bright light should be present. The pupillary light reflex is usually present after 31 weeks' gestational age, but it can be difficult to evaluate because of miosis in the newborn. At about 6 weeks of age, parent and baby should be able to make and keep eye contact, resulting in gratifying facial responses in a normal child. Horizontal saccades are slower than in an adult. Infants 2–3 months old should be interested in bright objects. Premature infants can be expected to reach these landmarks later, depending on their degree of prematurity.

Occasionally, disconjugate eye movements may be noted during the first several months, but they should not persist after 4 months of age. Skew deviation and "sunsetting" (tonic downward deviation of both eyes) have been observed as transient deviations in the newborn period. In contrast, signs of actual poor visual development include wandering eye movements, lack of response to familiar faces and objects, and nystagmus. Onset of nystagmus secondary to decreased sensory input usually occurs at 2–3 months of life, not at birth. Staring at bright lights in an otherwise visually disinterested infant and forceful rubbing of the eyes (oculodigital reflex) are other signs of poor visual development. The oculodigital reflex suggests an ocular etiology for the visual deficiency.

Approach to the Infant with Decreased Vision

When the ophthalmologist encounters an infant or young child with poor visual attention, inability to fixate on an object, or reduced response to light, many possible conditions should come to mind. A careful history is essential, beginning with a review of vision problems in the family. If the patient is male, the possibility of X-linked disorders should be explored. If a sibling has a similar condition not present in previous generations, an autosomal recessive disease is suggested. Details of the pregnancy should be reviewed, focusing on such factors as maternal infection, radiation, drugs, or trauma. Perinatal problems including prematurity, intrauterine growth retardation, fetal distress, bradycardia, meconium staining, and exposure to oxygen can be important. The clinician should also inquire about the presence of systemic abnormalities or delayed developmental milestones.

Examination of the infant begins with special attention to visual fixation, crispness and equality of pupillary light responses, ocular alignment and motility, and the presence of nystagmus or roving eye movements. An infant with a normal but visually immature visual system may be unresponsive to even a very bright light, appearing indistinguishable from a blind baby. Exotropia may be present, but nystagmus or roving eye movements are usually not seen. The clinician can sometimes observe a fixation and following response in an otherwise unresponsive infant by moving a red light horizontally or vertically in front of the infant.

Nystagmus implies a rhythmic pendular or jerk movement pattern and is a sign of decreased vision. It is not seen in total blindness, however, and thus does imply some visual function. Roving eye movements, on the other hand, imply total or near-total blindness. Congenital motor nystagmus (no organic eye abnormality), which causes only a mild to moderate reduction in visual acuity, may appear in the first month of life. Sensory nystagmus associated with eye abnormalities has a more delayed onset, usually at 2–4 months of age. Chapter XII discusses nystagmus in detail.

Sluggish pupillary responses are seen with anterior visual pathway disease such as optic nerve hypoplasia, optic atrophy, and optic nerve coloboma or morning glory disc anomaly. Paradoxical pupillary phenomenon, or constriction to darkness, implies diffuse retinal disease such as cone dystrophy. Infants with cortical visual impairment have normal pupillary responses.

A cycloplegic refraction is necessary, as is a detailed fundus examination that includes evaluation of the optic nerve, macula, and peripheral retina. A careful search for signs of optic nerve hypoplasia, optic atrophy, or foveal hypoplasia is necessary since these disorders can be subtle and difficult to detect in some cases. Additional testing might include an electroretinogram, visually evoked cortical potentials, ultrasonography, CT, or MRI. In some cases specialized laboratory studies may be indicated. Consultation with a pediatric neurologist, an endocrinologist, a neurosurgeon, or a geneticist may be needed.

When an infant presents with poor vision and ocular structures that appear normal, a number of retinal disorders should be considered, including Leber congenital amaurosis, achromatopsia, blue-cone monochromatism, and X-linked or autosomal recessive congenital stationary night blindness. Electroretinography can aid in the diagnosis of these disorders, and some investigators advocate ERG testing for all infants with visual inattentiveness and a normal examination of the eye structures. Others feel that ERGs in infancy should be reserved only for patients thought to have Leber congenital amaurosis. Obtaining quality ERGs in infants is difficult, and the examiner must be aware of the normal developmental variations that occur in these electrophysiological tests in the first year of life. Serial testing may be important before definitive diagnostic and prognostic information is provided.

Infants with reduced but not absent visual function should receive appropriate visual stimulation as part of early intervention services. These children are followed until the preschool years when quantitative visual acuity measurements can be made.

Children with generalized neurologic dysfunction may have severely delayed visual development and may appear blind in the first few months of life, although pupillary responses are generally normal. Differentiating these children from those with cortical visual impairment (previously referred to as *cortical blindness,* although these children usually have some visual function) may be difficult. The most common causes of reduced vision in infants are listed here and discussed individually below:

□ Anterior segment anomalies

□ Glaucoma

□ Cataract

□ Albinism

□ Leber congenital amaurosis

□ TORCH/congenital infection

□ Achromatopsia

□ Coloboma

□ Retinopathy of prematurity

□ X-linked retinoschisis

□ Optic nerve hypoplasia

□ Optic atrophy

□ Delay in visual maturation

□ Cortical visual impairment

□ Congenital motor nystagmus

Optic Nerve Hypoplasia

Optic nerve hypoplasia frequently causes reduced visual function in infants. It can range from minimal to complete absence of the nerve and accompanying retinal vessels. The nerve appears somewhat pale and small and may be circumscribed by a yellow-white ring, surrounded by pigmentation. This encircling ring has been described clinically as the double ring sign. The condition can be unilateral or bilateral, and there is no sex predilection. When unilateral, strabismus is often present. Nystagmus frequently accompanies bilateral disease. Visual reduction ranges from minimal to total blindness. Part of the loss may be secondary to a superimposed amblyopia.

An afferent pupillary defect is usually present with asymmetric involvement, and the ERG is commonly normal. The visually evoked cortical potential is subnormal. Radiologic study may demonstrate a small optic foramen or optic nerve.

Optic nerve hypoplasia occurs in association with other developmental abnormalities including hydrocephalus, hydrancephaly, anencephaly, and congenital tumors of the anterior visual pathways. Midline defects in the growth of the brain may be seen, including agenesis of the septum pellucidum and malformations of the fornix, with failure of the fornix to attach to the corpus callosum. In addition, the chiasmal cistern may be enlarged. Neuroimaging is recommended for children with bilateral optic nerve hypoplasia. When unilateral, the incidence of midline brain abnormalities is much smaller.

The de Morsier syndrome (septo-optic dysplasia) includes optic nerve hypoplasia, absence of the septum pellucidum, and pituitary dwarfism. Endocrine abnormalities may occur when the midline defect extends into the hypothalamus. Panhypopituitarism, growth hormone deficiency, diabetes insipidus, and hypoglycemia may be present. Recent studies have identified ectopia of the posterior pituitary gland as seen on MRI as a predictor of endocrine abnormalities in patients with optic nerve hypoplasia.

The etiology of optic nerve hypoplasia remains unknown, although maternal ingestion of phenytoin, quinine, and LSD has been associated. In addition, this finding is common in infants with fetal alcohol syndrome and has been reported in offspring of mothers with diabetes. A postulated cause of optic nerve hypoplasia is degeneration of ganglion cell axons. The insult occurs prior to the 13th week of gestation. See also pp 297–299.

Optic Atrophy

Various conditions, both inherited and noninherited, can cause optic atrophy. Congenital and acquired forms occur and can be an isolated defect or a facet of systemic disease. Secondary optic atrophy has been attributed to perinatal hypoxia, central nervous system malformations such as porencephaly, and toxins such as lead, quinine, and methyl alcohol. Acquired optic atrophy has been associated with metabolic storage diseases and with trauma, including child abuse. See also pp 300–301.

Leber Congenital Amaurosis

An estimated 10% of congenital blindness is a result of this disorder. Infants with Leber congenital amaurosis are blind or have severe visual impairment at birth, although the visual deficit may not be noted until 2–3 months of age with the onset of sensory nystagmus. A coarse, searching nystagmus is usually noted. The pupillary reactions are poor to direct light, and the pupils may paradoxically constrict in the dark. The oculodigital habit is common, with gouging of the eyes by a finger or fist, possibly in an effort to induce entoptic stimulation of the retina. The inheritance pattern is autosomal recessive.

Often, the fundus appears completely normal, although at times a diffuse pigmentary change and/or optic nerve pallor or hypoplasia may be noted. A blond fundus may be seen, and frequently, the macula appears atrophic. With time optic atrophy, narrowing of the retinal vessels, and diffuse retinal pigmentary changes are seen that may be indistinguishable from retinitis pigmentosa. Other findings may include cataracts, hyperopia, macular defects, and glaucoma. The ERG is abnormal, either completely flat or low voltage, and the base value of the electro-oculogram may be low, with no rise after light adaptation. Histologic examination reveals severe disorganization or absence of the rods and cones.

Associated neurologic conditions may include an abnormal electroencephalogram, microcephaly, hydrocephaly, seizures, and cerebral abnormalities. Skeletal changes that can be seen in combination are acrocephaly, hemifacial hypoplasia, polydactyly, kyphoscoliosis, arachnodactyly, and osteoporosis. Muscular hypotony and kidney abnormalities with oligophrenia may also be associated. Because of the associated renal abnormalities, a urinalysis should be obtained. See also pp 277–278.

Achromatopsia (Rod Monochromatism)

Achromatopsia is total color blindness inherited as an autosomal recessive trait. Photophobia, nystagmus, and visual acuity in the 20/200 range are frequently encountered. The amount of photophobia is variable, and the degree of nystagmus may decrease at near fixation, giving better visual acuity at near than at distance.

Fundus examination is usually normal when the child is young, although an abnormal foveal reflex may develop as the child gets older. A central scotoma can usually be demonstrated, and there are distinct abnormalities in color vision, with all colors perceived as various brightnesses of gray. The ERG usually shows a normal scotopic recording and an abnormal photopic response. The electro-oculogram is usually normal in achromatopsia.

Histopathologic examination reveals an absence of cones, abnormally structured cones, and, occasionally, some anatomically normal appearing cones. The rods are normal. The condition is nonprogressive and has no associated neurologic abnormalities. See also p 279.

Congenital Infection Syndrome/TORCH Syndrome

Marked reduction in visual acuity is often associated with congenital infections, primarily toxoplasmosis, rubella, cytomegalovirus, herpes simplex, and syphilis. Chapter XVII discusses these conditions in detail. Severe disruption of the visual pathways and decreased vision results from encephalitis, meningitis, arachnoiditis, optic neuritis, and chorioretinitis.

Congenital Motor Nystagmus

Congenital motor nystagmus is present at birth or shortly afterward. Most cases are not inherited, although it may rarely be transmitted as an X-linked recessive or autosomal dominant or recessive trait. The nystagmus is typically a pendular type but may have a jerk component as well. In some cases a null point is seen in specific fields of gaze, and head oscillation may be present. If the nystagmus is horizontal in primary position, it will remain horizontal in either upgaze or downgaze. The nystagmus may dampen on attempted convergence. A rotary component is often noted and may be the prominent eye movement. Visual acuity is reduced on the basis of the nystagmus. Oscillopsia is not commonly encountered.

Since congenital motor nystagmus is generally associated with less severe visual impairment, it is necessary to rule out organic ophthalmic causes such as optic nerve hypoplasia as well as neurologic disease when the nystagmus is associated with profound visual loss. Nystagmus is often associated with ocular defects that result in deprivation amblyopia.

Cortical Visual Impairment

Cortical visual impairment may be congenital or acquired. Prenatal and perinatal etiologies include intrauterine infection, cerebral dysgenesis, asphyxia, intracranial hemorrhage, hydrocephalus, and infection. Acquired causes of cortical visual impairment include trauma and child abuse, shunt malfunction, meningitis and encephalitis, and asphyxia.

Infants with cortical visual impairment may demonstrate a variable degree of visual attentiveness. Both the family and the ophthalmologist may be uncertain as to whether or not the baby can see. Examination reveals normal ocular structures, normal pupillary responses, and searching eye movements. However, descending optic atrophy (transsynaptic degeneration) may coexist with cortical visual impairment. The ERG is normal, while the visually evoked cortical potential may be normal or subnormal.

Neuroimaging with CT scan or MRI may reveal changes in the occipital cortex (striate or parastriate cortex) such as atrophy and porencephaly. Damage to the optic radiations and periventricular leukomalacia may also be noted. However, in some cases, no such findings are present on the scan, and the prognosis may be more favorable in these cases. Cortical visual impairment may be transient or permanent, and it can be an isolated finding or associated with multiple neurologic handicaps.

Delay in Visual Maturation

Some patients whose eye examination is totally normal but who demonstrate poor fixation may have a delay in maturation of the visual system. These children have a normal neurologic examination with the exception of poor visual attention. Visually evoked cortical potentials may be abnormal, only to improve between the ages of 4 and 12 months.

Albinism

Poor fixation in an infant or child may be a result of one of several forms of albinism. Ocular involvement in albinism conforms to one of two clinical patterns:

☐ True albinism, with subnormal visual acuity and nystagmus

☐ Albinoidism, with normal or minimally reduced visual acuity and no nystagmus

Subtypes of true albinism share common clinical features of photophobia, iris transillumination, and hypopigmentation of the fundus. This form has foveal hypoplasia, whereas albinoidism has a normal or nearly normal fovea. True albinism can be divided into two major types:

☐ Oculocutaneous albinism, in which both skin and eyes are involved

☐ Ocular albinism, in which the eyes are primarily involved

See also p 288.

Acquired Vision Loss in Childhood

When a child with normal visual development in infancy loses vision, the search for a treatable disorder is paramount. Table XXXI–1 lists many of the conditions that can lead to acquired amaurosis. Amblyopia, the most prevalent cause of treatable vision loss in children, is discussed in chapter IV and elsewhere in this volume. Childhood cataracts acquired as a developmental, familial, traumatic, or metabolic disorder are also discussed in chapter XXII.

Early diagnosis of acquired visual loss in childhood is extremely important. Vision-screening programs in schools, primary care medical offices, and community outreach programs should be supported and monitored. Visual recovery is often directly related to early, accurate detection of the visual loss. Table XXXI-2 lists resources for further information.

TABLE XXXI-1

ACQUIRED CHILDHOOD AMAUROSIS

Congenital Malformations

Congenital hydrocephalus
Encephalocele, particularly occipital type

Tumors

Retinoblastoma
Optic glioma
Perioptic meningioma
Craniopharyngioma
Chiasmal glioma
Posterior and intraventricular tumors when complicated by hydrocephalus

Neurodegenerative Diseases: Abiotrophies

Cerebral storage disease

Gangliosidoses, particularly Tay-Sachs disease (infantile amaurotic familial idiocy), Sandhoff disease, generalized gangliosidosis

Other lipidoses and ceroid lipofuscinoses, particularly the late-onset amaurotic familial idiocies such as those of Jansky-Bielschowsky and of Spielmeyer-Vogt

Mucopolysaccharidoses, particularly Hurler syndrome and Hunter syndrome

Leukodystrophies (dysmyelination disorders), particularly metachromatic leukodystrophy and Canavan disease

Demyelinating scleroses (myelinoclastic diseases) especially Schilder disease and Devic neuromyelitis optica

Special types: Dawson disease, Leigh disease, the Bassen-Kornzweig syndrome, Refsum disease

Retinal degenerations of obscure pathogenesis: retinitis pigmentosa and its variants, and Leber congenital type

Optic atrophies of obscure pathogenesis: congenital autosomal recessive type, infantile and congenital autosomal dominant types, Leber disease, and atrophies associated with hereditary ataxias—the types of Behr, of Marie, and of Sager-Brown

Infectious or Inflammatory Processes

Encephalitis, especially in the prenatal infection syndromes due to *Toxoplasma gondii*, cytomegalovirus, rubella virus, *Treponema pallidum*

Meningitis; arachnoiditis
Optic neuritis
Chorioretinitis

Hematologic Disorders

Leukemia with CNS involvement

Vascular and Circulatory Disorders

Collagen vascular diseases
Arteriovenous malformations: intracerebral hemorrhage, subarachnoid hemorrhage

Trauma

Contusion or avulsion of optic nerves or chiasm
Cerebral contusion or laceration
Intracerebral, subarachnoid, or subdural hemorrhage

Drugs and Toxins

Lead
Quinine
Methyl alcohol

Table adapted from Nelson LB, Calhoun JH, Harley RD, eds. *Pediatric Ophthalmology.* 3rd ed. Philadelphia: Saunders; 1991.

TABLE XXXI-2

SOURCES OF INFORMATION ON LOW VISION

NAPVI (National Association of Parents of the Visually Impaired)
(800) 562-6265
(Some areas have a state organization as well: NAPVI can direct the parent.)

Prevent Blindness America
160 East 56th Street
New York, NY 10022   (212) 980-2020 or (800) 331-2020

National Information Center for Children and Youth with Handicaps (NICCYH)
PO Box 1492
Washington, DC 20013   (800) 999-5599

National Association for the Visually Handicapped, Inc. (Western Office)
3201 Balboa Street
San Francisco, CA 94121   (415) 221-3201
(Large-print textbooks, library material on request. Sources of information and guidance on resources for the visually handicapped.)

National Association for the Visually Handicapped (NAVH)
22 West 21st St.
New York, NY 10010   (212) 889-3141

National Organization for Albinism and Hypopigmentation (NOAH)
1530 Locust St., #29
Philadelphia, PA 19102   (215) 545-2322
http://www.albinism.org

Recording for the Blind, Inc.
20 Roszel Road
Princeton, NJ 08540   (609) 452-0606

American Foundation for the Blind, Inc.
11 Pennsylvania Plaza, Suite 300
New York, NY 10001
(212) 502-7600 or (800) 232-5463
(For the publication *Reach Out and Teach,* call (800) 232-3044.)

Library of Congress National Library Service for the Blind and Physically Handicapped
1291 Taylor St. NW
Washington, DC 20542
(202) 707-5100 or (800) 424-8567
(Recorded poetry and literature talking books.)

American Printing House for the Blind
1839 Frankfort Avenue
PO Box 6085
Louisville, KY 40206   (502) 895-2405 or (800) 223-1839
Fax: (502) 899-2274
(Large-print textbooks, tapes, braille books, and tangible aids.)

Lighthouse for the Blind
(Independent organizations in every state; check local directories for listings.)

The Family Resource Coalition of America
200 S. Michigan Avenue
16th floor
Chicago, IL 60604   (312) 341-0900
(Provides identification of parent support groups all over the country.)

TABLE XXXI-2 (Cont.)

SOURCES OF INFORMATION ON LOW VISION

Retinoblastoma Support News (newsletter for families of children with retinoblastoma, and *Parent To Parent* (newsletter for families of blind and visually impaired children) published by:
The Institute for Families of Blind Children
Children's Hospital of Los Angeles
Division of Ophthalmology, Box 111
P.O. Box 54700
Los Angeles, CA 90054-0700   (213) 669-4649

National Toll-Free Numbers

American Council of the Blind   (800) 424-8666

Better Hearing Institute   (800) 327-9355 (EAR-WELL)

Epilepsy Information Line   (800) EFA-1000

Cystic Fibrosis Foundation   (800) 344-4823

National Down Syndrome Society   (800) 221-4602

Down Syndrome Information Center   (888) 999-3759

National Easter Seal Society   (800) 221-6827

National Health Information Clearinghouse   (800) 336-4797

Spina Bifida   (800) 621-3141

United Cerebral Palsy Association   (800) 872-5827

National Fragile X Foundation   (800) 688-8765

American Kidney Fund   (800) 638-8299

The Arc (formerly Association for Retarded Citizens)   (800) 433-5255

Sickle Cell Association   (800) 421-8453

Retinitis Pigmentosa (RP) Association International   (800) 344-4877

Sources of large-print books

New York Times Large Print Weekly
229 West 43rd Street
New York, NY 10036   (800) 631-2580

Library for the Blind
919 Walnut Street
Philadelphia, PA 19107   (215) 925-3213

Reader's Digest Large Print Edition
(800) 678-9746

CHAPTER XXXII

Learning Disabilities, Dyslexia, and Vision

Subnormal reading and learning skills may be the reason for an ophthalmic evaluation for a child or even an adult. The determination of subnormal educational performance is best left to educators, the professionals in this discipline. The role of the ophthalmologist is to determine if a visual abnormality is contributing to poor performance. The standard ophthalmic examination should be performed, with special attention given to visual function at near. If the ophthalmic examination is normal, the patient should be directed to the pediatrician or primary care physician for assistance in continuing the multidisciplinary approach to diagnosis and treatment.

Little evidence suggests that reading disabilities result from problems in the visual system. The American Academy of Ophthalmology, the American Association for Pediatric Ophthalmology and Strabismus, and the American Academy of Pediatrics have issued a joint policy statement, which is printed here in its entirety.

LEARNING DISABILITIES, DYSLEXIA, AND VISION

A Joint Statement of the American Academy of Pediatrics, the American Association for Pediatric Ophthalmology and Strabismus, and the American Academy of Ophthalmology

Policy

Learning disabilities are common conditions in pediatric patients. The etiology of these difficulties is multifactorial, reflecting genetic influences and abnormalities of brain structure and function. Early recognition and referral to qualified educational professionals is critical for the best possible outcome. Visual problems are rarely responsible for learning difficulties. No scientific evidence exists for the efficacy of eye exercises "vision therapy" or the use of special tinted lenses in the remediation of these complex pediatric neurological conditions.

Background

Learning disabilities have become an increasing personal and public concern. Among the spectrum of issues of concern in learning disabilities is the inability to read and comprehend, which is a major obstacle to learning and may have long-term educational, social, and economic implications. Family concern for the welfare of children with dyslexia and learning disabilities has led to a proliferation of diagnostic and remedial treatment procedures, many of which are controversial or without clear scientific evidence of efficacy. Many educators, psychologists, and medical specialists concur that individuals who have learning disabilities should:

1) receive early comprehensive educational, psychological, and medical assessment

2) receive educational remediation combined with appropriate psychological and medical treatment

3) avoid remedies involving eye exercises, filters, tinted lenses, or other optical devices that have no known scientific proof of efficacy

This policy statement addresses these issues.

Evaluation and Management

Reading involves the integration of multiple factors related to an individual's experience, ability, and neurological functioning. Research has shown that the majority of children and adults with reading difficulties experience a variety of problems with language[1–3] that stem from altered brain function and that such difficulties are not caused by altered visual function.[4–7] In addition, a variety of secondary emotional and environmental factors may have a detrimental effect on the learning process in such children.

Sometimes children may also have a treatable visual difficulty along with their primary reading or learning dysfunction. Routine vision screening examinations can identify most of those who have reduced visual acuity. Pediatricians and other primary care physicians, whose pediatric patients cannot pass vision screening according to the national standards,[8,9] should refer these patients to an ophthalmologist who has experience in the care of children.

1. *Role of the eyes.* Decoding of retinal images occurs in the brain after visual signals are transmitted from the eye via the visual pathways. Some vision care practitioners incorrectly attribute reading difficulties to one or more subtle ocular or visual abnormalities. Although the eyes are obviously necessary for vision, the brain performs the complex function of interpreting visual images. Currently no scientific evidence supports the view that correction of subtle visual defects can alter the brain's processing of visual stimuli. Statistically, children with dyslexia or related learning disabilities have the same ocular health as children without such conditions.[10–12]

2. *Controversies.* Eye defects, subtle or severe, do not cause the patient to experience reversal of letters, words, or numbers. No scientific evidence supports claims that the academic abilities of children with learning disabilities can be improved with treatments that are based on 1) visual training, including muscle exercises, ocular pursuit, tracking exercises, or "training" glasses (with or without bifocals or prisms);[13–15] 2) neurological organizational training (laterality training, crawling, balance board, perceptual training);[16–18] or 3) colored lenses.[18–20] These more controversial methods of treatment may give parents and teachers a false sense of security that a child's reading difficulties are being addressed, which may delay proper instruction or remediation. The expense of these methods is unwarranted, and they cannot be substituted for appropriate educational measures. Claims of improved reading and learning after visual training, neurological organization training, or use of colored lenses are almost always based on poorly controlled studies that typically rely on anecdotal information. These methods are without scientific validation.[21] Their reported benefits can be explained by the traditional educational remedial techniques with which they are usually combined.

3. *Early detection.* Pediatricians, primary care physicians, and educational specialists may use screening techniques to detect learning disabilities in preschool-age children but, in many cases, the learning disability is discovered after the child experiences academic difficulties. Learning disabilities can include dyslexia, problems with memory and language, and difficulty with mathematic computation. These difficulties are often complicated by attention deficit disorders. A family history of learning disabilities is common in such conditions. Children who are considered to be at risk for or suspected of having these conditions by their physician should be evaluated by more detailed study by educational and/or psychological specialists.

4. *Role of the physician.* Ocular defects in young children should be identified as early as possible, and when they are correctable, they should be managed by an ophthalmologist who is experienced in the care of children.[22] Treatable ocular conditions among others include refractive errors, focusing deficiencies, eye muscle imbalances, and motor fusion deficiencies. When children have learning problems that are suspected to be associated with visual defects, the ophthalmologist may be consulted by the primary care pediatrician. If no ocular defect is found, the child needs no further vision care or treatment and should be referred for medical and appropriate special educational evaluation and services. Pediatricians have an important role in coordination of care between the family and other health care services provided by ophthalmologists, optometrists, and other health care professionals who may become involved in the treatment plan.

5. *Multidisciplinary approach.* The management of a child who has learning disabilities requires a multidisciplinary approach for diagnosis and treatment that involves educators, psychologists, and physicians. Basic scientific and clinical research into the role of the brain's structure and function in learning disabilities has demonstrated a neural basis of dyslexia and other specific learning disabilities and not the result of an ocular disorder alone.[4–6]

6. *The role of education.* The teaching of children, adolescents, and adults with dyslexia and learning disabilities is a challenge for educators. Skilled educators use standardized educational diagnostic evaluations and professional judgment to design and monitor individualized remedial programs. Psychologists may help with educational diagnosis and classification. Physicians, including pediatricians, otolaryngologists, neurologists, ophthalmologists, mental health professionals, and other appropriate medical specialists, may assist in treating the health problems of these patients. Since remediation may be more effective during the early years, prompt diagnosis is paramount.[20,21] Educators with specialty training in learning disabilities ultimately play a key role in providing help for the learning disabled or dyslexic child or adult.

Recommendations

1. For all children, clinicians should perform vision screening according to national standards.[8,9]

2. Any child who cannot pass the recommended vision screening test should be referred to an ophthalmologist who has experience in the care of children.

3. Children with educational problems and normal vision screening should be referred for educational diagnostic evaluation and appropriate special educational evaluation and services.

4. Diagnostic and treatment approaches that lack objective, scientifically established efficacy should not be used.

Summary

Reading difficulties and learning disabilities are complex problems that have no simple solutions. The American Academy of Pediatrics, the American Academy of Ophthalmology, and the American Association for Pediatric Ophthalmology and Strabismus strongly support the need for early diagnosis and educational remediation. There is no known eye or visual cause for these learning disabilities and no known effective visual treatment.[23,24] Recommendations for multidisciplinary evaluation and management must be based on evidence of proven effectiveness demonstrated by objective scientific methodology.[23,24] It is important that any therapy for learning disabilities be scientifically established to be valid before it can be recommended for treatment.

The recommendations in this policy statement do not indicate an exclusive course of treatment of procedure to be followed. Variations, taking into account individual circumstances, may be appropriate.

References

1. Mattis T, French JH, Rapin I. Dyslexia in children and young adults: three independent neuropsychological syndromes. *Dev Med Child Neurol.* 1975;17:150–163.

2. Vellutino FR. Dyslexia. *Scientific American.* 1987;256(3):34–41.

3. Council on Scientific Affairs. Dyslexia. *JAMA.* 1989;261:2236–2239.

4. Petersen SE, Fox PT, Posner MI, et al. Positron emission tomographic studies of the cortical anatomy of single-word processing. *Nature.* 1988;331:585–589.

5. Galaburda A. Ordinary and extraordinary brain development: anatomical variation in developmental dyslexia. *Ann Dyslexia.* 1989;39:67–80.

6. Hynd GW, Semrud-Clikeman M, Lorys AR, et al. Brain morphology in developmental dyslexia and attention deficit disorder/hyperactivity. *Arch Neurol.* 1990;47:919–926.

7. Metzger RL, Werner DB. Use of visual training for reading disabilities: a review. *Pediatrics.* 1984;73:824–829.

8. American Academy of Pediatrics, Committee on Practice and Ambulatory Medicine and Section on Ophthalmology. Eye examination and vision screening in infants, children, and young adults. *Pediatrics.* 1996;98:153–157.

9. American Academy of Ophthalmology and American Association for Pediatric Ophthalmology and Strabismus. *Vision Screening for Infants and Children.* 1996.

10. Goldberg HK, Drash PW. The disabled reader. *J Pediatr Ophthalmol.* 1968;5:11–24.

11. Helveston EM, Weber JC, Miller K, et al. Visual function and academic performance. *Am J Ophthalmol.* 1985;99:346–355.

12. Levine MD. Reading disability: do the eyes have it? *Pediatrics.* 1984;73:869–870.

13. Keogh B, Pelland M. Vision training revisited. *J Learn Disabil.* 1985;18:228–236.

14. Beauchamp GR. Optometric vision training. *Pediatrics.* 1986;77:121–124.

15. Cohen HJ, Birch HG, Taft LT. Some considerations for evaluating the Doman-Delacato "patterning method." *Pediatrics.* 1970;45:302–314.

16. Kavale K, Mattson PD. One jumped off the balance beam: meta-analysis of perceptual-motor training. *J Learn Disabil.* 1983;16:165–173.

17. Black JL, Collins DWK, DeRoach JN, et al. A detailed study of sequential saccadic eye movements for normal and poor reading children. *Percept Mot Skills.* 1984;59:423–434.

18. Solan HA. An appraisal of the Irlen technique of correcting reading disorders using tinted overlays and tinted lenses. *J Learn Disabil.* 1990;23:621–623.

19. Hoyt CS. Irlen lenses and reading difficulties. *J Learn Disabil.* 1990;23:624–626.

20. Sedun AA. Dyslexia at New York Times: (mis)understanding of parallel vision processing. *Arch Ophthalmol.* 1992;110:933–934.

21. Bradley L. Rhyme recognition and reading and spelling in young children. In: Masland RL, Masland MW, eds. *Preschool Prevention of Reading Failure.* Parkton, MD: York Press; 1988:143–162.

22. Ogden S, Hindman S, Turner SD. Multisensory programs in the public schools: a brighter future for LD children. *Ann Dyslexia.* 1989;39:247–267.

23. Romanchuk KG. Skepticism about Irlen filters to treat learning disabilities. *CMAJ.* 1995; 153:397.

24. Silver LB. Controversial therapies. *J Child Neurol.* 1995;10 Suppl 1:S96–100.

Approved by:
American Academy of Pediatrics / January 1984
American Association for Pediatric Ophthalmology and Strabismus / February 1984
American Academy of Ophthalmology / February 1984

Revised and approved by:
American Academy of Pediatrics
American Association for Pediatric Ophthalmology and Strabismus
American Academy of Ophthalmology

September 1998

BASIC TEXTS

Pediatric Ophthalmology and Strabismus

Brodsky MC, Baker RS, Latif Hamed LM. *Pediatric Neuro-Ophthalmology.* New York: Springer-Verlag; 1995.

Buckley EG, Freedman S, Shields MB. *Atlas of Ophthalmic Surgery.* Vol III: *Strabismus and Glaucoma.* St Louis: Mosby; 1995.

Calhoun JH, Nelson LB, Harley RD. *Atlas of Pediatric Ophthalmic Surgery.* Philadelphia: Saunders; 1987.

Cibis GW, Tongue AC, Stass-Isern ML. *Decision Making in Pediatric Ophthalmology.* St Louis: Decker; 1993.

Del Monte MA. *Atlas of Pediatric Ophthalmology and Strabismus Surgery.* New York: Churchill Livingstone; 1993.

Helveston EM. *Surgical Management of Strabismus: An Atlas of Strabismus Surgery.* 4th ed. St Louis: Mosby; 1993.

Helveston EM, Ellis FD. *Pediatric Ophthalmology Practice.* 2nd ed. St Louis: Mosby; 1984.

Isenberg SJ, ed. *The Eye in Infancy.* 2nd ed. St Louis: Mosby-Year Book; 1994.

Jones KL. *Smith's Recognizable Patterns of Human Malformation.* 5th ed. Philadelphia: Saunders; 1997.

Leigh RJ, Zee DS. *The Neurology of Eye Movements.* 2nd ed. Philadelphia: FA Davis; 1991.

Miller NR, Newman NJ. *Walsh and Hoyt's Clinical Neuro-Ophthalmology.* 5th ed. Baltimore: Williams & Wilkins; 1997.

Nelson LB, ed. *Harley's Pediatric Ophthalmology.* 4th ed. Philadelphia: Saunders; 1998.

Pratt-Johnson JA, Tillson G. *Management of Strabismus and Amblyopia: A Practical Guide.* New York: Thieme; 1994.

Renie WA, eds. *Goldberg's Genetic and Metabolic Eye Disease.* 2nd ed. Boston: Little, Brown & Co; 1986.

Spencer WH, ed. *Ophthalmic Pathology: An Atlas and Textbook.* 4th ed. Philadelphia: Saunders; 1996.

Tasman W, Jaeger EA, eds. *Duane's Clinical Ophthalmology.* Philadelphia: Lippincott-Raven; 1996.

Taylor D. *Pediatric Ophthalmology.* 2nd ed. Cambridge, MA: Blackwell Science; 1997.

von Haam E, Helveston EM. *Strabismus: A Decision Making Approach.* St Louis: Mosby; 1994.

von Noorden GK. *Binocular Vision and Ocular Motility: Theory and Management of Strabismus.* 5th ed. St Louis: Mosby; 1996.

von Noorden GK. *von Noorden–Maumenee's Atlas of Strabismus.* 4th ed. St Louis: Mosby; 1983.

Wright KW, ed. *Color Atlas of Ophthalmic Surgery.* Vol 1, *Strabismus.* Philadelphia: Lippincott; 1992.

Wright KW, ed. *Pediatric Ophthalmology and Strabismus.* St Louis: Mosby; 1995.

RELATED ACADEMY MATERIALS

Focal Points: Clinical Modules for Ophthalmologists

Archer S. Esotropia (Module 12, 1994).

Beck AD, Lynch MG. Pediatric glaucoma (Module 5, 1997).

Borchert MS. Nystagmus in childhood (Module 8, 1991).

Dinning WJ. Uveitis and juvenile chronic arthritis (Module 5, 1990).

Dortzbach RK, Woog JJ. Diagnosis and management of congenital ptosis (Module 2, 1987).

Dunn JP. Uveitis in children (Module 4, 1995).

Haldi BA, Mets MB. Nonsurgical treatments of strabismus (Module 4, 1997).

Helveston EM. Management of dyslexia and related learning disabilities (Module 1, 1985).

Hoyt CS. Assessment of visually impaired infants (Module 7, 1987).

Hoyt CS. Management of congenital cataracts (Module 6, 1983).

Hutcheson KA, Drack AV. Diagnosis and management of the infant who does not see (Module 12, 1998).

Isenberg SJ. How to examine the eye of the neonate (Module 1, 1989).

Lambert SR, Boothe RG. Amblyopia: basic and clinical science perspectives (Module 8, 1994).

Levin AV. The ocular findings in child abuse (Module 7, 1998).

Metz HS. Adjustable suture techniques in strabismus surgery (Module 1, 1986).

Palmer EA. Current management of retinopathy of prematurity (Module 3, 1993).

Rapoza PA, Chandler JW. Neonatal conjunctivitis: diagnosis and treatment (Module 1, 1988).

Ruttum MS. Childhood cataracts (Module 1, 1996).

Scott WE, Arthur BW. Current approaches to superior oblique muscle surgery (Module 3, 1988).

Silkiss RZ. Craniofacial anomalies (Module 11, 1992).

Spencer JB. A practical approach to refraction in children (Module 4, 1993).

Stefanyszyn MA. Orbital tumors in children (Module 8, 1990).

Stevens JCL. Retinoblastoma (Module 1, 1990).

Sutula FC. Management of tearing in children (Module 11, 1989).

Walton DS. Childhood glaucoma (Module 10, 1990).

Wilson ME. Exotropia (Module 11, 1995).

Wright KW. Current approaches to inferior oblique muscle surgery (Module 6, 1986).

Publications

Edelman PM, ed. *Orthoptics: A Syllabus of Ocular Motility.* 2nd ed. (1992).

Lane SS, Skuta GL, eds. *ProVision: Preferred Responses in Ophthalmology,* Series 3 (Self-Assessment Program, 1999).

Skuta GL, ed. *ProVision: Preferred Responses in Ophthalmology,* Series 2 (Self-Assessment Program, 1996).

Wilson FM II, ed. *Practical Ophthalmology: A Manual for Beginning Residents* (1996).

Multimedia

Wright KW, Drack AV, McKeown CA, Repka MX. *LEO Clinical Update Course on Pediatric Ophthalmology and Strabismus* (CD-ROM, 1998).

Slide-Scripts

Day SH. *Understanding and Preventing Amblyopia* (Eye Care Skills for the Primary Care Physician Series, 1987).

Young SE. *Managing the Red Eye* (Eye Care Skills for the Primary Care Physician Series, 1994).

Continuing Ophthalmic Video Education

Bergin DJ. *Management and Surgery of Congenital and Acquired Ptosis* (1990).

Price RL, Beauchamp GR. *Strabismus Surgery: Oblique Procedures* (1989).

Price RL, Beauchamp GR. *Strabismus Surgery: Rectus Recession and Resection* (1989).

Smelser G, Ozanics V. *Embryology of the Eye* (1977).

Wilson ME. *Ocular Motility Evaluation of Strabismus and Myasthenia Gravis* (1993).

Wright KW. *Inferior Oblique Surgery;* John T. *Intraoperative Control of Corneal Astigmatism During Penetrating Keratoplasty;* and Goldberg RA. *The Transcaruncular Approach to the Medial Orbit* (1997).

Preferred Practice Patterns

Preferred Practice Patterns Committee, Pediatric Ophthalmology Panel. *Amblyopia* (1997).

Preferred Practice Patterns Committee, Pediatric Ophthalmology Panel. *Esotropia* (1997).

Preferred Practice Patterns Committee, Pediatric Ophthalmology Panel. *Pediatric Eye Evaluations* (1997).

LEO Clinical Topic Updates

Repka M. *Pediatric Ophthalmology and Strabismus* (1996).

> To order any of these materials, please call the Academy's Customer Service number at (415) 561-8540.

CREDIT REPORTING FORM

BASIC AND CLINICAL SCIENCE COURSE
Section 6

1999–2000

CME Accreditation

The American Academy of Ophthalmology is accredited by the Accreditation Council for Continuing Medical Education to sponsor continuing medical education for physicians.

The American Academy of Ophthalmology designates this educational activity for a maximum of 40 hours in category 1 credit toward the AMA Physician's Recognition Award. Each physician should claim only those hours of credit that he/she has actually spent in the educational activity.

If you wish to claim continuing medical education credit for your study of this section, you must complete and return the study question answer sheet on the back of this page, along with the following signed statement, to the Academy office. This form must be received within 3 years of the date of purchase.

I hereby certify that I have spent _____ (up to 40) hours of study on the curriculum of this section, and that I have completed the study questions. (The Academy, *upon request,* will send you a transcript of the credits listed on this form.)

☐ *Please send credit verification now.*

Signature _____
                                                             Date

Name:_____

Address: _____

City and State:_____ Zip: _____

Telephone: (_____) _____ *Academy Member ID# _____
            area code

*   *Your ID number is located following your name on any Academy mailing label, in your Membership Directory, and on your Monthly Statement of Account.*

Section Evaluation

Please indicate your response to the statements listed below by placing the appropriate number to the left of each statement.

1 = agree strongly
2 = agree
3 = no opinion
4 = disagree
5 = disagree
    strongly

_____ This section covers topics in enough depth and detail.

_____ This section's illustrations are of sufficient number and quality.

_____ The references included in the text provide an appropriate amount of additional reading.

_____ The study questions at the end of the book are useful.

In addition, please attach a separate sheet of paper to this form if you wish to elaborate on any of the statements above or to comment on other aspects of this book.

Please return completed form to: **American Academy of Ophthalmology**
P.O. Box 7424
San Francisco, CA 94120-7424
ATTN: Clinical Education Division

SECTION COMPLETION FORM

BASIC AND CLINICAL SCIENCE COURSE
ANSWER SHEET FOR SECTION 6

Question	Answer	Question	Answer	Question	Answer
1	a b c d	23	a b c d	44	a b c d
2	a b c d	24	a b c d	45	a b c d
3	a b c d	25	a b c d	46	a b c d
4	a b c d	26	a b c d	47	a b c d
5	a b c d	27	a b c d	48	a b c d
6	a b c d	28	a b c d	49	a b c d
7	a b c d	29	a b c d	50	a b c d
8	a b c d	30	a b c d	51	a b c d
9	a b c d	31	a b c d	52	a b c d
10	a b c d	32	a b c d	53	a b c d
11	a b c d	33	a b c d	54	a b c d
12	a b c d	34	a b c d	55	a b c d
13	a b c d	35	a b c d	56	a b c d
14	a b c d	36	a b c d	57	a b c d
15	a b c d	37	a b c d	58	a b c d
16	a b c d	38	a b c d	59	a b c d
17	a b c d	39	a b c d	60	a b c d
18	a b c d	40	a b c d	61	a b c d
19	a b c d	41	a b c d	62	a b c d
20	a b c d	42	a b c d	63	a b c d
21	a b c d	43	a b c d	64	a b c d
22	a b c d				

STUDY QUESTIONS

STUDY QUESTIONS

The following multiple-choice questions are designed to be used after your course of study with this book. Record your responses on the answer sheet (the back side of the Credit Reporting Form) by circling the appropriate letter. For the most effective use of this exercise, *complete the entire test* before consulting the answers.

Although a concerted effort has been made to avoid ambiguity and redundancy in these questions, the authors recognize that differences of opinion may occur regarding the "best" answer. The discussions are provided to demonstrate the rationale used to derive the answer. They may also be helpful in confirming that your approach to the problem was correct or, if necessary, in fixing the principle in your memory.

1. An infant is no longer at risk for developing retinopathy of prematurity when

    a. She is off the respirator
    b. The retinal vessels extend to the temporal ora serrata
    c. The iris vessels become dilated
    d. She reaches a weight of 2000 g

2. Which of the following statements is correct for aniridia?

    a. The majority of patients will develop Wilms tumor.
    b. It is an X-linked recessive condition occurring only in males.
    c. It usually is associated with good vision.
    d. It is often associated with glaucoma.

3. In craniofacial syndromes, which of the following statements is true?

    a. Amblyopia and refractive errors are rare.
    b. Oblique muscle dysfunction is very common, and it produces A- and V-pattern strabismus.
    c. Strabismus surgery should follow any orbital bone repositioning.
    d. Hydrocephalus as a result of suture closure is unusual.

4. Which of the following conditions is inherited?

    a. Retinopathy of prematurity
    b. Cortical visual impairment
    c. Albinism
    d. Graves ophthalmopathy

5. The development of ROP is highly correlated with which of the following?

    a. Asian descent
    b. Intrauterine growth retardation
    c. Younger gestational age at birth
    d. Immature retinal vasculature in zone III

6. Which of the following statements about ROP is true?

   a. The development of myopia associated with ROP can be prevented with the use of cryotherapy.
   b. Blindness from ROP has been eliminated with modern surgical techniques.
   c. Laser photocoagulation has some distinct advantages over cryotherapy and has had no complications.
   d. Threshold disease often occurs around the time the child would have been discharged from the hospital.

7. Oculocutaneous albinism is characterized by which of the following?

   a. Stereopsis
   b. Intellectual impairment
   c. Reduced fertility
   d. Nystagmus

8. Patients with Down syndrome are at higher than normal risk for all of the following except:

   a. Esotropia
   b. Exotropia
   c. Nystagmus
   d. High refractive errors

9. Which of the following has a low association with congenital esotropia?

   a. Dissociated strabismus
   b. Nystagmus
   c. Sixth nerve palsy
   d. Accommodative esotropia

10. Which of the following maternally transmitted congenital infections is least likely to be acquired transplacentally?

   a. Rubella
   b. Herpes simplex
   c. Toxoplasmosis
   d. Cytomegalic inclusion disease

11. A 3-month-old infant referred for evaluation of strabismus is found to have bilateral, diffuse pigmentary changes of the retina. His visual acuity appears normal. Which of the following is the most appropriate diagnostic test?

   a. Electroretinogram
   b. Serum antibody test
   c. Chromosome analysis
   d. CT scan of brain

12. Which of the following statements about diagnostic tests for ophthalmia neonatorum is true?

    a.   Multinucleate giant cells on Gram stain of a conjunctival swab are commonly found in chlamydial conjunctivitis.

    b.   Lymphocytes on Gram stain of a conjunctival swab indicate viral conjunctivitis.

    c.   Basophilic intracytoplasmic inclusions in conjunctival epithelial cells on a Giemsa stain indicate pneumococcal conjunctivitis.

    d.   Eosinophilic intranuclear inclusions in a Papanicolaou smear of conjunctival epithelial cells indicate herpetic conjunctivitis.

13. A 4-year-old girl has a 2-day history of unilateral eyelid edema and erythema, fever, and a runny nose. Examination shows normal visual acuity and unilateral proptosis. Appropriate initial management should consist of

    a.   Hospitalization (for intravenous antibiotics)

    b.   An MRI (to rule out a subperiosteal abscess)

    c.   Surgical drainage if a subperiosteal abscess is found

    d.   Broad-spectrum oral antibiotics

14. The type of childhood cataract usually associated with the worst visual prognosis is

    a.   Unilateral anterior polar cataract

    b.   Bilateral lamellar cataract

    c.   Unilateral posterior lenticonus cataract

    d.   Posterior hyperplastic primary vitreous cataract

15. Which of the following statements regarding management of aphakia in children is most compatible with common practice today?

    a.   A posterior chamber IOL should be used at the time of surgery for a unilateral (but not bilateral) cataract in a 1-month-old infant.

    b.   Bilateral congenital cataracts in a 3-month-old infant should be treated with contact lenses followed by sulcus fixation of a posterior chamber IOL at age 2 years.

    c.   Ciliary sulcus fixation of a posterior chamber IOL is preferred over capsular fixation until the child is at least 8 years old.

    d.   A posterior chamber IOL is useful in children with unilateral traumatic cataracts.

16. The risk of developing chronic uveitis is greatest with which of the following types of juvenile rheumatoid arthritis?

    a.   Polyarticular JRA with onset over age 7 years and positive antinuclear antibody test

    b.   Pauciarticular JRA with onset under age 7 years and negative antinuclear antibody test

    c.   Systemic JRA with onset under age 7 years and positive antinuclear antibody test

    d.   Pauciarticular JRA with onset under age 7 years and positive antinuclear antibody test

17. Which of the following is the most common cause of vision loss in intermediate uveitis?

    a. Band keratopathy
    b. Cystoid macular edema
    c. Amblyopia
    d. Optic neuritis

18. A 6-month-old girl with esotropia would be most likely to have

    a. Alternating fixation
    b. Strabismic amblyopia
    c. An accommodative component
    d. Dissociated vertical deviation

19. Surgery for congenital esotropia in a healthy child is generally recommended

    a. When the child is over 2 years old so that Inferior oblique overaction and dissociated vertical deviation can be treated simultaneously
    b. When the child starts to walk
    c. When amblyopia has been treated and the deviation is of stable magnitude
    d. When the child is 4 months old so as to maximize the chance for developing stereopsis

20. A 4-year-old boy has had onset of esotropia within the past year. Which of the following is a true statement about prism adaptation testing in this child?

    a. If the child is a responder to prism adaptation, a smaller amount of surgery than indicated for the initial amount of esotropia will be performed.
    b. Any accommodative component to the child's esotropia is ignored in planning the amount of surgery after prism adaptation.
    c. If the child does not respond to prism adaptation, surgery is unlikely to provide functional improvement.
    d. In prism adaptation responders, surgery based on the prism-adapted angle of esotropia significantly improves the motor and sensory outcome.

21. The correct order for fusional amplitudes as measured at a distance is

    a. Convergence > Divergence = Vertical
    b. Convergence > Divergence > Vertical
    c. Convergence > Vertical > Divergence
    d. Convergence = Divergence > Vertical

22. Horror fusionis

    a. Is common in children after strabismus surgery
    b. Is usually associated with a large angle of strabismus
    c. Often requires the presence of central suppression
    d. Often occurs after head trauma

23. Inferior oblique muscle overaction is characterized by

    a.   Depression of the adducted eye
    b.   Primary position extorsion of the fundus
    c.   Innervational as opposed to mechanical causes
    d.   Common association with A-pattern strabismus

24. Compared to magnocellular cells, parvocellular neurons are more sensitive to

    a.   Low-medium spatial frequencies
    b.   Fine two-point discrimination
    c.   Direction, motion, and speed
    d.   Flicker stereopsis

25. The vertical prism or induced tropia fixation test is useful

    a.   To measure cyclovertical deviations
    b.   To detect amblyopia in preverbal children without strabismus
    c.   To assess binocular cooperation
    d.   To measure vertical fusional vergences

26. The simultaneous prism-cover test is most useful to

    a.   Measure the total tropia plus phoria
    b.   Measure the phoria only
    c.   Measure the tropia only
    d.   Assess the binocular potential

27. The cardinal positions include

    a.   Primary position at distance
    b.   Straight up and down
    c.   The near point of convergence
    d.   Gaze up and left

28. Fusional vergences

    a.   Eliminate retinal disparity
    b.   Are usually voluntary
    c.   Can be measured even in patients with abnormal retinal correspondence
         (ARC)
    d.   Are usually larger in the vertical plane than in the horizontal plane

29. Which of the following procedures is useful for weakening a muscle only in
    its field of action?

    a.   Myotomy
    b.   Recession
    c.   Posterior fixation
    d.   Anteriorization

30. Which of the following is true of complications following strabismus surgery?

   a. Unsatisfactory alignment can occur with any surgical approach and therefore should not be considered a complication.
   b. Diplopia is most common in patients who develop a consecutive deviation.
   c. Scleral perforation requires prophylactic treatment for possible endophthalmitis or retinal detachment.
   d. Orbital cellulitis typically does not present until 2 or 3 weeks postoperatively.

31. Change in eyelid position following strabismus surgery

   a. Is rarely seen after inferior rectus muscle recession
   b. Is often a manifestation of the adherence syndrome
   c. Can be prevented by resecting the lower eyelid retractors
   d. Can be minimized by posterior dissection of the muscle

32. Which of the following is *not* an early sign of malignant hyperthermia?

   a. Sweating
   b. Blotchy discoloring of the skin
   c. Tachycardia
   d. High temperature

33. Botulinum toxin injection is least suitable for which of the following?

   a. Large-angle exotropia
   b. Small- to moderate-angle esotropia
   c. Postoperative residual strabismus
   d. Weakening of an antagonist muscle in acute paralytic strabismus

34. The most common complication of botulinum toxin injection is

   a. Eyelid ptosis
   b. Globe perforation
   c. Retrobulbar hemorrhage
   d. Vertical strabismus

35. An infant is suspected of being blind or having grossly reduced vision. The pupils are sluggish bilaterally, and pendular nystagmus is present. The fundus, however, appears normal. There are no signs or symptoms of other disease. The most likely diagnosis is

   a. Tay-Sachs disease
   b. Leber congenital amaurosis
   c. Anomalous development of the occipital cortex
   d. Congenital hydrocephalus

36. Acute orbital infections in young children are likely to arise from

    a. The maxillary sinuses
    b. The ethmoid sinuses
    c. The sphenoid sinuses
    d. The frontal sinuses

37. The optimal time to diagnose and treat dense, bilateral congenital cataracts is

    a. As soon as possible during the first 2 months of life
    b. Between 2 and 6 months of age
    c. Between 6 months and 1 year of age
    d. Between 1 and 2 years of age

38. The most practical and reliable method for diagnosing congenital toxoplas-mosis infection is

    a. Sabin-Feldman dye test on infant's serum
    b. Detection of IgM antibodies in infant's serum
    c. Indirect fluorescent antibody test on mother's serum
    d. Detection of scattered calcifications within the brain on CT scan

39. The most common congenital infection is

    a. Toxoplasmosis
    b. Herpes simplex
    c. Cytomegalovirus
    d. Rubella

40. Which of the following statements concerning congenital nasolacrimal duct obstruction is false?

    a. The major advantage in delaying surgical treatment until 1 year is that the canaliculus is larger and easier to dilate.
    b. Congenital impatency of the nasolacrimal system is present in about 5% of term infants.
    c. Delay of surgical intervention may make probing unnecessary.
    d. Early treatment may make general anesthesia unnecessary.

41. The most common identifiable cause of bilateral congenital cataracts is

    a. Autosomal recessive inheritance
    b. Autosomal dominant inheritance
    d. Galactosemia
    d. Intrauterine infection

42. Which of the following statements concerning retinoblastoma is true?

    a. Cataract is a common complication.
    b. Strabismus is a common clinical presentation.
    c. Tumors are bilateral in about two thirds of cases.
    d. There is a family history of retinoblastoma in 40% of cases.

43. Which of the following conditions is *not* associated with retinopathy of prematurity?

    a. Myopia
    b. Pseudoesotropia
    c. Glaucoma
    d. Cataract

44. You are asked to see a 2-day-old infant born prematurely at 26 weeks' gestation, weighing 1100 g at birth. Which of the following is true?

    a. All supplemental oxygen should be discontinued.
    b. This child is only minimally at risk for developing ROP.
    c. The first eye examination on this child should be performed at 4–6 weeks of age.
    d. This child is likely to require laser therapy and high doses of vitamin E.

45. Leukocoria may be caused by all of the following except:

    a. Retinoblastoma
    b. Adrenoleukodystrophy
    c. Persistent hyperplastic primary vitreous
    d. Retinopathy of prematurity

46. Which of the following is *not* a cause of pseudopapilledema?

    a. Optic nerve drusen
    b. Pseudotumor cerebri
    c. High hyperopia
    d. Prominent glial tissue on the disc

47. Congenital ptosis is frequently associated with all of the following except:

    a. Poor levator function
    b. Absent upper eyelid crease
    c. Occlusion amblyopia
    d. Chin-up posture

48. All of the following are common features of shaken baby syndrome except:

    a. Hyphema
    b. Vitreous hemorrhage
    c. Retinal hemorrhage
    d. Retinoschisis

49. All of the following statements are true of tuberous sclerosis except:

    a. Ocular findings include retinal hamartomas.
    b. It follows an autosomal dominant inheritance pattern.
    c. Mental retardation is always present.
    d. Angiofibromas occur over the nose and cheeks.

50. In an infant with poor vision and roving eye movements, which of the following diagnoses need *not* be considered?

    a. Leber congenital amaurosis
    b. Achromatopsia
    c. Leber optic atrophy
    d. Optic nerve hypoplasia

51. To which of the following does Hering's law *not* apply?

    a. Version movements
    b. Inhibitional palsy
    c. Primary and secondary deviations
    d. Cocontraction of the horizontal muscles in Duane syndrome

52. A 34-year-old man sustained closed head trauma and now complains of objects appearing tilted. The degree of tilting can be quantified by which of the following tests?

    a. Simultaneous prism-cover test
    b. Double Maddox rod test
    c. Careful analysis of ductions and versions together
    d. Lateroversion reflex test

53. All of the following are true with regard to jerk nystagmus with a null point in right gaze except:

    a. The head would be turned to the left.
    b. Visual acuity is poorest at the null point.
    c. Muscle surgery may improve visual acuity with the eyes in primary position.
    d. Prism therapy has been used to improve head posture.

54. After a 6-mm bilateral lateral rectus recession for an intermittent exotropia of 25 prism diopters, the patient develops an esotropia of 40Δ with constant diplopia and inability to abduct OD beyond the midline. The most likely cause is

    a. Muscle slippage or loss
    b. Accommodative spasm
    c. Surgical increase in AC/A ratio
    d. Inadvertent trauma to right sixth nerve during surgery

55. Paradoxic diplopia observed after strabismus surgery in a formerly esotropic patient is most likely caused by which one of the following?

    a. Surgical undercorrection
    b. Eccentric fixation
    c. Surgical overcorrection
    d. Persistence of abnormal retinal correspondence

56. Which of the following cannot be used to test for ARC?

   a. Worth four-dot test
   b. Major amblyoscope test
   c. Titmus stereo test
   d. Cuppers monocular afterimage test

57. Bilateral ametropic amblyopia

   a. May be seen with moderate degrees of myopia
   b. Is often treated with alternate patching
   c. Sometimes affects visual resolution only along certain meridians
   d. Usually does not improve with time

58. Which of the following is the *least* characteristic of monofixation syndrome?

   a. Small central scotoma
   b. Equal visual acuity
   c. Peripheral fusion
   d. Misalignment of 8Δ or less

59. A patient presents with a left superior oblique muscle paresis and the following measurements. Which of the operations listed is the most appropriate?

	30	15	0	
Right head tilt: LHT = 5	15	LHT = 10	0	Left head tilt: LHT = 15
	0	0	0	

Right gaze   Left gaze

   a. Tuck LSO
   b. Tuck LSO, recess LIO
   c. Recess LIO
   d. Recess RSR and LIR

60. A patient presents with the following measurements. Which of the following procedures is the most appropriate?

LHT = 25	0	RHT = 25	Double Maddox rod test:
LHT = 20	0	RHT = 20	OD = 9° extorsion
LHT = 18	ET = 20	RHT = 15	OS = 11° extorsion

   a. Recess IR OU, infraplace MR OU
   b. Tuck SO OU
   c. Recess SR OU
   d. Recess IO OU

61. A patient presents with the following measurements. Which of the following operations is the most appropriate?

		70		
RHT=10	40	ET = 40	40	LHT = 10
		10		

Right gaze   Left gaze

Versions: 3+ superior oblique overaction bilaterally

a. Tenotomy SO OU alone
b. Recess MR OU with infraplacement
c. Tenotomy SO OU, recess RMR with infraplacement and resect RLR with supraplacement
d. Tenotomy SO OU, resect LR OU with infraplacement

62. A patient presents with the following measurements. If surgery is performed, which of the following operations is the most appropriate?

	ET = 10	
RHT = 20	0	LHT = 20
	XT = 40	

Right gaze   Left gaze

a. Myectomy IO OU
b. Displace IR laterally OU
c. Tenotomy SO OU
d. Tuck SO OU

63. A patient presents with the following measurements. No obvious oblique muscle dysfunction is seen on version testing. Which of the following operations is the most appropriate?

	10	
20	XT = 20	20
	40	

a. Recess LR OU, tenotomy SO OU
b. Recess LR OU and infraplace
c. Recess LLR and supraplace, resect LMR and infraplace
d. Resect MR OU and infraplace

64. Which of the following is the least characteristic of spasmus nutans?

 a. Head nodding
 b. Conjugate nystagmus
 c. Torticollis
 d. Onset between 4 and 12 months of age

ANSWERS

1. Answer—b. Immature retinal vasculature is the basic substrate for ROP. Current weight and respirator dependency are not relevant and iris vessel dilatation is a serious harbinger of threshold ROP.

2. Answer—d. Aniridia is an autosomal dominant condition affecting both sexes, most often causing poor vision. Wilms tumor is a serious concern for the sporadic cases, occurring in about one third of these patients.

3. Answer—c. Orbital bone repositioning can have a marked effect on ocular position. Therefore, if possible, bone surgery should be done first. Amblyopia, refractive errors, and hydrocephalus are common and can cause profound visual loss.

4. Answer—c. Parents of a child with the most common forms of albinism have a 25% recurrence risk for each subsequent child.

5. Answer—-c. ROP is a disease of immature retinal vessels. The less gestational time the child has had, the more immature the retinal vessels are going to be. They thus have more potential for developing ROP.

6. Answer—d. Myopia and blindness can still occur even with treatment. Although laser photocoagulation has replaced cryotherapy as the treatment modality of choice in many centers, it is not without possible complications. Argon laser has been associated with cataract formation in some cases, especially when a prominent tunica vasculosa lentis is present.

7. Answer—d. Nystagmus and reduced visual acuity are characteristic of albinism. Stereopsis is prevented by the abnormally large number of crossed fibers in the optic chiasm. Intellectual ability is not affected in albinism. Fertility is also unaffected.

8. Answer—b. Exotropia. Down syndrome patients are at high risk for esotropia, nystagmus, and high refractive errors.

9. Answer—c. Sixth nerve palsy. It may be difficult to demonstrate full abduction and esotropia since these patients prefer to cross fixate. However, congenital sixth nerve palsy is very rare and is not associated with congenital esotropia. Dissociated deviations and latent nystagmus can be seen in more than 50% of congenital esotropia patients during childhood. In addition, many will develop an accommodative component to the esotropia in the toddler or preschool years.

10. Answer—b. Neonatal herpes simplex infection is most frequently acquired from passage through the genital tract of a woman with an active cervical herpetic infection.

11. Answer—b. Serum antibody test for rubella, syphilis, or other infectious agents may allow a specific diagnosis of congenital infection to be made as a cause of "salt-and-pepper" retinopathy. In a child with normal vision an ERG is unlikely to yield useful information. Chromosomal evaluation is nonspecific. Congenital rubella and luetic infections are not associated with intracranial calcification, and, therefore, a CT scan of the brain is not likely to aid in the diagnosis.

12. Answer—d. Multinucleate giant cells are seen in herpetic conjunctivitis, not chlamydial conjunctivitis. Lymphocytes are found on Gram stains in chemical, chlamydial, and viral conjunctivitis. Basophilic intracytoplasmic inclusions are seen in chlamydial conjunctivitis. Eosinophilic intranuclear inclusions are seen in herpetic conjunctivitis and can be demonstrated in a Pap smear of conjunctival epithelial cells.

13. Answer—a. Hospitalization for IV antibiotic treatment is indicated for presumed orbital cellulitis. A CT scan is superior to MRI for orbital imaging in orbital cellulitis and should be performed in the presence of proptosis. Surgical drainage of a subperiosteal abscess is indicated for acute visual loss or if the patient fails to respond to IV antibiotics over 24-48 hours. However, most patients in this age group respond well to medical management. Oral antibiotics are not sufficient for treatment of orbital cellulitis.

14. Answer—d. Cataracts associated with PHPV frequently have a poor prognosis because of microphthalmos, retinal or optic nerve abnormalities, and competition with the normal eye. The other types of cataracts are either nonamblyogenic in most cases (anterior polar cataract), are frequently developmental after a period of normal visual experience with the affected eye (posterior lenticonus and lamellar), or are only partial.

15. Answer—d. The least controversial indication for IOLs in children is correction of aphakia in unilateral traumatic cataracts. IOLs are still controversial in children less than 2 years old. Secondary IOLs are not performed routinely at any particular age but only if the child cannot or will not wear contact lenses or glasses. Capsular fixation is always preferred over sulcus fixation.

16. Answer—d. Pauciarticular JRA with early onset and positive ANA constitutes the greatest risk for developing chronic uveitis.

17. Answer—b. Band keratopathy can be treated, but vision loss still tends to occur from CME. Most patients with intermediate uveitis are beyond the amblyopia-sensitive age. The optic nerve is not typically involved in intermediate uveitis.

18. Answer—a. Most infants with congenital esotropia at this age have not yet developed significant amblyopia and will alternate fixation preference. An accommodative component is possible at this age but uncommon. DVD is unlikely at this age.

19. Answer—c. Better sensory outcomes are obtained in children whose eyes are aligned before 2 years of age. Most surgeons operate when preexisting amblyopia has been treated and the deviation is of stable magnitude. This often occurs at age 6 months or older. The age at which a child walks has no bearing on the age for surgery. Strabismus surgery at age 4 months or even younger is currently being studied but remains controversial.

20. Answer—d. If the child is a prism responder, a larger dose of surgery is often performed. Any accommodative esotropia is taken into account in planning surgery. Children who do not respond to prism adaptation still have a high rate of sensory and motor success from surgery.

21. Answer—b. Normal convergence amplitudes are much greater than divergence amplitudes. Vertical fusional amplitudes are very small except in patients with long-standing vertical deviation such as congenital superior oblique muscle paresis.

22. Answer—d. Horror fusionis produces intractable absence of fusion and absence of fusional amplitudes. It often occurs after head trauma or after long-standing sensory strabismus with diplopia.

23. Answer—b. The inferior oblique muscle is an extortor and may produce extorsion of the fundus in primary position when it is overacting. In addition, inferior oblique muscle overaction produces overelevation in adduction. It is commonly associated with V-pattern strabismus.

24. Answer—b. Parvocellular neurons are more sensitive to color, high spatial frequencies, fine two-point discrimination, and fine stereopsis. They project to areas of central visual field and fovea.

25. Answer—b. The vertical prism or induced tropia fixation test creates an artificial strabismus so the preferred eye can be determined. In this way amblyopia can be detected in the absence of strabismus.

26. Answer—c. The simultaneous prism-cover test is used to measure a tropia in monofixation syndrome where a tropia and an overlying phoria may coexist.

27. Answer—d. In the six cardinal positions, one muscle is the primary mover in each eye and can be tested for under- and overaction. The nine *diagnostic* positions include the six cardinal positions with the addition of primary position, straight up, and straight down.

28. Answer—a. Fusional vergences eliminate retinal disparity. They are usually involuntary and are larger in the horizontal plane as compared to the vertical plane. Patients with large-angle strabismus and ARC do not have measurable fusional vergences.

29. Answer—c. Placing a posterior fixation suture on a muscle will weaken it only in its field of action.

30. Answer—b. Diplopia is common in patients who are overcorrected and develop a consecutive deviation. Unsatisfactory alignment is the most common complication of strabismus surgery. Scleral perforation from a deep needle pass may or may not require treatment depending on the severity of the injury. Orbital cellulitis following strabismus surgery typically presents 2 or 3 days postoperatively.

31. Answer—d. Changes in eyelid position are often seen after inferior rectus recession. The adherence syndrome is usually not present. Lower eyelid retractor release or recession can be done as a treatment for lower eyelid malposition with scleral show after inferior rectus muscle recession. The problem is minimized by careful dissection of the posterior surface of the inferior rectus muscle when it is operated.

32. Answer—d. High temperature. This is usually a later sign. Ideally, the hyperthermia is diagnosed before the temperature reaches high levels. The earliest sign is often tachycardia. Other early signs include tachypnea, sweating, muscle rigidity, blotchy discoloration of skin, cyanosis, and dark urine.

33. Answer—a. Botulinum toxin injection is least suitable for large-angle deviations or restrictive or mechanical strabismus.

34. Answer—a. Eyelid ptosis is the most common complication of botulinum toxin injection. It is slightly more common for medial rectus injections as compared to lateral rectus injections. Induced secondary strabismus occurs less commonly than ptosis, but both are almost always temporary. Scleral perforation and retrobulbar hemorrhage are very rare.

35. Answer—b. Only Leber congenital amaurosis will present in infancy with sluggish pupils, pendular nystagmus, and a normal fundus. All the other conditions listed either have fundus changes (Tay-Sachs disease and congenital hydrocephalus) or present with no nystagmus or a searching sensory type, not a pendular type, of nystagmus.

36. Answer—b. Orbital cellulitis in young infants may arise from infection in the ethmoid sinuses. The maxillary and frontal sinuses are not well developed in infants and young children. Infections in the sphenoid sinus are relatively uncommon and, therefore, not a frequent cause of orbital infection in young children.

37. Answer—a. Dense, bilateral congenital cataracts will cause bilateral amblyopia and nystagmus if not treated in early infancy.

38. Answer—b. The finding of specific IgM antibodies in the newborn's serum is diagnostic for congenital toxoplasmosis. IgM antibodies do not cross the placenta and, therefore, cannot be passively transferred from the mother. The Sabin-Feldman dye test is not practical because it requires live toxoplasma organisms, and so it is seldom used. Although fluorescent antibody tests are frequently employed and effective, positive titer in the mother does not necessarily mean congenital infection has occurred. Finally, although scattered calcifications can be found within the brain on CT scan, this finding is not diagnostic of toxoplasmosis infection.

39. Answer—c. Of all of the TORCHS infections, cytomegalovirus is certainly the most common and is, in fact, the most common congenital infection of humans.

40. Answer—a. Although the canaliculus is larger in older infants, this presents no technical advantage, as probing even a 1-week-old is generally not difficult. The remainder of the answers are correct.

41. Answer—b. Although bilateral cataracts can be inherited in autosomal dominant, autosomal recessive, and X-linked patterns, the most common inheritance pattern is autosomal dominant.

42. Answer—b. Although leukocoria is the most common clinical presentation of retinoblastoma, strabismus is the next most common, especially if the tumor involves the macula. Cataract is not a common complication of retinoblastoma. Tumors are bilateral in one third of cases, and a family history is present in only 5%–10% of cases.

43. Answer—b. Because the macula can be dragged temporally in ROP, a very positive angle kappa can be seen, giving the appearance of an exotropia, not an esotropia.

44. Answer—c. This child is at high risk for developing ROP. The first examination should be performed at 6 weeks of age, although it can be performed sooner. High doses of vitamin E are controversial in ROP.

45. Answer—b. Only adrenoleukodystrophy does not result in a median opacity with leukocoria.

46. Answer—b. Pseudotumor cerebri causes true papilledema, associated with increased intracranial pressure.

47. Answer—c. Although occlusion amblyopia must be carefully sought in any patient with congenital ptosis, it is rarely encountered.

48. Answer—a. Only hyphema is not commonly seen either acutely or late in shaken baby syndrome, since hyphema generally requires direct blunt ocular trauma.

49. Answer—c. Severe mental retardation is present in 50% of tuberous sclerosis patients, but intelligence is normal in many affected persons.

50. Answer—c. Poor vision and nystagmus during infancy are presenting signs for Leber congenital amaurosis, achromatopsia, and optic nerve hypoplasia. Leber optic atrophy presents much later, usually during the second or third decade.

51. Answer—d. According to Hering's law, equal and simultaneous innervation flows to synergistic muscles (or muscle groups) concerned with the desired direction of gaze. In cocontraction of the medial and lateral rectus muscles, as it occurs on adduction in a typical case of Duane syndrome, innervation flows to these muscles simultaneously. Normally, the medial and lateral rectus muscles are antagonists, which are not innervated simultaneously.

52. Answer—b. "Tilted vision" after closed head trauma is usually a result of superior oblique palsy. The double Maddox rod test is the easiest way to quantify the resulting cyclotropia. Patients are sometimes unable to describe or call attention to the tilted images after trauma. For this reason the double Maddox rod test should be employed routinely on all adults who complain of vertical tropia. In certain cases patients may complain of tilted objects with one eye occluded.

53. Answer—b. Patients with jerk nystagmus put their eyes in the field of least nystagmus, and their heads usually are turned in the opposite direction. Vision is improved at the null point because the eyes move less. Surgery and prisms can be employed to improve head position.

54. Answer—a. Although an overcorrection of an intermittent exotropia may occur, the inability to abduct the eye past the midline most likely is a result of a slipped lateral rectus muscle. Trauma to the sixth nerve during a lateral rectus recession is unlikely.

55. Answer—d. Diplopia in the postoperative phase is disturbing to both the patient and the surgeon. It may be caused by an overcorrection, undercorrection, or persistence of ARC during the immediate postoperative phase. Crossed diplopia in a surgically aligned, formerly esotropic patient clearly identifies the diplopia as being paradoxic and thus a result of persisting ARC. It is comforting to know that this symptom is usually transient and will disappear spontaneously as normal retinal correspondence establishes itself.

56. Answer—c. The Titmus stereo test cannot be used to detect ARC.

57. Answer—c. Bilateral ametropic amblyopia results from high degrees of myopia, hyperopia, or astigmatism in both eyes. It frequently presents as loss of resolving ability (blurring) limited to certain meridians. Treatment generally involves correction of the refractive error, and patching is usually not required.

58. Answer—b. A small 3°–5° central scotoma along with peripheral fusion and a misalignment of 8Δ or less is characteristic of monofixation syndrome. However, amblyopia, either slight or profound, is present in most patients.

59. Answer—c. This is a superior oblique paresis with the deviation being greatest in the opposite up field of gaze. It is of only moderate amount in primary position, and a weakening procedure on the left inferior oblique is the indicated operation.

60. Answer—b. The patient has evidence for bilateral superior oblique palsy with V-pattern esotropia in downgaze, no vertical deviation in primary position, and greater than 10° extorsion. The best procedure would be a bilateral superior oblique tuck. Bilateral inferior oblique recession could also be considered but would not help the esotropia in downgaze.

61. Answer—d. This patient has A-pattern esotropia. A superior oblique tenotomy would lessen the A but would not affect the esotropia in primary position. The horizontal recti can be offset by supraplacing the medial rectus or infraplacing the lateral recti. Only answer d includes all correct approaches.

62. Answer—c. This is an A-pattern strabismus with no deviation in primary position. The right gaze right hypertropia and the left gaze left hypertropia are the result of overaction of both superior oblique muscles. A superior oblique tenotomy would be expected to normalize the A pattern and have the least effect on primary position.

63. Answer—b. Recess LR OU and infraplace. This patient has an A-pattern exotropia with no obvious oblique muscle dysfunction of version testing. To help correct the A pattern, the lateral rectus muscles would need to be infraplaced or the medial rectus muscles would need to be supraplaced.

64. Answer—b. Head nodding, torticollis, and nystagmus are the triad of signs in spasmus nutans. However, the nystagmus is of a disconjugate type.

INDEX

Atropine
  for amblyopia, 50
  for cycloplegic refraction, 72, 72t
  in refractive accommodative esotropia
    management, 78
Axenfeld anomaly. See Axenfeld-Rieger
  syndrome
Axenfeld-Rieger syndrome, 211,
    211i, 212i
  posterior embryotoxon in, 210, 211
  pseudopolycoria in, 225, 225i
Axes of Fick, 23, 23i

Bacteria. See also specific organism
  conjunctivitis caused by, 184–186
Baerveldt implant, for childhood
    glaucoma, 235
Bagolini lenses
  retinal correspondence tested with, 42,
    42i, 43i
  suppression tested with, 40, 43i
Band keratopathy, in juvenile rheumatoid
    arthritis, 253, 254i
  surgery for, 254
Base-in prisms
  for intermittent exotropia, 88
  for undercorrection of intermittent
    exotropia, 89
Base-out prism test (4Δ), for
    monofixation syndrome, 44
Base-out prisms
  for monofixation syndrome evaluation,
    44
  for nystagmus, 132
  for overcorrection of intermittent
    exotropia, 89
Bassen-Kornzweig syndrome, Leber
    congenital amaurosis and, 278
Bear tracks, 323
Behr optic atrophy, 300
Bergmeister's papilla, 297
Bernheimer-Seitelberger disease (GM$_2$ type
    III gangliosidosis), 292, 361t
  enzyme defect in, 361t
  ocular findings in, 292, 361t
Best vitelliform dystrophy, 281–282, 282i
Beta blockers, for childhood glaucoma,
    235–236
Bielschowsky head-tilt test, 70, 71i

Bifixation, in monofixation
    syndrome, 42
Bifocal lenses
  for nonrefractive accommodative
    esotropia, 79, 80
  for refractive accommodative esotropia,
    78, 80
Bilateral acoustic neurofibromatosis, 330.
    See also Neurofibromatosis
Binocular eye movements, 28–31. See also
    specific type
  conjugate (versions), 28–31, 30i
  disjugate (vergences), 31
  in infants, 372
Binocular field of fixation, testing,
    69, 69i
Binocular fixation pattern, for amblyopia
    detection, 48
Binocular vision
  abnormalities of, 38–44. See also
    specific type
  physiology of, 33–36
Binocular Visual Acuity Test (BVAT), 69
Biomicroscopy, slit-lamp, for pediatric
    cataract, 244–247, 245i, 246i
Birth weight, retinopathy of prematurity
    and, 268, 273
Blepharitis, congenital nasolacrimal duct
    obstruction differentiated from, 201
Blepharoconjunctivitis, herpes simplex,
    186
  in newborn, 182
Blepharophimosis, with epicanthus
    inversus, telecanthus, and ptosis, 171,
    171i
Blepharoptosis. See Ptosis
Blepharospasm
  botulinum toxin for, 160
  in primary congenital
    glaucoma, 228
Blindness. See also Low vision;
    Visual loss
  cortical, 374
  Leber congenital amaurosis causing,
    375–376
  night, congenital stationary, 279
  primary congenital glaucoma causing,
    232, 236–237
Blink reflex, in newborn, 372

Cavernous sinus thrombosis, 191
Ceftriaxone, for gonococcal conjunctivitis
in newborn, 183
Cellulitis, 190–193
orbital, 191–193, 192*i*
fungal (mucormycosis), 193, 194*i*
preseptal, 190–191
after strabismus surgery,
149–150, 151*i*
Center of rotation, 23, 23*i*
Central cysts (pupillary cysts), 221
Central fusional disruption (horror
fusionis), 38, 91
Central neurofibromatosis, 330. *See also*
Neurofibromatosis
Central posterior keratoconus (posterior
corneal depression), 211–212
Central suppression, 39
Central vision loss, in leukemia, 287
Ceroid lipofuscinosis, 361*t*
Chalazia, 322
CHARGE association, 220
Check ligaments, 18
CHED. *See* Congenital hereditary
endothelial dystrophy
Chédiak-Higashi syndrome, 288, 291*t*
Chemical injury (burns), 367
Chemodenervation. *See also* Botulinum
toxin
for eyelid disorders, 160
for strabismus, 159–160
Chemotherapy, for
retinoblastoma, 328
Cherry-red spot,
in gangliosidoses, 292
myoclonus syndrome, 360*t*
Chickenpox. *See* Varicella
Child abuse, ocular trauma and, 363–366
Children
abuse of, ocular trauma and, 363–366
examination of
checklist for, 3–5, 4*i*
rapport and, 3–6
for strabismus, 5–6

intraocular lens implantation
in, 249
normal eye in, 163–164, 165*i*, 165*t*
nystagmus in, 125–135. *See also*
Nystagmus, childhood
Chlamydia, conjunctivitis caused by, in
neonates, 182, 183
Chloroma, of orbit, 310
Chlorpheniramine, for seasonal allergic
conjunctivitis, 194
Cholesteatoma, orbital, 315–316
Cholinesterase inhibitors
accommodative convergence affected
by, 66
for nonrefractive accommodative
esotropia, 79
Chondrosarcoma, orbital, 308
Chorioretinitis
syphilitic, 181, 181*i*, 258
in toxoplasmosis, 175
Choristomas, orbital, 315
Choroid
hemangioma of, 324
in leukemia, 286
in neurofibromatosis, 333
osteoma of, 324
retinoblastoma involving, 328
in Sturge-Weber syndrome, 343–344,
344*i*
tumors of, 323–324
Choroiditis
in ocular histoplasmosis, 262
posttraumatic, 255
Chromosomal abnormality, iris coloboma
associated with, 219
Chronic cyclitis. *See* Intermediate uveitis
Chronic progressive external
ophthalmoplegia, 119*t*, 121
CHRPE. *See* Congenital hypertrophy of
retinal pigment epithelium
CHSD. *See* Congenital hereditary stromal
dystrophy
Ciancia syndrome, 76*t*, 77
CID. *See* Cytomegalic inclusion disease
Ciliary arteries, anterior, 17

Cover-uncover test, 59, 60*i*
CPEO. *See* Chronic progressive external ophthalmoplegia
Cranial nerve III, palsy of. *See* Third nerve palsy
Cranial nerve IV, palsy of. *See* Fourth nerve palsy
Cranial nerve VI, palsy of. *See* Sixth nerve palsy
Craniofacial malformations, 349–357. *See also specific type*
   approach to child with, 349–350
   craniosynostosis, 350–353
   in fetal alcohol syndrome, 356, 357*i*
   in fetal hydantoin syndrome, 357
   Goldenhar syndrome. *See* Goldenhar syndrome
   Hallerman-Streiff syndrome, 354
   hemifacial microsomia, 353, 354*i*
   hypertelorism, 353
   intrinsic ocular pathology in, 349
   mandibulofacial dysostosis (Treacher Collins–Franceschetti syndrome), 354–355, 355*i*
   Pierre Robin sequence (anomaly/deformity), 354
   secondary ocular complications in, 349–350
   Waardenburg syndrome, 353
Craniopharyngiomas, nystagmus caused by, 125*t*
Craniosynostosis, 350–353
Credé prophylaxis (silver nitrate prophylaxis), 182, 183
Cromolyn
   for seasonal allergic conjunctivitis, 194
   for vernal keratoconjunctivitis, 195–196
Cross syndrome, 290*t*
Crossed diplopia, 41
Crouzon syndrome, 351*i*
   V pattern associated with, 109–110
Crowding bars, for amblyopia evaluation, 48, 48*i*
Crowding phenomenon, 45–46
Cryotherapy
   for retinal angiomas, 332
   for retinoblastoma, 328

for retinopathy of prematurity, 273, 274*i*
Cryptophthalmos, 168, 168*i*
CSM method, for visual acuity assessment, 57–58
Cup/disc ratio
   in megalopapillae, 297
   in primary congenital glaucoma, 231
Cyclitis, chronic. *See* Intermediate uveitis
Cycloablation, for childhood glaucoma, 235
Cyclocryotherapy, for childhood glaucoma, 235
Cyclodeviations, double Maddox rod test in evaluation of, 63
Cyclomydril. *See* Cyclopentolate
Cyclopentolate
   for cycloplegic refraction, 70–72, 72*t*
   for fundus evaluation of premature infant, 271
Cycloplegic refraction, 70–72, 72*t*
   in classic congenital (essential infantile) esotropia, 75
   in infant with decreased vision, 373
Cycloplegics
   for hyphema, 369
   for refraction, 70–72, 72*t*. *See also* Cycloplegic refraction
   side effects of, 72
Cyclovertical muscle palsies, three-step test in, 70, 71*i*
Cyclovertical strabismus, surgery planning and, 141
Cystinosis, 361*t*
   cysteamine for, 216
   ocular findings in, 216, 217*i*, 361*t*
Cytomegalovirus, congenital infection caused by (cytomegalic inclusion disease), 178–179

Dacryocystitis, congenital dacryocystocele and, 200
Dacryocystocele/dacryocele, congenital, 200, 201*i*
Dacryocystorhinostomy, for nasolacrimal duct obstruction, 207

Dantrolene, for malignant hyperthermia, 157, 158t
Daraprim. *See* Pyrimethamine
DCR. *See* Dacryocystorhinostomy
de Morsier syndrome (septo-optic dysplasia), 298
Deformation, definition of, 167
Dellen, after strabismus surgery, 152–153, 153i
Dendritic keratitis
  herpes simplex, 186, 187i
  herpes zoster, 256
Dendritic keratoconjunctivitis, herpes simplex, 187i
Denervation and extirpation, 138t
Deorsumduction/Deorsumversion. *See* Depression
Depression (of gaze), 27, 28
  inferior rectus muscle in, 11, 12i, 25t
  superior oblique muscle in, 13, 13i, 25t
Deprivation amblyopia, 38, 47
  pattern, P-cell abnormalities and, 37
Depth perception
  stereo acuity testing and, 68
  stereopsis differentiated from, 36
Dermoids (dermoid cysts/tumors), 215
  epibulbar, 320
  infantile corneal opacities in, 214t, 215
  limbal, 320, 321i
    Goldenhar syndrome and, 215, 320, 321i, 353, 354i
  orbital, 315–316, 315i
Dermolipomas (lipodermoids)
  conjunctival, 320, 320i
  Goldenhar syndrome and, 320, 321i, 353, 354i
Derry disease (GM$_1$ type II gangliosidosis), 292, 361t
  enzyme defect in, 361t
  ocular findings in, 292, 361t
Descemet's membrane, injuries to, infantile corneal opacities and, 213–214, 214t
Desmoid tumors, of orbit, 314
Developmental field, definition of, 167

Developmental glaucoma, 233–234. *See also* Glaucoma, pediatric
Deviation. *See also specific type and* Esodeviations; Exodeviations
  alternate cover (prism and cover) test in assessment of, 59–60, 61i
  comitant (concomitant), 55, 93
  horizontal, dissociated, 91, 92i, 94
  incomitant (noncomitant), 55
  primary, 29
  secondary, 29
  vertical, 93–106. *See also* Vertical deviations
Dextrocycloversion, 28
Dextrodeorsumversion, yoke muscles in, 29t
Dextrosursumversion, yoke muscles in, 29t
Dextroversion, 28
  yoke muscles in, 29t
DHD. *See* Dissociated horizontal deviations
Diabetes mellitus, 285–286
  cataracts associated with, 285
  insulin-dependent (type 1/IDDM), 285–286
Diabetic retinopathy, 285–286
  nonproliferative (background), 285
Diagnostic positions of gaze, 65, 65i
Diamox. *See* Acetazolamide
Diktyoma (medulloepithelioma), 323
Diode laser
  cycloablation with, for childhood glaucoma, 235
  hyperthermia with, for retinoblastoma, 328
Dipivefrin, for childhood glaucoma, 236
Diplopia, 38
  crossed, 41
  heteronymous, 41
  homonymous, 41
  Panum's area and, 34i, 35
  after strabismus surgery, 148–149
  strabismus surgery for elimination of, 137
  testing for, 40–41. *See also* Red filter/red lens test
  uncrossed, 41

strengthening procedures in, 139
techniques for, 137–140
transposition procedures in, 140
weakening procedures in,
137, 138t
Extraocular muscles. *See also specific type
and* Eye movement; Ocular motility
actions of, 9, 9–15, 15t, 24–25
anatomy of, 9–22
blood supply of, 17
surgery and, 21–22
contraction of, physiology of, 27
fascial relationships of, 18–19, 19i
fiber types in, 17
fine structure of, 17
innervation of, 9–15, 15t
surgery and, 136, 158t
insertions of, 9–15, 15t
advancing, as strengthening
procedure, 139
lost, in strabismus surgery, 155, 155i
orbital relationships of, 18–19, 19i
origin of, 9–15, 15t
relationships of, 16i
secondary actions of, 9
slipped, in strabismus surgery, 155–156,
156i
surgery of. *See* Extraocular muscle
surgery; Strabismus surgery
tertiary actions of, 9
venous system of, 17
Eye
color of, age affecting, 163
development of, 163–165
dimensions of, 163, 164i, 165t
injury to. *See* Trauma
Eye movements, 27–31. *See also specific
type and* Ocular motility
assessment of, 59–73
binocular, 28–31
conjugate (versions), 28–31, 30i
disjugate (vergences), 31, 372
in infants, 372–373
monocular (ductions), 27–28
recruitment after, 27
supranuclear control systems for, 32
Eye muscles. *See* Extraocular muscles

Eye patches. *See* Patching
Eyelids
disorders of
botulinum toxin for, 160
congenital, 168–172
drooping. *See* Ptosis
lacerations of, 367–368
strabismus surgery affecting position of,
153–154, 154i
tumors of, 319–322

Fabry disease, 360t
Facial angiofibromas, in tuberous sclerosis,
338, 338i
Facial defects. *See* Cleft syndromes;
Craniofacial malformations
Facultative suppression, 39
Fadenoperation (posterior fixation suture),
138t
Fallen eye syndrome, 97
False passage, probing of nasolacrimal
duct obstruction and, 205
Familial drusen, 282–283
Familial dysautonomia (Riley-Day
syndrome), corneal manifestations
of, 217
Familial exudative
vitreoretinopathy, 284
Familial iridoplegia, 224
Familial oculorenal syndromes, 289
Familial renal-retinal dystrophy, 289
Fanconi syndrome, corneal manifestations
of, in childhood, 216, 217i
FAS. *See* Fetal alcohol syndrome
Fascia bulbi. *See* Tenon's capsule
Felderstruktur muscle fibers, 17
Fetal alcohol syndrome, 356, 357i
Fetal hydantoin syndrome, 357
FEVR. *See* Familial exudative
vitreoretinopathy
FHS. *See* Fetal hydantoin syndrome
Fibrillenstruktur muscle fibers, 17
Fibrin clots, after penetrating
trauma, 367
Fibroma/fibromatosis
juvenile, of orbit, 314
molluscum, in neurofibromatosis,
334–335
ossifying, of orbit, 314

Hering's law of motor correspondence, 28–31, 30*i*
Hermansky-Pudlak syndrome, 288, 290*t*
Herpes simplex viruses, 179–181, 257
  conjunctivitis caused by, 180, 182, 186–187, 187*i*
  iridocyclitis caused by, 257
  iritis caused by, 257
  perinatal infection caused by, 180–181, 183
  type 1, 180, 187
  type 2, 180, 187
  uveitis caused by, 257
Herpes zoster, 256–257. *See also* Varicella-zoster virus
  conjunctivitis in, 187–188, 188*i*
  uveitis in, 256–257
Hess screen test, 64
  in superior oblique muscle palsy, 97
Heterochromia iridis, 222, 223*i*, 223*t*
  in leukemia, 287
Heteronymous diplopia, 41
Heterophoria, 53
Heterophoria method, for accommodative convergence/accommodation ratio measurement, 66
Heterotropia, 53
  alternating, 59
  simultaneous prism-cover test in assessment of, 60–61
Hirschberg test, 61, 62*i*
Histiocytosis X (Langerhans cell histiocytosis), orbital involvement in, 310–311, 311*i*
Histo spots, 262
Histocompatibility antigens (HLA antigens), in juvenile rheumatoid arthritis, 253
Histoplasmin skin test, 262
Histoplasmosis (*Histoplasma capsulatum*), ocular, 261–262, 262*i*
History
  in amblyopia, 56
  in infant with decreased vision, 373
  in intermittent exotropia, 86–87
  in strabismus, 56

HIV infection/AIDS, cytomegalovirus retinopathy and, 178
HLA antigens. *See* Histocompatibility antigens
Holes, optic (optic pits), 299, 299*i*
Homatropine, for cycloplegic refraction, 72, 72*t*
Homocystinuria, 241–242, 242*i*, 361*t*
Homonymous diplopia, 41
Horizontal deviations, dissociated, 91, 92*i*, 94
Horizontal incomitance, strabismus surgery planning and, 140
Horizontal rectus muscles
  action of, 9, 10*i*, 24, 25*t*
    gaze posltion and, 26, 26*t*
  anatomy of, 9, 10*i*
  surgery of, for A- and V-pattern deviations, 110–111, 111*i*, 146
  V pattern associated with dysfunction of, 109
Horner syndrome, in neuroblastoma, 309, 309*i*
Horopter, empirical, 34–35, 34*i*
Horror fusionis (central fusional disruption), 38, 91
HSV. *See* Herpes simplex viruses
Human immunodeficiency virus infection. *See* HIV infection/AIDS
Human leukocyte antigens (HLA antigens). *See* Histocompatibility antigens
Hunter syndrome, 360*t*
Hurler syndrome, 360*t*
  infantile corneal opacities in, 214, 214*t*, 215*i*
Hutchinson's triad, 181
Hyaloid system, persistent, 297
Hydantoin, anomalies associated with maternal use of, 357
Hyperlysinemia, 242
Hyperplasia, definition of, 166
Hypertelorism, 353
  telecanthus differentiated from, 171
Hypertensive retinopathy, in renal disease, 289
Hyperthermia
  diode laser, for retinoblastoma, 328
  malignant, 156–157, 158*t*

Latanoprost, for childhood
    glaucoma, 236
Latent nystagmus, 77, 129
    manifest, 76*t*, 77, 129, 130*i*
Lateral incomitance, strabismus surgery
    planning and, 141
Lateral muscular branch, of ophthalmic
    artery, extraocular muscles supplied
    by, 17
Lateral rectus muscles, 15*t*
    action of, 9, 10*i*, 15*t*, 25*t*
    anatomy of, 9, 10*i*, 15*t*
    surgery of, 146–147
        for A- and V-pattern deviations,
            110–111, 111*i*, 112, 113
Law of motor correspondence, Hering's,
    28–31, 30*i*
Law of reciprocal innervation,
    Sherrington's, 28
Learning disabilities, vision and, 382–385
Leash phenomenon, 114, 115, 116*i*
Leber congenital amaurosis, 277–278,
    278*i*, 375–376
Leber hereditary optic neuropathy,
    300–301
Leber idiopathic stellate neuroretinitis,
    301, 302*i*
Left gaze (levoversion), 28
    yoke muscles in, 29*t*
Lens (crystalline), 238
    absence of (aphakia), 238
    colobomas of, 238, 238*i*
    congenital anomalies/defects of,
        238–242
    dislocation of, 239–240. *See also*
        Ectopia lentis
    disorders of, 238–250. *See also specific*
        type
    in homocystinuria, 241–242, 242*i*
    in hyperlysinemia, 242
    in Marfan syndrome,
        240–241, 241*i*
    opacities of. *See* Cataract
    removal of, 248
    structural or positional abnormalities of,
        238–242
    in sulfite oxidase deficiency, 242
    in Weill-Marchesani syndrome, 242
Lensectomy, 248

Lenticonus, 239
    anterior, 239
        in Alport syndrome, 239, 289
    posterior (lentiglobus), 239, 239*i*,
        245–247, 246*i*
Letterer-Siwe disease, orbital involvement
    in, 310
Leucovorin (folinic acid), for
    toxoplasmosis, 175, 261*t*
Leukemia
    orbital involvement in, 287, 310
    retinal manifestations of, 286–287,
        286*i*, 287*i*
    uveitis differentiated from, 264*t*
Leukocoria, 266–276. *See also specific*
    cause
    differential diagnosis of, 327*t*
    in retinoblastoma, 324, 324*i*
Leukodystrophy, metachromatic, 360*t*
Levator palpebrae superioris
    muscle, 15*t*
    anatomy of, 14, 15*t*
Levocabastin, for seasonal allergic
    conjunctivitis, 194
Levocycloversion, 28
Levodeorsumversion, yoke muscles
    in, 29*t*
Levosursumversion, yoke muscles
    in, 29*t*
Levoversion (left gaze), 28
    yoke muscles in, 29*t*
LHON. *See* Leber hereditary optic
    neuropathy
Ligaments
    check, 18
    Lockwood's, 18
Ligneous conjunctivitis,
    phlyctenular, 322
Limbal dermoids, 320, 321*i*
    Goldenhar syndrome and, 215, 320,
        321*i*, 353
Limbal incision, for extraocular muscle
    surgery, 147–148
Limbus, vernal keratoconjunctivitis
    affecting, 195
Lipidoses, 360*t*
Lipodermoids (dermolipomas)
    conjunctival, 320, 320*i*
    Goldenhar syndrome and, 320, 321*i*,
        353, 354*i*

Median facial cleft syndrome (frontonasal dysplasia), 353
Median plane, 23, 24*i*
Medullated (myelinated) nerve fibers, 296, 296*i*
Medulloblastoma, nystagmus caused by, 125*t*
Medulloepithelioma (diktyoma), 323
Megalocornea, 209
Megalopapillae, 297
Megalophthalmos, anterior, 209
Melanocytic lesions, in neurofibromatosis, 332
Melanocytoma, 324
Melanocytosis
    ocular (melanosis oculi), 321
    oculodermal (nevus of Ota), 321
Melanoma, uveitis differentiated from, 264*t*
Meningioma
    optic nerve sheath, optic glioma differentiated from, 335
    orbital, 314
Meningocele, orbital, 317
Meriodional amblyopia, 47
Mesectodermal dysgenesis. *See* Anterior segment, dysgenesis of
Mesenchymal dysgenesis. *See* Anterior segment, dysgenesis of
Metabolic disorders. *See* Inborn errors of metabolism
Metachromatic leukodystrophy, 360*t*
Metastatic disease of orbit, 309–311
Microcoria (congenital miosis), 224
Microcornea, 209, 210*i*
Microphthalmos
    in congenital rubella, 176
    with cyst (colobomatous cyst), 317, 318*i*
Microsomia, hemifacial, 353, 354*i*. *See also* Goldenhar syndrome
Microtropias, 42
Midline positions of gaze, 65
Minimal pigment albinism, 291*t*
Miosis, congenital (microcoria), 224
Miotic agents
    for childhood glaucoma, 236
    for refractive accommodative esotropia, 78
Mitomycin-C, with trabeculectomy, for childhood glaucoma, 235

Mittendorf's dot, 297
Möbius syndrome, 116–117
Modified Snellen technique, in amblyopia evaluation, 48
Molteno implant, for childhood glaucoma, 235
Monochromatism
    blue-cone, 279
    rod (achromatopsia), 279, 376
Monocular cover-uncover test, 59, 60*i*
Monocular deprivation, 37–38
Monocular elevation deficiency (double elevator palsy), 100–101, 100*i*
Monocular eye movements (ductions), 27–28. *See also specific type*
Monocular fixation, 55
Monocular nystagmus, 131
Monocular recess-resect procedures
    for esodeviation, 142, 143*t*
    for exodeviation, 144, 144*t*
Monocular suppression, 39
Monofixation syndrome, 42–44
Mononucleosis, infectious, conjunctivitis in, 188
Morning glory disc, 295, 295*i*
Morquio syndrome, 360*t*
de Morsier syndrome (septo-optic dysplasia), 298
Motility examination. *See* Ocular motility, assessment of
Motor correspondence, Hering's law of, 28–31, 30*i*
Motor fusion, 35, 36*t*
Motor nystagmus, congenital, 128, 376–377
Motor physiology, 23–32
    basic principles and terms related to, 23–27
    eye movements and, 27–31
    strabismus and, 23–32
    supranuclear control systems and, 32
Motor tests, special, 69
Motor units, in extraocular muscle contraction, 27
MPS. *See* Mucopolysaccharidoses
MPS IH. *See* Hurler syndrome
MPS IS. *See* Scheie syndrome
MPS II. *See* Hunter syndrome
MPS III. *See* Sanfilippo syndrome

Optic disc (optic nerve head). *See also* Optic nerve
  anomalies of, in fetal alcohol syndrome, 356
  coloboma of, 295–296, 296*i*
  edema of, 302–304, 303*t*
    in leukemia, 286–287, 287*i*
  enlarged diameter of, in megalopapillae, 297
  hypoplasia of, 297–299, 298*i*
    in fetal alcohol syndrome, 356
  in leukemia, 286–287, 287*i*
  morning glory, 295, 295*i*
  tilted (Fuchs coloboma), 296–297, 297*i*
Optic nerve (cranial nerve II). *See also* Optic disc
  anomalies of, 295–299
    in fetal alcohol syndrome, 356
  aplasia of, 299
  atrophy of. *See* Optic atrophy
  coloboma of, 295–296, 296*i*
  disorders of, 295–304. *See also specific type*
  evaluation of, in nystagmus, 127, 128*t*
  glioma of. *See* Optic nerve glioma
  hypoplasia of, 297–299, 298*i*, 374–375
  in leukemia, 286–287, 287*i*
  in primary congenital glaucoma, 231, 233*i*
  retinoblastoma affecting, 328
Optic nerve glioma, 314
  in neurofibromatosis, 335–336, 335*i*
  orbital involvement in, 314
Optic nerve sheath meningioma, optic glioma differentiated from, 335
Optic neuritis, 301–302, 301*i*
Optic neuropathy, Leber hereditary, 300–301
Optic pits/optic holes, 299, 299*i*
Optical degradation, for amblyopia, 50
  complications of, 50–51
Optokinetic nystagmus response, in congenital motor nystagmus, 128

Orbit
  floor of, fracture of, 104–105, 105*i*
    vertical deviations and, 104–105, 105*i*
  leukemic involvement of, 287, 310
  myositis affecting, 318–319
  roof of, fracture of, 370–371, 371*i*
  tumors of, 307–319
    benign, 311–315
    bony, 314
    connective tissue, 314
    differential diagnosis of, 305–307, 306*t*
    ectopic tissue masses, 315–318
    inflammations simulating, 318–319
    malignant
      metastatic, 308–311
      primary, 307–308
    neural, 314
    vascular, 314
Orbital cellulitis, 191–193, 192*i*
  fungal (mucormycosis), 193, 194*i*
  intracranial extension of, 191
  preseptal cellulitis differentiated from, 191
Orbital inflammation, childhood, 318–319, 319*i*
Orbital pseudotumor, 318, 319*i*
Orbital subperiosteal abscess, 191, 192*i*
Orbital varices, 314
Orbital veins, 17
Orthophoria, 53
Orthoptics
  fusional vergences and, 67
  for intermittent exotropia, 88
  for suppression, 40
  for undercorrection of intermittent exotropia, 89
Ossifying fibroma, of orbit, 314
Osteoma, choroidal, 324
Osteomyelitis, maxillary, 193
Osteosarcoma, orbital, 308
Ovoid bodies, in neurofibromatosis, 336
Oxygen, supplemental, in retinopathy of prematurity, 268

Phakoma, retinal, in tuberous sclerosis, 339–340, 340*i*

Phakomatoses, 330–348, 331*t*. *See also* specific type

Pharyngeal conjunctival fever, 186

Phenylephrine, and fundus evaluation of premature infant, 271

Phlyctenular keratoconjunctivitis, 322

Phoria, 54

    alternate cover (prism and cover) test in assessment of, 59–60, 61*i*

    cover-uncover test in assessment of, 59, 60*i*

Phospholine. *See* Echothiophate

Photocoagulation

    for retinal angiomas, 332

    for retinopathy of prematurity, 273

Photophobia, in primary congenital glaucoma, 228

PHPV. *See* Persistent hyperplastic primary vitreous

Phytanic acid storage disease, infantile (Refsum disease), 361*t*

    enzyme defect in, 278, 361*t*

    ocular findings in, 361*t*

    Leber congenital amaurosis, 278

Pierre Robin sequence (anomaly/deformity), 354

    Stickler syndrome and, 283, 354

Pilocarpine, for childhood glaucoma, 236

Pineoblastoma, 326

Plagiocephaly, 352

Pleomorphic rhabdomyosarcoma, 308

Plexiform neurofibromas, 314, 334–335, 334*i*

Plica semilunaris, incorporation of during strabismus surgery, 152, 152*i*

Plus disease, 269, 269*t*, 270*i*

Pneumococcus. *See* Streptococcus, pneumoniae

Poland syndrome, Möbius syndrome and, 117

Polycoria, 225

Port-wine stain (nevus flammeus), 321

    in Sturge-Weber syndrome, 321, 331*t*, 342, 343, 343*i*

Position maintenance system, 32

Position of rest, 27

Positions of gaze. *See* Gaze, positions of

Positive angle kappa, 64, 65*i*

Posterior capsulorrhexis with optic capture, 249

Posterior chamber intraocular lenses, 249

Posterior corneal depression (central posterior keratoconus), 211–212

Posterior embryotoxon, 210, 210*i*

Posterior fixation suture (Fadenoperation), 138*t*

Posterior keratoconus, central (posterior corneal depression), 211–212

Posterior lenticonus/lentiglobus, 239, 239*i*, 245–247, 246*i*

Posterior synechiae, 226

Posterior uveitis, 251, 252*t*, 259–264

    differential diagnosis of, 264*t*

    histoplasmosis and, 261–262, 262*i*

    laboratory tests for, 265*t*

    toxocariasis and, 262–263, 263*i*

    toxoplasmosis and, 259–261, 261*t*

Postoperative adjustable (two-stage) techniques, 139–140

Povidone-iodine, for neonatal conjunctivitis prophylaxis, 183–184

PPM. *See* Persistent pupillary membranes

Prednisone

    for capillary hemangioma, 312

    for hyphema, 370

    for toxoplasmosis, 175, 261*t*

Pregnancy

    cytomegalovirus infection during, 178–179

    herpes simplex virus infection during, 179–181

    rubella during, 176–177

    syphilis during, 181–182

    toxoplasmosis during, 173–175

Prematurity, retinopathy of, 268–275

    angle kappa and, 64

Pupils, abnormalities in size/shape/
  location of, 224–225, 225*i*
Pursuit eye movements, 32
Pyogenic granuloma, 322
Pyrimethamine, for toxoplasmosis, 175,
  261, 261*t*

Racemose angioma (Wyburn-Mason
  syndrome), 331*t*, 348, 348*i*
Railroad-track sign, in Sturge-Weber
  syndrome, 342
Random dot animals, stereopsis tested
  with, 68
Randot circles, stereopsis tested
  with, 68
Recess-resect procedures, monocular
  for esodeviation, 142, 143*t*
  for exodeviation, 144, 144*t*
Recession (extraocular muscle), 138*t*
  and anteriorization, 138*t*
Reciprocal innervation, Sherrington's law
  of, 28
Recruitment, 27
Rectus muscles. *See also specific muscle*
  action of, 9–11, 10*i*, 11*i*, 12*i*, 15*t*,
    24–25, 25*t*
  anatomy of, 9–11, 10*i*, 11*i*, 12*i*, 15*t*
    surgery and, 20–21*i*, 21
  fascial capsules of, 18
  horizontal
    action of, 9, 10*i*, 24, 25*t*
      gaze position and, 26, 26*t*
    anatomy of, 9, 10*i*
    surgery of, 146
      for A- and V-pattern deviations,
        110–111, 111*i*, 146
    V pattern associated with dysfunction
      of, 109
  insertion relationships of, 15, 16*i*
  intermuscular septum of, 18
  lateral, 15*t*
    action of, 9, 10*i*, 15*t*, 25*t*
    anatomy of, 9, 10*i*, 15*t*
    surgery of, 146–147
      for A- and V-pattern deviations,
        110–111, 111*i*, 112, 113

surgery of, 146–147
  for A- and V-pattern deviations,
    110–111, 111*i*, 112, 113
  anatomy and, 20–21*i*, 21
  for congenital nystagmus,
    134, 134*t*
  for Duane syndrome, 115
  for hypotropia and hypertropia,
    145–146
vertical
  action of, 10–11, 11*i*, 12*i*,
    24–25, 25*t*
    gaze position and, 26, 26*t*
  anatomy of, 10–11, 11*i*, 12*i*
  surgery of, for hypotropia and
    hypertropia, 145–146
  V pattern associated with dysfunction
    of, 109
Red filter/red lens test
  in eye movement assessment, 63
  in monofixation syndrome, 44
  retinal correspondence evaluated with,
    40–41
  for suppression, 40
Red-green test, Lancaster, 64
  in superior oblique muscle
    palsy, 97
Red reflex test, for pediatric
  cataract, 244
Refraction, clinical
  in congenital glaucoma, 229
  cycloplegic, 70–72, 72*t*
    in infant with decreased
      vision, 373
Refractive accommodative esotropia, 76*t*,
  78–79
Refractive errors
  changes in, after strabismus
    surgery, 148
  correction of. *See also* Spectacles
    in amblyopia treatment, 49
Refsum disease (infantile phytanic acid
  storage disease), 361*t*
  enzyme defect in, 278, 361*t*
  ocular findings in, 361*t*
    Leber congenital amaurosis, 278
Renal disease, ocular findings in, 289

Rieger anomaly/syndrome. *See* Axenfeld-Rieger syndrome
Right gaze (dextroversion), 28
  yoke muscles in, 29*t*
Riley-Day syndrome (familial dysautonomia), corneal manifestations of, 217
Rod monochromatism (achromatopsia), 279, 376
ROP. *See* Retinopathy, of prematurity
Rosenmüller, valve of, 199
Rosettes, in retinoblastoma, 326
Rotation, center of, 23, 23*i*
RPE. *See* Retinal pigment epithelium
Rubella, 176–177
  congenital, 176–177, 177*i*
Rubeola, conjunctivitis in, 188

Sabin-Feldman dye test, for toxoplasmosis, 261
SAC. *See* Seasonal allergic conjunctivitis
Saccades, 32
  horizontal, in infants, 372
  muscle contraction physiology in, 27
  testing, in orbital floor blowout fractures, 105
Saccadic system, 32
Saccadic velocity, 69
  increased, in myasthenia gravis diagnosis, 121
Salmon patch, in interstitial keratitis secondary to syphilis, 217
Salt-and-pepper fundus/retinopathy
  in congenital rubella syndrome, 177, 177*i*
  in congenital syphilis, 181, 181*i*, 258
Sandhoff disease (GM$_2$ type II gangliosidosis), 292, 361*t*
  enzyme defect in, 361*t*
  ocular findings in, 292, 361*t*
Sanfilippo syndrome, 360*t*
Sarcoidosis, pediatric, 256
  iris nodules and posterior synechiae associated with, 226
  uveitis in, 256

Sarcoma
  Ewing, 310
  granulocytic, 310
  orbital, 308
  reticulum cell, uveitis differentiated from, 264*t*
Satellite lesions, in toxoplasmosis, 261
Scheie syndrome, 360*t*
  infantile corneal opacities in, 214, 214*t*
Schwannoma (neurilemoma, neurinoma), orbital, 314
Sclera, extraocular muscle surgery and, 22
  perforation of, 149, 150*i*
Scleral plaque, for retinoblastoma, 328
Sclerocornea, 213, 214*t*
Scopolamine, for cycloplegic refraction, 72, 72*t*
Seasonal allergic conjunctivitis, 193–194
Secondary glaucoma, 227. *See also* Angle-closure glaucoma; Glaucoma
Secondary positions of gaze, 24
See-saw nystagmus, 130–131
Sensory defect nystagmus, 128
Sensory deprivation esodeviation, 82
Sensory exotropia, 91
Sensory fusion, 35
Sensory visual system, 33–44
  abnormalities of binocular vision and, 38–34
  neurophysiological aspects of, 36–38
  physiology of normal binocular vision and, 33–36
Septo-optic dysplasia (de Morsier syndrome), 298
Shagreen patch, in tuberous sclerosis, 338–339
Shaking injury (shaken baby syndrome), 363–366
  ocular involvement in, 364–366, 365*i*
Sherrington's law of reciprocal innervation, 28
Sialidoses, 360*t*

Sickle cell disease, traumatic hyphema and, 369, 369*i*

Silicone intubation, for congenital lacrimal duct obstruction, 206–207

Silver nitrate prophylaxis, 182, 183

Simple megalocornea, 209

Simulated divergence excess exotropia, 87

Simultaneous prism-cover test, 60–61

Sinusitis, paranasal, orbital cellulitis caused by, 191, 192*i*

Sixth nerve (abducens) palsy
  congenital, 114
  incomitant esodeviation caused by, 76*t*, 83–84, 114
  strabismus in, 114

Skew deviation, in infants, 372

Sleep test, for myasthenia gravis diagnosis, 121

Slipped muscle, in strabismus surgery, 155–156, 156*i*

Slit-lamp biomicroscopy, for pediatric cataract, 244–247, 245*i*, 246*i*

Sly syndrome, 360*t*

Smooth pursuit system, 32

Snellen chart, modified, for amblyopia evaluation, 48

Snowbank formation, in pars planitis, 258, 259*i*

Spasmus nutans, 129–130

Spectacles
  for intermittent exotropia, 87–88
  for nonrefractive accommodative esotropia, 79, 80
  for overcorrection of intermittent exotropia, 89
  for partially accommodative esotropia, 81
  for refractive accommodative esotropia, 78–79, 80

Spherophakia, 238, 238*i*

Spielmeyer-Vogt disease, 361*t*

Spiral of Tillaux, 15, 16*i*

Staphylococcus aureus
  conjunctivitis caused by, 184–185
  orbital cellulitis caused by, 191
  preseptal cellulitis caused by, 190

Staphyloma, peripapillary, 299

Stargardt disease (juvenile macular degeneration), 281, 281*i*

Stay (pull-over) sutures, 140

Stereo acuity testing, 68–69

Stereopsis, 34*i*, 35, 35–36
  depth perception differentiated from, 36
  in monofixation syndrome, 44
  testing, 68–69

Steroids. *See* Corticosteroids

Stevens-Johnson syndrome (erythema multiforme), 196–197, 197*i*

Stickler syndrome, 283–284
  Pierre Robin sequence (anomaly/deformity) and, 283, 354

Still disease (systemic juvenile rheumatoid arthritis), 253, 253*t*, 255*t*

Stimulus accommodative convergence/accommodation ratio, 66

Strabismic amblyopia, 46–47

Strabismus, 7–160
  A-pattern, 66, 107–113
  accommodative convergence/accommodation ratio abnormalities and, 31
  acquired, 55
  amblyopia and, 45–52
  botulinum toxin in treatment of, 159–160
  in chronic progressive external ophthalmoplegia, 119*t*, 121
  classification of, 54–55
  congenital, 55
  in congenital fibrosis syndrome, 122, 123*i*
  in congenital ocular motor apraxia, 123–124
  in congenital sixth nerve palsy, 114
  in craniosynostosis, 352
  cyclovertical, surgery planning and, 141
  definition of, 53
  dissociated, 91, 92*i*. *See also* Dissociated horizontal deviations; Dissociated vertical deviations
  in Duane syndrome, 114–116
  esodeviations, 74–84
  examining child for, 5–6, 56–73
  exodeviations, 85–92

extraocular muscle anatomy and, 9–22
fascial anatomy and, 9–22
in fetal alcohol syndrome,
  356, 357*i*
fixus, 122
in Graves eye disease (thyroid
  ophthalmology), 118–120, 119*t*
hemangiomas and, 312
history/presenting complaint in, 56
infantile, 55
in internuclear
  ophthalmoplegia, 123
M-cell abnormalities in, 37
in Möbius syndrome, 116–117
motor physiology and, 23–32
in myasthenia gravis, 119*t*,
  121, 122*i*
nystagmus and, 125–135. *See also*
  Nystagmus blockage syndrome
in orbital rhabdomyosarcoma,
  308, 308*i*
paralytic, Hering's law and,
  29–31, 30*i*
in retinoblastoma, 324
secondary, botulinum toxin injections
  causing, 160
sensory physiology and pathology and,
  33–44
terminology related to, 53–54, 53*t*
in third nerve palsy, 117–118
treatment of
  chemodenervation, 159–160
  surgical, 136–157, 158*t. See also*
    Strabismus surgery
V-pattern, 66, 107–113
vertical deviations, 93–106
  botulinum toxin injections causing,
    160
Strabismus surgery, 136–157, 158*t. See
  also* Extraocular muscle surgery
adjustable suture techniques for,
  139–140
anesthesia for, 147
complications of, 148–157, 158*t*
conjunctival incisions for, 147–148
for esodeviations, 142, 143*t*
for exodeviations, 142, 143*t*, 144*t*

extraocular muscle anatomy and,
  19–22, 20–21*i*, 136
guidelines for, 142–147
indications for, 137
planning, 140–142
prior surgery and, 141
strengthening procedures in, 139
techniques for, 137–140
transposition procedures in, 140
weakening procedures in,
  137, 138*t*
  oblique muscle, 144–145
Strengthening procedures, 139
Streptococcus
  pneumoniae (pneumococcus)
    conjunctivitis caused by, 184
    orbital cellulitis caused by, 191
    preseptal cellulitis caused by, 190
  pyogenes, orbital cellulitis caused
    by, 191
Stroma, iris, cysts of, 222
Stromal dystrophy, congenital hereditary,
  corneal opacities and, 214*t*, 215
Sturge-Weber syndrome (encephalofacial
  angiomatosis), 331*t*, 342–345,
  343*i*, 344*i*
  nevus flammeus in, 321, 331*t*, 342,
    343, 343*i*
Subjective visual space, 33
Subluxation, lens, 239–240. *See also*
  Ectopia lentis
Subperiosteal abscess, orbital,
  191, 192*i*
Sudoriferous cyst, orbital, 317
Sulfadiazine, for toxoplasmosis, 175,
  261, 261*t*
Sulfite oxidase deficiency, 242
"Sunsetting," in infants, 372
Superior oblique muscles, 15*t*
  action of, 12–13, 13*i*, 15*t*, 25*t*
  anatomy of, 12–13, 13*i*, 15*t*
  overaction of, 95–96, 96*i*
    A pattern associated with, 109
  paresis of, 96–98, 98*i*
    Hering's law and, 29, 30*i*
  weakening procedures for, 95–96,
    99, 145
    for A-pattern esotropia, 112, 145
    for A-pattern exotropia, 113, 145

Superior oblique tendon sheath syndrome (Brown syndrome), 101–103, 104*t*

Superior orbital vein, 17

Superior rectus muscles, 15*t*
  action of, 10, 11*i*, 15*t*, 25, 25*t*
  anatomy of, 10, 11*i*, 15*t*
  surgery and, 20–21*i*, 21

Supernumerary puncta, 200

Suppression, 38–40
  Worth four-dot testing in evaluation of, 39–40, 67–68

Supraduction. *See* Elevation

Supranuclear control systems, for eye movement, 32

Suprofen, for vernal keratoconjunctivitis, 196

Sursumduction/sursumversion. *See* Elevation

Sutures (surgical)
  adjustable, for strabismus surgery, 139–140
  allergic reaction to, in strabismus surgery, 150, 151*i*
  pull-over (stay), 140

Sympathetic ophthalmia, 257

Syndrome (genetic), definition of, 166

Synechiae, posterior, 226

Synergist muscles, 28

Synkinetic reflex, near, spasm of, esotropia and, 76*t*, 83

Syphilis, 181–182, 258
  congenital, 181–182, 181*i*, 258
    corneal manifestations of, 216–217, 217*i*
    toxoplasmosis differentiated from, 175
  uveitis and, 258

Taches de bougie, 256

Tangent screen, field of binocular fixation measured with, 69

Tarsal kink, congenital, 169, 169*i*

Tay-Sachs disease (GM$_2$ type I gangliosidosis), 292, 361*t*
  enzyme defect in, 361*t*
  ocular findings in, 292, 361*t*

Tearing (epiphora)
  in congenital nasolacrimal duct obstruction, 201

  in primary congenital glaucoma, 228
  in punctal atresia, 199

Telangiectasia, 275
  of conjunctiva, in ataxia-telangiectasia, 345, 346*i*

Telecanthus, 171
  with blepharophimosis, epicanthus inversus, and ptosis, 171, 171*i*
  in fetal alcohol syndrome, 356, 357*i*

Tenacious proximal fusion, in intermittent exotropia, 87

Tenectomy, 138*t*

Tenon's capsule, 18, 19, 19*i*
  extraocular muscle surgery and, 22
  scarring of after strabismus surgery, 151, 152

Tenotomy, 138*t*

Tensilon test, for myasthenia gravis diagnosis, 121, 122*i*

Teratogen, definition of, 167

Teratomas, orbital, 316–317, 316*i*

Terfenadine, for seasonal allergic conjunctivitis, 194

Tertiary positions of gaze, 24

Tetracycline, for neonatal conjunctivitis prophylaxis, 183

Thermal injury (burns), 367

Thermochemotherapy, for retinoblastoma, 328

Third nerve (oculomotor) palsy, 117–118
  exodeviation in, 117–118
  inferior oblique muscle paresis caused by, 104

Three-step test, 70, 71*i*
  in superior oblique muscle palsy, 97

Threshold disease, in retinopathy of prematurity, 271, 273

Thyroid ophthalmopathy (Graves disease), 118–120, 119*t*, 120*i*
  proptosis and, 318, 319*i*
  strabismus and, 118–120, 119*t*, 120*i*

Tillaux, spiral of, 15, 16*i*

Tilted disc syndrome (Fuchs coloboma), 296–297, 297*i*

Timolol, for childhood glaucoma, 236

ILLUSTRATIONS

The authors submitted the following figures for this revision. (Illustrations that were reproduced from other sources or submitted by contributors not on the committee are credited in the captions.)

Edward G. Buckley, MD: Fig XXI-3, XXV-7

Jane D. Kivlin, MD: Fig XX-5, XX-7

Mark S. Ruttum, MD: Fig XVII-11

John W. Simon, MD: Fig XX-6, XX-8

M. Edward Wilson, MD: Fig VIII-1, VIII-2, VIII-3